PLAY THERAPY

A Psychodynamic Primer for the Treatment of Young Children

PLAY THERAPY

A Psychodynamic Primer for the Treatment of Young Children

Pamela Meersand, Ph.D.

Karen J. Gilmore, M.D.

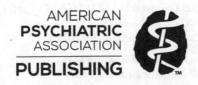

AMERICAN
PSYCHIATRIC
ASSOCIATION
PUBLISHING

Copyright © 2018 American Psychiatric Association Publishing
ALL RIGHTS RESERVED
First Edition

Manufactured in the United States of America on acid-free paper
21   20   19   18   17   5   4   3   2   1

American Psychiatric Association Publishing
1000 Wilson Boulevard
Arlington, VA 22209-3901
www.appi.org

Library of Congress Cataloging-in-Publication Data
Names: Meersand, Pamela, author. | Gilmore, Karen J., author. | American Psychiatric Association Publishing, issuing body.
Title: Play therapy : a psychodynamic primer for the treatment of young children / Pamela Meersand, Karen J. Gilmore.
Description: Arlington, Virginia : American Psychiatric Association Publishing, [2018] | Includes bibliographical references and index.
Identifiers: LCCN 2017028373 (print) | LCCN 2017029477 (ebook) | ISBN 9781615371440 (ebook) | ISBN 9781615370436 (paperback : alk. paper)
Subjects: | MESH: Play Therapy | Child | Psychotherapy, Psychodynamic | Child Development | Case Reports
Classification: LCC RJ505.P6 (ebook) | LCC RJ505.P6 (print) | NLM WS 350.4 | DDC 618.92/891653—dc23
LC record available at https://lccn.loc.gov/2017028373

British Library Cataloguing in Publication Data
A CIP record is available from the British Library.

Contents

PART I
Theory of Play and Play Therapy

PART II
Technique of Play Therapy

About the Authors

Pamela Meersand, Ph.D., is Associate Professor of Psychology in the Department of Psychiatry at Columbia University College of Physicians and Surgeons, and Director of the Child Division at the Columbia University Center for Psychoanalytic Training and Research. She is in private practice in Manhattan.

Karen J. Gilmore, M.D., is Clinical Professor of Psychiatry at Columbia University College of Physicians and Surgeons, and Senior Consultant to the Columbia University Center for Psychoanalytic Training and Research. She is in private practice in Manhattan.

Preface

Psychodynamic play therapy is the premier medium for the treatment of young children. As a therapeutic modality, it comprises elements of both science and art: the practitioner is guided by a set of theoretical principles and informed by a vast reserve of developmental research, while the playing state between child and adult is fueled by their unique subjectivities, affective reciprocity, and creative potential. Indeed, the simultaneous cognitive and emotional challenges of play therapy—engaging fully in the spontaneous, rapidly unfolding imaginary action while retaining the capacity to evaluate and reflect—require the clinician's substantial knowledge, preparation, and personal resourcefulness. Despite this, contemporary training programs for child clinicians in all disciplines rarely provide in-depth education in the theory and practice of play therapy; fellowships and internships are far more likely to emphasize brief, evidence-based modalities with highly specific methods for eliciting and guiding children's participation in treatment. During our many years as teachers and supervisors of aspiring child practitioners, we have experienced first-hand the frustration of young trainees who feel ill-equipped to approach play from a more exploratory, less directive stance even as they recognize its function as the most natural and revealing and potentially the most growth-promoting form of self-expression for young patients.

Ideas for the current book developed during our interactions with students as they began to immerse themselves in working and playing with children; along with our trainees, we grappled with theoretical questions (How do we conceptualize major psychodynamic ideas, such as transference and resistance, in work with young children? What is the role of play in the mental development of the child?), questions of technique (What are effective ways to work with parents while maintaining the integrity and privacy of the child's treatment? How does the child clinician begin to make meaning out of play characters and narratives?), and pragmatic concerns (How do early-career practitioners seek referrals for a child-focused practice? What are the best ways to set up an office that will facilitate imaginary play?). As we searched for resources to supplement supervision and teaching, the paucity of writings on the basic principles and practice of psychodynamic play therapy further convinced us of the need for a volume that provides broad but coherent foundational information as well as pragmatic guidance. Our theoretical vantage point, best described as modern ego psychology, represents an integration of classical with more pluralistic, post-1970s psychoanalytic thinking (described by Marcus [1999]); this viewpoint nonetheless leads us to privilege the child's inner world—affects, conflict and defense, fantasies about self and relationships—as it is structured, shaped, and reorganized throughout the course of development by biological endowments, maturation of body and brain, emerging ego capacities, interactions with others, the pressures and expectations of each developmental phase, and serendipitous life events. We therefore sought works that would help students learn to think in complex and nonlinear ways about children and their play, keeping in mind conscious and unconscious forces as well as past and present influences. In particular, we wanted students to be schooled in how to focus on children's affective states and self-protective mechanisms, detect central relational paradigms, maintain awareness of their own emotional reactions, and discern the meanings of children's play with an eye toward developmental pressures and vulnerabilities.

The psychoanalytic literature embodies a rich tradition of wonderfully illustrative child case studies and vignettes (accessible and helpful papers for students of play therapy include those by Altman [1997]; Birch [1997]; Mahon [2000]; and Yanof [2000]). However, examination of individual cases functions best when readers possess at least rudimentary conceptual knowledge of the play process. Moreover, this body of literature is geared toward the practice of child psychoanalysis, a form of treatment that is closely related to and has profoundly influenced psychodynamic play therapy but that represents a separate modality distinguished by the intensity of the treatment and the relative emphasis given to certain areas of work, such as transference and defense. Other valuable resources include books that describe play treatments from a multitude of theoretical perspectives (e.g., Schaefer 2011) or those that elaborate a particular process in child therapy, such as use of the child–clinician relationship to facilitate development of reflective capacities (Tuber and Caflisch 2011).

In writing this volume, our goal has been to present a basic, coherent framework for how to conceptualize, initiate, sustain, deepen, and terminate psychodynamic play therapy. Moreover, we hope to fulfill the need for a decisively modern guide to play therapy that reflects recent shifts in psychoanalytic theory and incorporates relevant information from neighboring fields, such as developmental science. In many ways, the practice of play therapy embodies an organic integration of traditional ego-psychological approaches to treatment (working with the child's evolving ego capacities to elaborate inner conflicts and ameliorate rigid modes of defense) and more recent relational perspectives (drawing on the unfolding, here-and-now, implicit aspects of child–clinician interactions to seek opportunities for shifts in interpersonal patterns). Another integral component of contemporary thinking involves twenty-first century changes in the very nature of children's play and in their modes of self-expression; our relationships with children require that we constantly push ourselves out of the zone of familiarity, embrace novel ideas, and adapt to cultural innovations such as the proliferation of digital-based games that our young patients take in stride but that often leave clinicians feeling hopelessly outmoded.

To address both theoretical and more practical issues, we have divided the book into two distinct but interconnected sections. Part I provides a conceptual background for play, both as a normative developmental capacity and as a form of psychodynamic therapy with a distinct set of concepts and principles. The first seven chapters provide discussions of the following: an introduction to contemporary thinking about the purpose and nature of psychodynamic play therapy; the role of play in mental life; the emergence of play during early childhood and its function in development; basic psychoanalytic concepts and their application to working with young children; the impact and potential of technological play both in and outside of therapy; the mutative, growth-promoting aspects of play therapy; and the role of play therapy in certain childhood disorders. In these chapters, play therapy vignettes form the basis for discussion, highlighting various aspects of the play process and the child–clinician relationship.

Part II emphasizes the practice of play therapy. To illustrate technical and pragmatic issues, we provide multiple vignettes demonstrating how a hypothetical group of child practitioners of diverse disciplines handle typical but challenging situations, including their own countertransference reactions. Chapters include the following topics: setting up a child-focused practice and beginning to see child patients; initiating play therapy, developing the child–clinician relationship, and responding to the child's inevitable anxieties about treatment; working with parents across a range of circumstances; working with play narratives to deepen the treatment and soften the child's rigid modes of relating and maladaptive defenses; preparing for and carrying out the process of termination; and working with specific child populations.

Throughout the volume, we have utilized boldfaced terms to alert the reader to important labels and concepts; these boldfaced items are defined in the Key Terms section located at the end of every chapter. In addition, a Key Points section, also positioned at the conclusion of each chapter, provides a brief summary of major theoretical and technical points.

This book functions both as an introduction for young therapists and as a guide for more experienced child clinicians who wish to expand their knowledge of play and its therapeutic potential. Although those with an interest in psychodynamic ideas will find that the volume fits naturally with their theoretical orientation, cognitive-behavioral practitioners also may benefit from increased awareness of the ways in which children's play reflects key aspects of their mental lives. Readers from any background may find that our previous work, *Normal Child and Adolescent Development: A Psychodynamic Primer* (Gilmore and Meersand 2014), serves as a useful companion to this volume; it elaborates the underlying developmental pressures, fantasies, capacities, and tasks that powerfully shape children's experience of their environments, including the therapeutic situation. Such knowledge further equips the therapist to create a secure playing space, target interventions at the level of the child's understanding, and interpret the meanings of behavior and play scenarios.

REFERENCES

Altman N: The case of Ronald: oedipal issues in the treatment of a seven-year-old boy. Psychoanal Dialogues 7(6):725–739, 1997

Birch M: In the land of counterpane: travels in the realm of play. Psychoanal Study Child 52:57–75, 1997 9489461

Gilmore K, Meersand P: Normal Child and Adolescent Development: A Psychodynamic Primer. Washington, DC, American Psychiatric Publishing, 2014

Mahon E: A "good hour" in child analysis and adult analysis. Psychoanal Study Child 55:124–142, 2000 11338985

Marcus ER: Modern ego psychology. J Am Psychoanal Assoc 47(3):843–871, 1999 10586403

Schaefer CE: Foundations of Play Therapy, 2nd Edition. Hoboken, NJ, Wiley, 2011

Tuber S, Caflisch J: Starting Treatment With Children and Adolescents: A Process Oriented Guide for Therapists. New York, Routledge, 2011

Yanof JA: Barbie and the tree of life: the multiple functions of gender in development. J Am Psychoanal Assoc 48:1439–1465, 2000 11212196

Acknowledgments

This volume represents over a decade of collaborative teaching at the Columbia University Center for Psychoanalytic Training and Research, as well as many years supervising candidates of child psychoanalysis and trainees in child psychiatry and psychology. We are constantly inspired by our students' dedication to learning, and by their openness and creativity in the face of treatment dilemmas; unfailingly, they help clarify our thinking and cause us to question our underlying assumptions.

As clinicians ourselves, we are grateful for all the children who allow us entry into their imaginary worlds and for the parents who entrust us with their care. It is our great privilege to witness and participate in the developmental and therapeutic processes with so many youngsters.

Our editors' encouragement and guidance, and their patience as we identified needed additions to the book, provided support throughout the writing of this volume. Inevitably, the process of writing about child treatment brings us back to our own numerous mentors, whose wisdom and generosity shaped our personal identities as child workers and teachers. Finally, we would like to express our appreciation for our families, who tolerated our frequent absences and managed to stay supportive through it all, and for our valued assistants, whose contributions are everywhere.

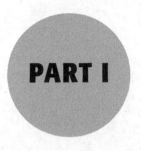

PART I

Theory of Play and Play Therapy

1

Why Play Therapy?

Introduction to the Psychodynamic Treatment of Young Children

Six-year-old Sophia was referred to Dr. Graber, a child psychologist, because of her difficulties adjusting to the routines of kindergarten. At school, she often resisted group activities such as joining her peers for circle time; teachers reported that she increasingly refused to try out new skills and became easily frustrated when her first efforts were not quickly successful. Her parents were baffled and concerned, because Sophia had enjoyed her previous 2 years of preschool and participated happily in all aspects of the classroom. With considerable regret, they described to Dr. Graber their choice of a kindergarten that both subsequently feared was "too academic" but that Sophia's former teacher had recommended, based on the girl's verbal maturity and lively interest in learning her numbers and letters. In her initial meeting with the parents, Dr. Graber focused on reducing their distress, gathering information about the girl's early development, and formulating an assessment plan; a school observation was soon arranged that confirmed Sophia's reluctance to engage in kindergarten activities. Play therapy was then initiated; after insisting that her mother accompany her into the playroom for her first meeting with Dr. Graber, Sophia settled easily into pretend play.

On their third session together, Sophia bounded into Dr. Graber's playroom, barely acknowledging the therapist as she headed for a bin of small dolls and furniture; these were quickly configured into a traditional classroom scene. "We're gonna play school, and you be the teacher," Sophia asserted, "but be a kind of teacher." "What kind?" the

3

therapist asked. "A kind of teacher named Miss Shell," responded the child. Dr. Graber recalled that this was the name of Sophia's current head teacher, whom the parents described as "nice but rather strict." Then, Sophia impatiently announced that it was art class and that the children would be learning how to draw stars and flowers. Somewhat imperiously, she demanded drawing paper and began to direct the action: "You do Miss Shell's drawings, and I'll do the kids' drawings"; then, she hastily cut a sheet of paper into smaller squares and handed one piece to the therapist, along with a few carefully selected crayons of dull brown and gray shades. With a slight smile, she eagerly picked out pinks, blues, and oranges and distributed them to her doll students. "I wish I could pick the bright colors," the "teacher" murmured. Sophia looked pleased and assumed the role of one student, whom she named "Mia": "Are you super mad?" Mia asked the teacher. She did not wait for an answer, however, and the play moved on: "Alright, Miss Shell, time for you to test us on our art. You do a picture and I do a picture, then we decide whose is best and they get a sticker. Do yours sort of messy," Sophia suggested helpfully to Dr. Graber, providing guidance as to her desired outcome. Sophia covered her character's paper with her hand and invited the teacher to "try and spy on me"; Miss Shell complied, and this attempt was met with the student's indignation, followed by more energetic hiding. Sophia then placed a bin between herself and the therapist so that her student's drawing was fully concealed. In her role as teacher, Dr. Graber vehemently protested the unfairness of dull colors, secrets, and the difficulty of art class. In accordance with Sophia's strongly implied preferences, she contrived to have her character ultimately produce a poorly executed, brownish-gray flower. Sophia appeared very satisfied, and her student-doll triumphantly swept aside the bin to reveal a bright, multicolored tulip. Next, Sophia introduced a new character, the school principal, who entered the scene, ceremoniously placed a sticker on the student's work, and scolded Miss Shell for poor artistic ability.

AN OVERVIEW OF PLAY THERAPY

The brief vignette that opens this chapter captures the essence of imaginary play and its privileged position within psychodynamic child therapy. The child's private fantasies and anxieties, along with the meanings and interpretations she attributes to her daily experience, are vividly portrayed via action and narration. In the safe, nonconsequential setting of pretense with a trusted adult, wherein reality is mutually suspended, Sophia's potentially unacceptable wishes and impulses can achieve full expression. Disavowed affects and unwanted roles are assigned to the therapist, who animates and elaborates them through her participation in the play. Sophia's overall absorption and pleasure in playing is unmistakable. Indeed, both child and therapist are fully immersed in their imaginary activities, but Dr. Graber attempts to maintain a reflective stance as well, thinking about the play in the context of what is known about Sophia's history and current situation.

Like Sophia, who is struggling with the social and learning expectations at her school, young children are generally brought to therapy because of their inability to negotiate age-salient tasks and advance along an expected developmental trajectory. Such difficulties may result from internal conflict, rigid defenses, maladaptive interpersonal patterns, environmental pressures, learning challenges, or more serious impairments in ego functioning; most often, it is a confluence of various factors that interfere with the child's forward progression. In the case of Sophia, certain play themes emerge quickly and clarify her subjective experience of 6-year-old life. The contents of play reflect a sense of inadequacy, fear of failure and exposure, a perceived lack of power and control, and anger at exclusion from adults' secret lives; these unwanted affects, outcast self-states, and perceptions of others are taken up by Dr. Graber, who vocalizes and clarifies them via the role of Miss Shell. Through the joint pretense with Dr. Graber, Sophia is helped to transform the passive, anxiety-laden experience of the classroom learner into a far more desirable role of student-achiever who ultimately turns the tables on the educator. At the same time, this narrative reflects Sophia's ongoing attachment to and dependency on adults; at the end of her story, a new authority figure appears to take control of the classroom and pronounce judgment. Such diverging representations of adults and interpersonal affects—anger and resentment at figures who make demands on children, but the need and desire for grown-ups who restore order and provide moral guidance—reflect painful underlying conflicts, as Sophia struggles with loving and negative feelings about important people in her life. The girl's easy entry into pretense, the richness of her scenarios, and the fluidity of child–therapist mutuality (co-creating narratives, sharing verbal and emotional communication) suggest well-developed symbolic and relational capacities. At the manifest level of playing, Dr. Graber is able to evaluate the level of Sophia's language, self-regulatory, fine motor, and preacademic skills, including her ability to take another's perspective, plan and organize a complex scenario, maintain the narrative during exciting moments, and demonstrate knowledge of classroom routines and standards.

Although Sophia and her therapist jointly create the play, inevitably contributing their unique subjectivities to the narratives and character animations, Dr. Graber allows the child to take the lead. She accepts assignments and directions, permitting Sophia to shape the arc of the pretense. Dr. Graber tolerates the attendant ambiguity, frustration, and confusion as the girl alternately suggests, demands, and ignores, but does not impose adult-like levels of logic and clarity before Sophia's meanings begin to emerge. Once the meanings are clearer, Dr. Graber does not prematurely link the play to the child's personal struggles or introduce comments that reach beyond the material of the pretend scenarios. While fully engrossed in the action of the play, Dr. Graber maintains the role of participant-observer, noting dominant themes, shifts in Sophia's affective states, and any disruptions in the ongoing activity. She does not seek to reassure, teach, or prohibit beyond what is necessary to maintain safety and preserve the boundaries of the treatment.

Psychodynamic work with young children is synonymous with play therapy. As an organically emerging capacity, play represents a natural mode of self-expression and an ideal medium for communicating and building relationships with children between ages 3 and 8 or so. Indeed, play *is* the language of childhood, with its unique integration of action and verbal narration. Passions and avid curiosities are best expressed through play scenarios; similarly, uncomfortable feelings and conflicts are better tolerated and more easily elaborated when children are invited to play, in contrast to when they are required to engage in exclusively verbal interactions or confronted with direct questions about their inner states.

Although play by its nature is a creative, spontaneous, and often pleasurable activity, play as a form of therapy represents a coherent theory with an accompanying set of techniques that, like other psychoanalytically derived treatments, require of the clinician substantial knowledge and personal resourcefulness. Certain intellectual and emotional challenges are unique to the play therapy experience. These include understanding the need to adapt interventions for the child's developmental vulnerabilities and capacities; handling the pressures of functioning as an emotional container for the child's disavowed affects; maintaining sufficient openness and availability during play in order "to be animated by the child's imagination" (Birch 1997, p. 63); becoming accustomed to the level of stimulation in the playroom and managing one's own reaction to the child's immature ego controls; maintaining tolerance for the ambiguity and confusion of play; resisting the urge to impose adult-like levels of logic and linearity as the child's comments, play narratives, and scenarios "zig zag to the point of bewilderment" (Kronengold 2010, p. 10); and balancing therapeutic aims, such as resolving past conflicts, with the naturally forward pull of development and the child's future orientation (Abrams et al. 1999; Galatzer-Levy 2008; Warshaw 2010). Moreover, the clinician must manage the inevitable tension between the joint roles of fully engaged play participant and thoughtful interpreter of play meanings; children's normative proclivity toward action, their limited verbal sophistication, and their lack of self-regulatory capacity create an environment in which the therapist is perpetually immersed in the immediacy of here-and-now interactions but must nonetheless retain an inwardly reflective stance.

We have found, during our many years of supervising play treatments, that trainees' most pressing questions often arise within the fast-paced, unfolding action of the play session when there is scant opportunity to stop and think. These involve familiar dilemmas such as how to handle direct aggressive behavior; what to do when the child climbs into the therapist's lap, refuses to enter or leave the playroom, runs out mid-session, or insists on bringing home the therapist's materials; whether or not to respond to children's personal questions about the clinician's age and marital or parental status; or how to react therapeutically when the child presses the therapist to assume a sexual or sadistic role in play. Other less immediate questions involve the value of insight in the treatment of young children, the importance of the therapeutic relationship given children's ongoing attachment to and dependence on their parents, and the benefit of making comments within the play as opposed to directly about the child. Finally, work with young children always involves individuals beyond the patient–therapist dyad, most notably parents but often additional caregivers and educators who are intimately engaged in the young child's life; as a result, the clinician must hold in mind multiple subjectivities and manage complex interpersonal reactions. Issues often arise around how to create a strong alliance with parents and achieve a balance between meeting their needs and safeguarding the child's privacy. The child therapist frequently needs to make decisions about the following: handling parents' questions about their child's sessions; responding to pressure, from patient or parent, that the therapist take sides in family conflicts or deliver counsel about particular behaviors (e.g., how many hours per day of screen time should be allowed); and reacting to information that parents provide to the therapist but wish to keep secret from the child (e.g., impending marital separation, illness of a family member).

We hope that this volume will provide a framework for child practitioners at different phases of career development who encounter these and many other challenges while sharing our fascination for the exciting, demanding, and creative world of play therapy. Of course, books and papers represent only one form of the resources that child clinicians need in order to work effectively. We highly recommend to our readers that they seek opportunities for additional experiential learning (advanced training programs with clinical components, exposure to diverse child populations), pursue emotional and professional support in various forms (peer supervision groups, mentoring relationships), and continue to foster self-understanding (via personal psychotherapy or psychoanalysis).

WHAT IS PLAY, WHEN DOES IT APPEAR, AND WHY IS IT IMPORTANT?

This book is about the form of play that is commonly referred to as *pretend play* (we may also use the terms *fantasy, imaginary, dramatic,* or *make-believe play,* or *pretense*). Defining features of pretend play include the following:

- A unique combination of both mental fantasy and physical action
- An inherent "as-if" quality
- The capacity to inhabit the play fully while maintaining awareness of pretending
- The inherently safe and nonconsequential nature of the playing situation

A number of writers have postulated a highly distinctive condition of ego or consciousness, known as the **playing state**, in which the child manifests intense absorption, spontaneity, unrestricted use of playthings and props, and unimpeded access to internal fantasy; indeed, a key component of play therapy involves the mutual playing state that arises between child and adult in which they jointly suspend reality, share meanings, and co-create imaginative narratives (Gilmore 2005, 2011; Keable 2001; Neubauer 1987; Ritvo 1978; Slade 1994; Solnit 1987). In these multiple ways, imaginary play is readily distinguishable from the infant's exploratory and sensorimotor play, from rule-bound pastimes such as board games and sports, and from the vast array of playful but nonpretend behaviors and activities (jokes, teasing, plays on words) of children and adults.

Contemporary research suggests that pretense is an innate human capacity, demonstrable from the earliest months of life via the baby's response to the parent's playful mock affects and expressions (Gergely 2000). In Chapters 2, "Play, Playfulness, and the Sequence of Play Forms in Development," and 3, "Pretend Play," we more fully elaborate the evolutionary aspects and developmental course of play. Pretend play follows a specific trajectory: it emerges between ages 1 and 2, achieves ascendance between the ages of 3 and 6 years, and then gradually recedes over the course of middle childhood (Fein 1981; Piaget 1962). In the toddler phase, children begin to enact simple self- and other-directed acts of make-believe that subsequently develop into more complex, multiple-step sequences (e.g., pretending to drink milk from an empty cup; later, pretending to pour milk into an empty cup and then offer it to mother); these are generally accompanied by positive affect and by a shared awareness of pretense (Emde et al. 1997; Fein 1981). Within a confluence of emerging psychological pressures and symbolic capacities (narrative language, imaginative fantasy, **mentalization**), pretend play behaviors begin to peak during the **oedipal phase**, between ages 3 and 6 years. During this period, children engage in increasingly complex and creative play, both in solitary and in sociodramatic forms (Fein 1981; Howe et al. 2005; Piaget 1962); their unique, individual narratives and scenarios provide a window into the role of naïve cognition in children's perceptions of reality-based situations while revealing their internal dilemmas and wishful solutions. More structured, reality-based games and rule-bound activities progressively gain importance during the **latency phase**, as the academic and social demands of external life interface with an explosion of cognitive capacities.

Psychoanalytic clinicians have long privileged the role of imaginary play in the assessment and treatment of young children, as well as in a child's overall mental development (e.g., Birch 1997; Cohen and Solnit 1993; Marans et al. 1991; Mayes and Cohen 1993; Neubauer 1987). Notions about play have evolved, however, in tandem with broader shifts in the field of psychoanalysis; these changing views have been influenced by the increased integration of relational and attachment theories with more traditional psychoanalytic concepts, as well as by inclusion of findings from developmental research. Prior conceptualizations emphasized the potential of play as a vehicle for drive and affective discharge, an enactment of wish fulfillment, and a psychological respite from the demands of reality (Neubauer 1987; Piaget 1962). Contemporary views of play are broader and reflect increased understanding of the link between the child's mental functioning, including imaginary potential, and the quality of early attachment relationships (Fonagy and Target 1996a; Lyons-Ruth 2006; Slade 1987). In current psychoanalytic theory, play is conceived as a naturally occurring growth-promoting capacity that contributes to a profound expansion of a child's psychological resources; pretense is correlated with emotional self-regulation, mental state knowledge, and the deepening of relationships (Fonagy and Target 1996a; Gilmore 2011; Tessier et al. 2016; Tuber and Caflisch 2012). Indeed, a number of theorists have noted that children at play demonstrate a level of social and emotional understanding that exceeds that of their nonplaying state (Fonagy and Target 1996a; Vygotsky 1978).

The potential developmental functions of play are hypothesized to include consolidation of self and other boundaries; enhanced concentration and problem solving; mastery of distressing experiences through transformation of passive into active; and practice assuming and shifting multiple roles, gender identifications, and social perspectives (Birch 1997; Piaget 1962; Tuber and Caflisch 2012; Yanof 2000). Children's natural use of play to rework and gain mastery over lived experience is easily observable in typical play scenarios; ordinary examples include engaging a parent in the playful reenactment of familiar but stressful separations, such as the moment of drop-off at preschool, or in the re-creation of a painful medical procedure wherein the child assumes the role of doctor. The construction of play narratives and scenarios helps the child organize experience, modulate potentially overwhelming affects, and make sense of emotionally laden interpersonal events; moreover, in the presence of an important adult, play functions as an interpersonal communication and an opportunity for the co-creation of shared meanings (Bucci 1997; Emde et al. 1997; Slade 1994; Tuber and Caflisch 2012). Dramatic play with peers offers additional developmental opportunities; during shared pretense, children verbally negotiate and plan, freely exchange roles and identities, and engage in mutual narrative building (Bretherton 1989; Howe et al. 2005).

THE THERAPEUTIC USE OF PLAY

In the treatment of young children, imaginary play serves as the primary medium for communication, relationship building, and therapeutic action. Our purview in this book is the practice of psychodynamic play therapy, in which the clinician privileges elements of the child's inner life (e.g., affect, conflict, defense, fantasy); attends to indirectly obtained information (e.g., the meanings of the child's behaviors and play narratives, or dawning awareness of unconscious reactions to the child); and assumes a highly engaged but nondirective stance, allowing the child to take the lead in devising storylines and assigning play roles to the therapist. Such fundamental principles distinguish psychodynamic play therapy from short-term or cognitive-behavioral treatments with specific goals, such as reduction of anxiety or promotion of age-appropriate social behaviors, even though these therapies often utilize play to develop an alliance, create a comfortable environment for the child, and present interventions in an age-appropriate fashion (Knell and Desai 2010). The psychodynamic clinician works from within the mutual playing state, functioning as a participant-observer who facilitates emotional expression, discovers and elaborates the child's unique play meanings and perspectives, increases the child's tolerance for uncomfortable affects, and ultimately promotes greater flexibility and novel solutions.

EARLY HISTORY OF PLAY AS A FORM OF TREATMENT

Psychoanalysts initially envisioned play as serving functions such as drive discharge, wish fulfillment, assimilation of reality, and mastery over developmental anxieties (Peller 1954; Waelder 1932); this somewhat limited view of play reflects the major tenets of early psychoanalytic theorizing as well as restricted knowledge about the mental capacities and interpersonal needs of very young children. Freud's (1962) account of the "fort-da" game, in which a toddler repeatedly casts away and then joyfully reclaims a toy reel, represents one of the earliest documented efforts at uncovering the symbolic meanings of play; in this instance, Freud postulated that the game provided the child with an illusory sense of mastery over painful separations from the mother.

Subsequently, a number of psychoanalytic practitioners began to observe and treat young children directly, gradually gaining a broader sense of the child's inner life; readers who desire a more thorough review of influential contributions might consider consulting works by Klein (1926, 1932), Spitz (1945, 1946), and Fairbairn (1954). A greater appreciation for the developmental role and therapeutic potential of play evolved as clinicians began to write about their work with younger patients. Hermione Hug-Hellmuth (1921), an educator and follower of Freud, promoted the use of play to gain access to children's internal worlds; her work served as foundational for later theorists who began incorporating play into psychoanalytic technique, most notably Melanie Klein and Anna Freud (Brinich 2013). These latter thinkers, both luminous figures in the history of child analysis, pursued divergent approaches to the use of play: Klein hypothesized that play provides direct access to the young child's fantasies, and she advocated that the clinician should elucidate such unconscious contents, whereas Anna Freud, more skeptical about the treatment of very young children, advised a gradual uncovering of the child's interior life (Aguayo 2000; Brody 1974; Klein 1926; Salomonsson 1997; Sandler et al. 1980). Berta Bornstein (1949, 1951) further refined A. Freud's more measured approach; recognizing young children's acute sensitivity to personal exposure, she developed a tactful, gentle technique for the exploration of affects, defense mechanisms, and play meanings. Some years later, Winnicott (1968) theorized about the essential role of play in the mental life of both children and adults. Indeed, he asserted that "playing is itself a therapy" during childhood; in his view, children's play is intrinsically exciting and precarious due to its unique position on the border of subjective experience and objective reality. His famous account of "The Piggle" (Winnicott 1980), frequently read by aspiring child psychoanalysts, demonstrates how a clinician might allow play to emerge and develop at its own pace, along with the child's deep investment and pleasure, before attempting verbal interpretive work.

Additional theories and techniques, related to but distinct from psychoanalytically oriented play therapy, have emerged as well. The development of "child-centered play therapy" (also referred to as "nondirective play therapy") in the 1940s helped popularize play treatment beyond the psychoanalytic community and increased the accessibility of play techniques for a wide range of therapeutic and educational practitioners. Basic principles of the child-centered approach emphasize the clinician's accepting and nonjudgmental attitude, full engagement in the child's play activity, minimal prohibition of children's behavior, and respect for the child's inherent tendency toward growth and autonomy (Axline 1969; Moustakas 1997).

PLAY IN CURRENT PSYCHODYNAMIC CHILD THERAPY

Contemporary theorizing about the role of play in psychodynamic child treatment reflects groundbreaking research into the minds and brains of infants and young children, as well as trends within the field of psychoanalysis. A traditional emphasis on patients' intrapsychic lives (conflicts, defenses, fantasies, memories) has broadened, with greater inclusion of pivotal patient–clinician relational processes such as intersubjectivity, the interplay of language and implicitly understood meanings, and other conscious and unconscious components of here-and-now interactions (Bruschweiler-Stern et al. 2007; Lyons-Ruth 2006; Vivona 2014). Within this more comprehensive view, children's play metaphors retain significance as representations of their unique subjectivity but are also seen as reflecting the mutuality of the child–clinician dyad as the pair collaboratively construct narratives and meanings, jointly moving the play toward greater complexity; co-created play characters and scenarios are viewed as inevitably containing elements of both the child's and the therapist's conscious and unconscious experience (First 2010; Frankel 1998; Harrison and Tronick 2011; Lyons-Ruth 2006; Slade 1994).

Many contemporary writers view the child therapist's traditional role—understanding and **interpretation** of the child's modes of relating and defensive patterns—as only one part of an expanded, multidimensional set of functions. For example, the clinician's provision of **developmental assistance** has received renewed attention as an inevitable and essential part of the therapeutic process (Neubauer 2001); this function includes interventions that directly support the child's ego capacities, such as setting limits, containing aggressive impulses, and modeling pretend play (Barish 2004; Frankel 1998; Neubauer 2001; Sugarman 1994, 2003). Although previously viewed as belonging to a preparatory phase of therapy, or as applicable only to children with serious ego deficits, these growth-promoting interventions are increasingly seen as a central component of any ongoing child therapeutic process (Miller 2013; Neubauer 2001). Mayes and Cohen (1993) observed that the widening scope of psychoanalytic treatment, to include children with significant social and self-regulatory impairments, has contributed to these gradual reformulations of therapeutic principles and techniques. Indeed, many children begin treatment without the capacity to engage in play or benefit from the therapist's insight-oriented verbal remarks; for these youngsters, the clinician may need to scaffold affect tolerance, self-control, and imaginary play. The therapist's ego-supporting functions—maintaining calm and consistent attitudes, setting limits, helping to organize the child's actions, and beginning to make meaning of seemingly chaotic behaviors—serve as necessary building blocks for the treatment dyad's later joint communication through conversation and shared pretense (Gilmore 2005; Sugarman 1994, 2003; Yanof 2012).

We consider these multiple aspects of play therapy—the clinician's verbal interventions and direct developmental assistance, the emerging child–therapist conversation about affects and inner states, their mutual playing, and their continuous implicit communications—as essential psychodynamic processes that represent the complexity of the treatment situation. However, we continue to view language-based processes as cornerstones of psychodynamic play therapy; this includes naming feelings, linking behaviors to inner states, verbally elucidating aspects of the therapeutic relationship, and beginning to talk with the child about defenses against uncomfortable affects. Indeed, language functions as a major developmental contributor to the transformation and amelioration of the child's intense bodily and emotional experience (Bucci 1997; Cohen and Solnit 1993; Downey 1987; Mayes and Cohen 1993; Scott 1998). In work with young children, verbal interventions and shared discussions are often organically embedded within the play itself; moreover, the therapist's comments are always delivered in a manner that follows closely the play material and the child's signals, reflects existing ego capacities, avoids causing feelings of exposure and intrusion, and minimizes the likelihood of disruptions to the flow of child–therapist communication (Bornstein 1951; Hoffman 2007). This approach finds parallels in adult clinical theories that emphasize expansion of patients' awareness and strengthening of their ego capacities without prematurely interpreting unconscious wishes or transgressing the patients' verbal communications (Busch 2000). Therapists' tact and sensitivity to their patients' level of conscious understanding are fundamental to effective child treatment. Most child clinicians have experienced firsthand, often through a child's sudden action or withdrawal, the intense responses that children evince when deep wishes or urges are prematurely exposed (Chused 1996; Hoffman 2007); these include fleeing the room, demanding the therapist's silence, immediately disrupting play, and covering ears in an effort to ward off the adult's verbal commentary. In Chapter 6, "Therapeutic Action and the Multiple Functions of Play Therapy," we discuss more fully the role of the clinician's verbal interventions and the way in which these are adjusted to meet the child's developmental needs and vulnerabilities.

PERSPECTIVES FROM DEVELOPMENTAL STUDIES

Within the empirical literature, studies of pretend play tend toward an emphasis on the child's measurable cognitive and social competencies. Research definitions of *pretense* distinguish imaginary play from exploratory or skills-practicing activities; essential elements of pretend play include the child's intentional projection of a mental representation onto reality and an awareness of the state of pretense (Burghardt 2011; Lillard 2002). Numerous studies link play to diverse developmental capacities such as narrative competence, social perspective-taking, problem solving, and attentional and behavioral self-control (e.g., Howe et al. 2005; Lindsay and Colwell 2013; Pelligrini 1985; Sutherland and Friedman 2013). However, a meta-review of 50 years of empirical work clarifies the correlational rather than causal connection between pretend play and the above-mentioned developmental competencies (Lillard et al. 2013); this analysis supports the notion of a complex, nonlinear relationship between play and other emerging mental systems, closely paralleling contemporary psychodynamic notions of play and its role in child development (Gilmore 2011).

Well-controlled outcome studies on play therapy are far less abundant; unfortunately, the paucity of such work has hampered meta-reviews of therapeutic efficacy. Despite this, a number of analyses suggest that play therapy is an effective treatment for children with a wide range of emotional and behavioral symptoms, particularly when parents are involved and the duration of treatment is at least several months (Bratton and Ray 2000; Bratton et al. 2005; Eresund 2007; Leblanc and Ritchie 2001). Broader studies on the success of psychodynamic and psychoanalytic treatments for children, which include the use of play for younger participants, also tend to be limited by their small-scale nature and lack of carefully selected subject groups (Midgley and Kennedy, 2011). Nonetheless, reviews of this body of work point to the value of dynamic interventions for an array of childhood disorders, with some evidence that such therapies produce more gradual but longer-lasting gains when compared with behaviorally based treatments (Fonagy and Target 1996b; Midgley and Kennedy 2011).

Studies of play therapy suggest an important role for play during the evaluation phase of treatment, when pretense yields abundant information about a child's level of ego organization, the relative richness or impoverishment of inner life, feelings and perceptions about important relationships, capacities for emotional regulation, and potential to engage in treatment. In addition, play provides insight into the quality of the child's early relationships and affect-laden experiences; the inhibition, perseveration, and disruptions that typify the play of traumatized children, along with attendant negative affect, are well documented (Myers et al. 2011; Terr 1981). Moreover, children with secure parental relationships are more likely to engage in richly developed play themes; a history of **disorganized attachment** is correlated with poorly organized narratives, chaotic play scenarios, and the presence of frightening contents (Lyons-Ruth 2006; Slade 1987; Valentino et al. 2011).

Pretend play measures, such as the Children's Play Therapy Instrument (Chazan and Cohen 2010; Chazan and Wolf 2002, Kernberg et al. 1997, 1998), function as effective tools for measuring therapeutic change in young children; such instruments capture the quality and flow of play, the child's use of defensive strategies, the developmental level of play, and the presence of affects and narrative themes. Such measures may be used to elucidate qualitative aspects of children's functioning, such as relational patterns, and also shed light on their problem-solving capacities; assessment of dominant play contents reflects the presence of age-salient themes and anxieties (Marans et al. 1991; Nash and Schaefer 2010).

A CONTEMPORARY PSYCHODYNAMIC VIEW OF PLAY THERAPY

Psychodynamic theories in the postmodern era reflect an increasingly pluralistic approach to modes and techniques of treatment, as well as to conceptualizations about mental development throughout the lifespan. Indeed, it is rare to find current psychodynamic writings that are not profoundly influenced by developmental science, particularly the field of infant research, or that do not incorporate contemporary notions about the primacy of relational processes. In many ways, the unique challenges of working with young children necessitate a natural integration of classical psychoanalytic principles (having a keen interest in a child's emerging ego capacities, defenses, conflicts, and unconscious fantasies; finding representations of the child's central relationships and perceptions of past experience within play narratives) with more recent approaches (emphasis on the unfolding child–therapist relationship and on their here-and-now interactions, many of which occur outside the realm of verbal interventions; realization that play scenarios inevitably reflect the therapeutic dyad's co-created fantasies and meanings).

In our view, a contemporary psychodynamic theory of play therapy encompasses the following defining features:

- Recognition of play as the premier language of childhood, and as the main medium for relating and communicating in the treatment of young children.
- Realization that the themes and contents of play reflect key aspects of children's intrapsychic life (past and current conflicts; defensive mechanisms; modes of relating; the child's memories, including naïve interpretations of affect-laden events, and fantasies about the self and relationships) but also inevitably represent aspects of the therapist's unconscious and meanings that are co-created within the therapeutic dyad.
- A focus on working within the interface of children's unfolding ego capacities and psychodynamic technique. This implies that the thera-

pist intervenes with attunement to the child's developmental vulnerabilities (e.g., normative susceptibility to overstimulation, difficulty tolerating uncomfortable affects, tendency toward shame and feelings of exposure) and cognitive abilities; the latter powerfully determine and may limit the child's potential to comprehend and benefit from certain therapeutic techniques, such as verbal insight-oriented comments. Moreover, a developmentally sensitive approach to working with young children means balancing the child's naturally progressive, future-oriented tendencies with such treatment goals as resolving past conflicts and modifying old relational patterns.

- A broad, multidimensional view of the potential therapeutic functions of play, including the child–clinician mutual playing state, their reciprocal verbal and nonverbal interactions, and the clinician's direct provision of developmental assistance.
- Acknowledgment of the complex role of specific biological and environmental challenges, such as learning problems or difficult environments, in derailing developmental progression. An initial assessment of the child's endowment, attachment relationships, and learning settings may reveal additional areas that require the therapist's attention (e.g., the child may benefit from a recommendation for psychological testing, or referrals for the parents to receive individual or couples therapy).
- An emphasis on collaborative work with parents and other caregivers and helping figures in the child's life who are intimately involved in developmental outcome.
- Maintaining scholarly interest in neighboring fields, such as developmental research.
- An open attitude toward learning about the child's cultural surround and other important influences, including family, community, ethnicity, and the impact of technology on the child's developing fantasy life.
- A receptive stance toward shifts in the nature of children's play, such as the increasing role of digital media in the lives of children of all ages.

SUMMARY

Play therapy is the premier medium for the psychodynamic treatment of young children. Psychoanalysts view play as a unique window into the child's inner life and as a normative growth-promoting capacity that facilitates the following: making meaning of affect-laden events, organizing and modulating intense emotions, converting passive experience into active mastery, trying out numerous roles and identifications, and practicing emerging skills. During play therapy, child and therapist achieve a mutual playing state in which reality is jointly suspended as they co-construct meanings and narratives. Contemporary psychodynamic theory proposes a multidimensional view of the play therapy process; potentially mutative components include the child's and therapist's shared play, implicit aspects of their relationship, the therapist's verbal interventions, elaboration of the child's defensive and interpersonal patterns, and the therapist's provision of direct developmental assistance to bolster the child's evolving ego functions. Attunement to the child's developmental status and cultural surround is an essential therapeutic principle. In addition, the child therapist works collaboratively with parents and other central attachment figures in the child's life to restore developmental progression.

KEY POINTS

- Pretend play is a natural developmental capacity that provides a window onto age-salient anxieties and fantasies, and illuminates the child's subjective interpretation of environment and events. As a therapeutic process, play is uniquely suited to function as the major mode for communication, assessment, and treatment in work with young children.

- Play emerges during the oedipal phase, as do other symbolic functions such as narrative language and mentalization, and serves the following developmental functions: transforming passive experience into active mastery; modulating intense affects; making meaning of emotionally laden events; trying on others' perspectives; and sampling roles and identifications.

- A contemporary view of play therapy reflects shifts in psychoanalytic theory and incorporates information from neighboring fields, such as developmental research. Major principles of a modern approach include integrating traditional with more recent thinking about therapeutic processes, acknowledging the multidimensional therapeutic functions of play therapy, and attending to biological factors, central attachment relationships, and cultural influences in the child's life.

KEY TERMS

Developmental assistance   The therapist's multiple functions that support children's emerging capacities; these functions often center on scaffolding children's vulnerable self-regulation through interventions such as labeling affects, facilitating play, and setting limits.

Disorganized attachment   A particular form of insecure parent–child relationship wherein the child fails to derive comfort from the parental presence and manifests inconsistent, incoherent strategies for managing distress.

Interpretation   Verbal, insight-oriented interventions in which the therapist attempts to make conscious the patient's defensive and relational patterns.

Latency phase   The period of development that corresponds roughly with the grade-school years (i.e., ages 6 through 10 or 11), wherein most children manifest a significant increase in cognitive, social, and emotional maturation as demonstrated by greater autonomous self-regulation, awareness of reality, a capacity for logical thinking, and a decisive turn toward the peer group.

Mentalization   A developmental capacity that emerges at around age 4 years in which children begin to grasp mental states, differentiate inner and outer experience, and connect people's behavior to their beliefs and emotions. In the empirical literature, this capacity is often referred to as *theory of mind*.

Oedipal phase   The period of development, roughly between ages 3 and 6 years, when symbolic capacities proliferate, including narrative language, mentalization, and imaginary play. Within psychoanalytic theory, the oedipal phase also marks a time when children begin to grasp triadic relationships, develop intense feelings of possessiveness and jealousy toward a parent, and manifest avid curiosity about adults' sexual lives.

Playing state   The special consciousness or ego state that accompanies play during which reality is suspended and the child is fully engrossed in pretense.

●━━━━━━━━━━━━━━━●

REFERENCES

Abrams S, Neubauer PB, Solnit AJ: Coordinating the developmental and psychoanalytic processes: three case reports. Introduction (discussion). Psychoanal Study Child 54:19–24, discussion 87–90, 1999 10748626

Aguayo J: Patronage in the dispute over child analysis between Melanie Klein and Anna Freud, 1927–1932. Int J Psychoanal 81(Pt 4):733–752, 2000 11028236

Axline VM: Play Therapy. New York, Ballantine Books, 1969

Barish K: What is therapeutic in child therapy? I. Therapeutic engagement. Psychoanal Psychol 21(3):385–401, 2004

Birch M: In the land of counterpane: travels in the realm of play. Psychoanal Study Child 52:57–75, 1997 9489461

Bornstein B: The analysis of a phobic child: some problems of theory and technique in child analysis. Psychoanal Study Child 3:181–226, 1949

Bornstein B: On latency. Psychoanal Study Child 6:279–285, 1951

Bratton SC, Ray D: What the research shows about play therapy. International Journal of Play Therapy 9:47–88, 2000

Bratton SC, Ray D, Rhine T, et al: The efficacy of play therapy with children: a meta-analysis review of treatment outcomes. Professional Psychol Research and Practice 36(4):376–390, 2005

Bretherton I: Pretense: the form and function of make-believe play. Dev Rev 9:383–401, 1989

Brinich PM: Weaving child psychoanalysis: past, present, and future. Psychoanal Study Child 67:149–172, 2013 26072562

Brody S: Contributions to child analysis. Psychoanal Study Child 29:13–20, 1974 4614299

Bruschweiler-Stern N, Lyons-Ruth K, Morgan AC, et al: The foundational level of psychodynamic meaning: implicit process in relation to conflict, defense and the dynamic unconscious. Int J Psychoanal 88(Pt 4):843–860, 2007 17681896

Bucci W: Psychoanalysis and Cognitive Science: A Multiple Code Theory. New York, Guilford, 1997

Burghardt GM: Defining and recognizing play, in Oxford Handbook of the Development of Play. Edited by Pellegrini A. New York, Oxford University Press, 2011, pp 9–18

Busch F: What is a deep interpretation? J Am Psychoanal Assoc 48(1):237–254, 2000 10808479

Chazan S, Cohen E: Adaptive and defensive strategies in post-traumatic play of young children exposed to violence. Journal of Child Psychotherapy 36(2):133–151, 2010

Chazan SE, Wolf J: Using the Children's Play Therapy Instrument to measure change in psychotherapy: the conflicted player. J Infant Child Adolesc Psychother 2(3):73–102, 2002

Chused JF: The therapeutic action of psychoanalysis: abstinence and informative experiences. J Am Psychoanal Assoc 44(4):1047–1071, 1996 8987010

Cohen PM, Solnit AJ: Play and therapeutic action. Psychoanal Study Child 48:49–63, 1993 7694307

Downey TW: Notes on play and guilt in child analysis. Psychoanal Study Child 42:105–125; 1987 3438361

Emde R, Kubicek L, Oppenheim D: Imaginative reality observed during early language development. Int J Psychoanal 78(Pt 1):115–133, 1997 9104635

Eresund P: Psychodynamic psychotherapy for children with disruptive disorders. Journal of Child Psychotherapy 33:161–180, 2007

Fairbairn W: An Object Relation Theory of the Personality. New York, Basic Books, 1954

Fein GG: Pretend play in childhood: an integrative review. Child Dev 52(4):1095–1118, 1981

First E: Playing who we are together: commentary on Henry Kronengold's "Hey Toy Man." J Infant Child Adolesc Psychother 9(1):25–32, 2010

Fonagy P, Target M: Playing with reality, I: theory of mind and the normal development of psychic reality. Int J Psychoanal 77(Pt 2):217–233, 1996a 8771375

Fonagy P, Target M: Predictors of outcome in child psychoanalysis: a retrospective study of 763 cases at the Anna Freud Centre. J Am Psychoanal Assoc 44(1):27–77, 1996b 8717478

Frankel JB: The play's the thing: how the essential processes of therapy are seen most closely in child therapy. Psychoanal Dialogues 8(1):149–182, 1998

Freud S: Beyond the pleasure principle (1920), in The Standard Edition of the Complete Psychological Works of Sigmund Freud, Vol 20. Translated and edited by Strachey J. London, Hogarth, 1962, pp 1–64

Galatzer-Levy R: The nuts and bolts of child psychoanalysis. Annual of Psychoanalysis 36:189–202, 2008

Gergely G: Reapproaching Mahler: new perspectives on normal autism, symbiosis, splitting and libidinal object constancy from cognitive developmental theory. J Am Psychoanal Assoc 48(4):1197–1228, 2000 11212188

Gilmore K: Play in the psychoanalytic setting: ego capacity, ego state, and vehicle for intersubjective exchange. Psychoanal Study Child 60:213–238, 2005 16649681

Gilmore K: Pretend play and development in early childhood (with implications for the oedipal phase). J Am Psychoanal Assoc 59(6):1157–1182, 2011 22080503

Harrison AM, Tronick E: "The noise monitor": a developmental perspective on verbal and nonverbal meaning-making in psychoanalysis. J Am Psychoanal Assoc 59(5):961–982, 2011 21980139

Hoffman L: Do children get better when we interpret their defenses against painful feelings? Psychoanal Study Child 62:291–313, 2007 18524096

Howe N, Petrakos H, Rinaldi CM, et al: "This is a bad dog, you know...": constructing shared meanings during sibling pretend play. Child Dev 76(4):783–794, 2005 16026496

Hug-Hellmuth H: On the technique of child analysis. Int J Psychoanal 2:287–305, 1921

Keable H: From alloplay to play to transference—followed by a transference jewel. Journal of Clinical Psychoanalysis 10:403–444, 2001

Kernberg PF, Chazan SE, Normandin L: The Children's Play Therapy Instrument: Manual and Scale, unpublished paper, 1997

Kernberg PF, Chazan SE, Normandin L: The Children's Play Therapy Instrument (CPTI): description, development, and relationship studies. J Psychother Pract Res 7(3):196–207, 1998 9631341

Klein M: The psychological principles of infant analysis, in Contributions to Psycho-Analysis, 1921–1945. Edited by Klein M. London, Hogarth, 1926, pp 140–151

Klein M: The Psychoanalysis of Children. London, Hogarth, 1932

Knell SM, Desai M: Cognitive-behavioral play therapy for preschoolers: integrating play and cognitive-behavioral interventions, in Play Therapy for Preschool Children. Edited by Schaefer CE. Washington, DC, American Psychological Association, 2010, pp 155–178

Kronengold H: Hey toy man. J Infant Child Adolesc Psychother 9(1):3–17, 2010

Leblanc M, Ritchie M: A meta-analysis of play therapy outcomes. Couns Psychol Q 14(2):149–163, 2001

Lillard AS: Just through the looking glass: children's understanding of pretense, in Pretending in Animals and Children. Edited by Mitchell R. Cambridge, UK, Cambridge University Press, 2002, pp 102–114

Lillard AS, Lerner MD, Hopkins EJ, et al: The impact of pretend play on children's development: a review of the evidence. Psychol Bull 139(1):1–34, 2013 22905949

Lindsay EW, Colwell MJ: Pretend and physical play: links to preschoolers' affective social competence. Merrill-Palmer Q 59(3):330–360, 2013

Lyons-Ruth K: Play, precariousness and the negotiation of shared meaning: a developmental research perspective on child psychotherapy. J Infant Child Adolesc Psychother 5(2):142–159, 2006

Marans S, Mayes L, Cicchetti D, et al: The child-psychoanalytic play interview: a technique for studying thematic content. J Am Psychoanal Assoc 39(4):1015–1036, 1991 1800550

Mayes LC, Cohen DJ: Playing and therapeutic action in child analysis. Int J Psychoanal 74(Pt 6):1235–1244, 1993 8138367

Midgley N, Kennedy K: Psychodynamic psychotherapy for children and adolescents: a critical review of the evidence base. Journal of Child Psychotherapy 37:232–260, 2011

Miller JM: Developmental psychoanalysis and developmental objects. Psychoanal Inq 33(4):312–322, 2013

Moustakas C: Relationship Play Therapy. Northvale, NJ, Jason Aronson, 1997

Myers CE, Bratton SC, Hagen C, et al: Development of the trauma play scale: comparison of children manifesting a history of interpersonal trauma with a normative sample. International Journal of Play Therapy 20(2):66–78, 2011

Nash JB, Schaefer CE: Clinical and developmental issues in psychotherapy with preschool children: laying the groundwork for play therapy, in Play Therapy for Preschool Children. Edited by Schaefer CE. Washington, DC, American Psychological Association, 2010, pp 15–28

Neubauer PB: The many meanings of play: introduction. Psychoanal Study Child 42:3–9, 1987 3438372

Neubauer PB: Some observations about changes in technique in child analysis. Psychoanal Study Child 56:16–26, 2001 12102011

Peller LE: Libidinal phases, ego development and play. Psychoanal Study Child 9:178–198, 1954

Pelligrini AD: The effects of exploration and play on young children's associative fluency. Imagin Cogn Pers 41(1):29–40, 1985

Piaget J: Play, Dreams and Imitation. New York, WW Norton, 1962

Ritvo S: The psychoanalytic process in childhood. Psychoanal Study Child 33:295–305, 1978 715107

Salomonsson MW: Transference in child analysis: a comparative reading of Anna Freud and Melanie Klein. Scandinavian Psychoanalytic Review 20:1–19, 1997

Sandler S, Kennedy H, Tyson RH: The Technique of Child Psychoanalysis: Discussions With Anna Freud. Cambridge, MA, Harvard University Press, 1980

Scott ME: Play and therapeutic action: multiple perspectives. Psychoanal Study Child 53:94–101, 1998 9990825

Slade A: Quality of attachment and early symbolic play. Dev Psychol 23(1):78–85, 1987

Slade A: Making meaning and making believe: their role in the clinical process, in Children at Play: Clinical and Developmental Approaches to Meaning and Representation. Edited by Slade A, Wolf D. New York, Oxford University Press, 1994, pp 81–107

Solnit AJ: A psychoanalytic view of play. Psychoanal Study Child 42:205–219, 1987 3438366

Spitz RA: Hospitalism; an inquiry into the genesis of psychiatric conditions in early childhood. Psychoanal Study Child 1:53–74, 1945 21004303

Spitz RA: Hospitalism; a follow-up report. Psychoanal Study Child 2:113–117, 1946 20293627

Sugarman A: Toward helping child analysands observe mental functioning. Psychoanal Psychol 11(3):329–339, 1994

Sugarman A: A new model for conceptualizing insightfulness in the psychoanalysis of young children. Psychoanal Q 72(2):325–355, 2003 12718248

Sutherland SL, Friedman O: Just pretending can be really learning: children use pretend play as a source for acquiring generic knowledge. Dev Psychol 49(9):1660–1668, 2013 23148938

Terr LC: "Forbidden games:" post-traumatic child's play. J Am Acad Child Psychiatry 20(4):741–760, 1981 7328250

Tessier VP, Normandin L, Ensink K, et al: Fact or fiction? A longitudinal study of play and the development of reflective functioning. Bull Menninger Clin 80(1):60–79, 2016 27028339

Tuber S, Caflisch J: Starting Treatment With Children and Adolescents. New York, Routledge, 2012

Valentino K, Cicchetti D, Toth SL, et al: Mother-child play and maltreatment: a longitudinal analysis of emerging social behavior from infancy to toddlerhood. Dev Psychol 47(5):1280–1294, 2011 21744951

Vivona JM: Speech as the confluence of words, body, and relationship: discussion of Harris, Kirshner, and Spivak. J Am Psychoanal Assoc 62(6):1081–1086, 2014 25503760

Vygotsky L: Mind in Society: The Development of Higher Psychological Processes. Cambridge, MA, Harvard University Press, 1978

Waelder R: The psychoanalytic theory of play. Psychoanal Q 2:208–224, 1932

Warshaw SC: Missing pieces and incoherence: an interpersonal/relational perspective on Dr. Kronengold's clinical material. J Infant Child Adolesc Psychother 9(1):37–40, 2010

Winnicott DW: Playing: its theoretical status in the clinical situation. Int J Psychoanal 49(4):591–599, 1968 4180041

Winnicott DW: The Piggle: An Account of the Psychoanalytic Treatment of a Little Girl. London, Hogarth, 1980

Yanof JA: Barbie and the tree of life: the multiple functions of gender in development. J Am Psychoanal Assoc 48(4):1439–1465, 2000 11212196

Yanof JA: Treating children with affective dysregulation. Discussion of Dr. Wendy Olesker's analysis of Matt. Psychoanal Study Child 66:109–121, 2012 26020994

2

Play, Playfulness, and the Sequence of Play Forms in Development

When Jimmy was 2 years old, he was fascinated by trucks—garbage trucks, fire trucks, big container trucks, and even pickup trucks. He would shout, "Look, look!" whenever he and his mother passed by a truck and would drag his mother to the firehouse across the street from his apartment building every day until he became the firefighters' "mascot" and was allowed to sit in the cab of the big fire engine. He had a collection of pocket-sized cars and trucks, which he loved to line up. Whenever possible, he would persuade his father to race the vehicles with him. He also loved an electronic toy garage that parked his little cars and announced their parking fees as the cars drove out the exit ramp. For his third birthday, he received a large fire engine, replete with flashing lights, siren sounds, ladders, hose, and three firefighters.

His much older sister had abandoned her old dollhouse in their shared play space; it was still in good shape with three floors, furniture, and a family of five inside. Jimmy was told to ask her permission if he wanted to play with it, which he was careful to do; she actually helped him set up the furniture and place the dolls, narrating and playing out the stories she used to love to enact with them. She showed him which doll she usually identified as her character and the one who was the little brother. Jimmy began to create a story in which a fire broke out in the house, spinning a series of scenarios about how this happened and who was responsible; the kids were often to blame because they built up too big a fire in the fireplace or wanted to make a fire outside the house on the "lawn." Jimmy got the idea of how to make it really look like a fire. He begged for a roll of orange plastic wrap and crumpled it up. His sister was very impressed and complimented him on his imagination; he was speechless with joy. The plots thickened: In some scenarios, the father made a fire in the fireplace but it quickly flamed out of control; this was either a mistake due to ignorance or impulsivity or maybe there was something wrong with the chimney. Inevitably the fire engine was dispatched and the three firefighters arrived on the scene with considerable panache. His many narratives included saving the family, rescuing the mom who was trying to save the children, finding the cat, sliding down the chimney to fix the "block in the chimney" (which Jimmy made by putting a block in it), and, in still later iterations, discovering a criminal or careless culprit who started the fire and bringing in the police who arrested him, and so on. This was the play he most gravitated to and enjoyed for the following year. His play was given new life by a birthday present at age 4. At his sister's urging (and her contribution of a week's allowance), his parents got him a big toy firehouse that accommodated his engine. He became completely absorbed in exploring this new toy. He frequently called in his mother to observe the flames and the feats of the firefighters, particular the handsome Firefighter Sam, Badge 239.

Jimmy continued to love the actual firehouse and the firefighters across the street, spending many afternoons watching their activities. When he was age 8, he was offered the "job" of polishing the lower part of the engine when it was being cleaned. He worked on a "book" that included photos he took using his sister's cell phone (until he got his own at age 10) and descriptions of all the gizmos on the engine, the daily life of the firehouse, and the "brave people who fought fires." He attended the division commander's talks for children about fire safety and, when in fifth grade, got his school to invite the division commander and crew to do an assembly about fire prevention. He proudly introduced the commander to the whole school as his good friend whom he had known for his whole life.

The developmental arc of Jimmy's play shows the typical evolution of play forms during the first decade of life. His early pleasure in gazing at work trucks is one version of toddler boys' interest in things big, powerful, and capable. At home, he enjoyed his toy cars and trucks, but as a toddler he did little pretending. He was fortunate to have a firehouse nearby to nurture his interest and to help people the world of big trucks with real heroes. As he moved into the era of pretend play, his affectionate older sister provided **scaffolding** for his steps forward into symbolic play, both by offering her old dollhouse and then by heightening its glow with her own stories from earlier in her life; her compliments and support added to Jimmy's pride in his play. Her suggestion of the perfect gift for his fourth birthday was a brilliant exercise of her own **mentalization** skills. Oedipal themes dominated his stories, with an array of male figures representing facets of his complex feelings toward his father: admiration, identification, rivalry, devaluation. Jimmy identified with the brave Firefighter Sam who participated in the rescue of the mother and children, while the father of the endangered family only made foolish mistakes. The idealizing side of his ambivalence was also expressed in his hero worship of the real firefighters next door. As Jimmy moved into latency, his interest became more reality oriented and associated with actual achievements, as he helped out with the engine at the fire station and learned about fire safety. This trend took an entrepreneurial turn when he developed an assembly program that allowed him to shine at his school. Much as it might complete his story to say he grew up to become a firefighter, he did not; he actually followed his basic scientist father's footsteps and majored in environmental science in college. He did, however, join the volunteer firefighters and emergency medical technician (EMT) service as a student at his university in a small midwestern town; to his surprise, as he neared graduation he began to think about a career in medicine.

PRETEND PLAY IN CONTEXT

Although pretend play is only one of a series of play forms that emerge over the course of human development, it has a special status for researchers and play theorists for several reasons:

1. Pretend play is limited to a relatively brief period of ascendance in early childhood through mid-latency; although derivatives of pretending in adult creative activities have been suggested by many scholars, its duration as a distinct spontaneous play form is remarkably short (Gilmore 2011).
2. The consistent presence of pretend play across cultures among all children within this time frame has led researchers to propose a "neuropsychological timetable and biological basis" for symbolic play (Harris 1994, p. 256; 1996).
3. Pretend play is unique to humans as an invariant step in the small series of human play forms occurring early in development (explor-

atory, imitative, functional, pretend, rough-and-tumble) that has no counterpart in the juvenile phase of other young mammals (Pellegrini and Smith 2005).

4. Pretend play is the therapeutic medium for child therapy because, alone among all play forms, it is constructed de novo every day in every child; although it is tethered to its contemporaneous culture by virtue of toys, popular heroes, technology, and play equipment, it is essentially a newly created or improvised narrative that unfolds over hours, days, or months; follows its own set of rules; and is sustained by the individual child's or playmates' imagination.

For these and many other reasons, pretend play has garnered a position of prominence as a research focus and a presumed developmental engine.

Notably, the term *play* has many different forms over the course of the lifespan, encompassing "this little piggy," chess, video games, improvisational theater, baseball card collecting, and innumerable other play variants. In this chapter, we briefly extend our focus beyond pretend play to consider play in a broader sense, as a plastic but recognizable activity that is observed in humans of all ages and in many species of animals. This lens illuminates the complexity and breadth of the play concept and highlights its vast variation and incarnations. We describe play forms in their typical developmental progression and consider the scholarly debates that surround this untidy and chameleon phenomenon.

THE STUDY OF PLAY

The subject of play is a relative latecomer to scholarly study. Despite its long-documented history and celebration in human civilization (Parsons 1999), play only acquired sufficient gravitas to merit scientific interest in the twentieth century (Johnson et al. 1987). Play's conceptual unwieldiness may have contributed to this delay, but perhaps a more likely explanation is its association with childhood. Like many child-linked phenomena, play had to overcome a significant "triviality barrier" (Sutton-Smith 1997) to first attract serious scholarly interest. From the moment of that recognition forward, play has been claimed by an array of disciplines, from evolutionary scientists to public policy makers. Because it is so multiform and interfaces with so many fields of study, play is subject to the "three blind men and the elephant" phenomenon: different thinkers think about play differently, based on the way they think and what aspect of play they are considering. Like many other complex behavioral phenomena with a strong developmental arc and a formative interface with every culture, play is an unwieldy entity whose boundaries are blurry and whose features are both timeless and endlessly changing (Mechling 2000; Sutton-Smith 1997).[1]

Indeed, rather than wrestle play into one discipline with comprehensive theoretical propositions, many contemporary scholars reject the possibility of a singular definition sustained by a unifying theory and instead welcome the multiplicity of theories from all interested disciplines (Burghardt 2005; Pufall and Pufall 2008). Others suggest that play refers to a frame, a mode of experiencing, or an attitude that can be brought to bear on other phenomena, transforming them and creating new meaning (Handelman 2001). One of the earliest scholars to grant play significance, Huizinga (1955), offered the first version of this notion of frame, calling it a "**magic circle**" that contains the play, granting the player the opportunity to "step...out of real life into a temporary sphere of activity with a disposition all of its own" (p. 9). The notion of play as an orientation toward the activity at hand and a means of managing "real life" is grounded in its origins in infancy (see section "The Developmental Chronology of Play Forms" later in this chapter) and is fundamental to the parental attribute of **playfulness**, arguably the birthplace of a child's play.

DEFINITIONS OF PLAY

Although scholars from myriad disciplines agree that a comprehensive definition of *play* is elusive and perhaps even unnecessary, they also concur that play is self-evident; typically, the onlooker immediately knows whether an activity is serious and consequential or a version of the many play forms in the repertoire of the animal observed. In humans, these forms take such disparate shape as pretend play, struc-

---

[1]Play is clearly not the exclusive domain of childhood, but it is important to remember that childhood itself is a cultural concept that differs across societies and changes over the course of human history.

tured board or card games, athletic competitions, electronic games, and ritual (at least for some—see Huizinga 1955). An overarching definition of *human play* must encompass this broad range of play forms and must be flexible enough to apply to play in ancient cultures, contemporary societies, and both children and adults; presumably it would apply in some modified form to other species as well.

The list that follows is distilled from thinkers representing many approaches and stretching to encompass many play forms, conceptual systems, cultures, and the inevitable developmental transformations across the lifespan (Ablon 2001; Bateson 2005; Bateson and Martin 2013; Fein 1981; Graham and Burghardt 2010; Huizinga 1955; Johnson et al. 1987; Pellegrini and Bjorklund 2004; Winnicott 1971). Play is

1. Pleasurable, but not fueled directly by instinctual drives.
2. Symbolic (nonliteral), and therefore:
   a. Meaningful and yet not real.
3. Associated with activity, mental and/or physical, and with a more or less altered state of mind.
4. Process rather than product oriented.
5. Voluntary and self-perpetuating.
6. Possessed of idiosyncratic rules.

The pleasurable aspect of play is foundational; it is the presumed motive force for the player. Interestingly, although pleasure, "fun," and/or joy can be observed during some types of play, it is by no means a prominent aspect of all play for either spectator or player (Huizinga 1955). In fact, it may be more accurate to describe the emotional state associated with play as an altered state of consciousness, with a unique deployment of attention, altered experience of space and time, and apparent total immersion. This state is governed by play-specific rules and regulations and shows varying degrees of permeability to intrusions of reality (Gilmore 2011; Winnicott 1971).

Jimmy's dreamy state of mind as he played with his toy firehouse and his sharp, dedicated focus when performing his "jobs" in the real firehouse demonstrate versions of the intense absorption of play, composed of fantasy, pragmatic interest, and enjoyment of mastery. Other examples are the full absorption and suspended sense of time and space described by athletes playing their sport, the impenetrable engagement of the late-latency child playing Minecraft, and the rapt attention, intuitive communication, and immersion in an imaginary world typical of a group of kindergartners collaborating in **sociodramatic play**.

Play is "satisfying" (Winnicott 1971, p. 52) but does not involve real physical arousal or drive satisfaction, either sexual or aggressive. Affects during play are "virtual" (or intended to be virtual) in that they occur in safe and modulated settings (Sutton-Smith 2003). Indeed, the interface with reality in the playing state is complex and highly variable, but it is never fully absent; play occurs in the "potential space" between inner and outer reality (Winnicott 1971) and inevitably involves real objects and/or other people. This component of external reality augments over the arc of development, from the almost full suspension of reality in the make-believe world of the young child to the competitive stakes in sports and games that bring play into the professional arena. Indeed, play features have gradations, because the activity, derived from many aspects of inner life, evolving motor and cognitive capacities, and cultural affordances, can teeter on the domains of real-life need satisfaction, work, learning, and relationships. This is obviously the case with competitive sports, where the outcome becomes increasingly consequential over the course of development: money, fame, status, and power draw the activity away from pure "play" and toward reality. Nonetheless, even professional athletes describe some of the features associated with the altered state of play: "Time really does slow down for athletes" (Condliffe 2012).

In childhood play, the introduction of urgency, reality demands, or enforced agendas usually transforms the experience of the individuals involved. Coercion, real desire, the pursuit of drive satisfaction, or intentional, serious instruction can intrude, more or less, on the playing state. Perhaps paradoxically, the opposite is also true: "making something into a game" can help to ease the pain of reality. This device is intuitively exploited by parents who use varying degrees of playfulness to help their children through the tribulations of daily life.

A gradient similar to that pertaining to proximity to reality also applies to the quality of purposelessness emphasized in some definitions. In this regard, it is important to distinguish between the felt experience of the player and the purpose of play in a larger sense, such as its role in evolution, culture, or development. Ever since play accrued the gravitas to merit study, its function has been a topic of great interest. But its function as understood by any discipline or conceptual system has no particular relationship to the player's motivation and/or goal. Even in play where stakes, such as winning and losing, are emphasized, the players are at least consciously aware that the criteria for success are arbitrary, albeit shared by other participants. Most types of play require sufficient detachment from real purpose in order to feel like play. For the player then, the only consistent purpose of play is playing, underscoring the fact that play imparts meaning to itself.

PERSPECTIVES ON PLAY IN HUMAN DEVELOPMENT

Stepping back from the player's experience of "just playing," the purpose or function of play has been explored from different vantage points for the last century. Here we offer a brief overview of the fields that would appear to have bearing on the role of play in human development.

Play in Evolution

Ethological studies, which place a given behavior in evolutionary context, have generated a wealth of ideas about play in animal development, identifying the requisite conditions for its appearance and its development over a given individual's lifetime (ontogeny), while theorizing about its evolutionary consequences and tracing its evolutionary history (Burghardt 2005, p. 10; Pellegrini et al. 2007). The detailed elucidation of specific features of play within orders and species is only just beginning. Given that play is such a multifaceted category and that, even within species, play forms can differ in observed affective state, content, cognitive demand, developmental trajectory, and overall complexity, evolutionary research concerning the function of different types of play within and between species is in its infancy.

According to Robert Fagen (1981), a pioneer in the field of animal play, play is seen primarily in large-brained species with environmental circumstances that include the prerequisite conditions of safety, resilience, and surplus for the pursuit of pleasure. Although some of his assertions have been challenged by subsequent research, especially in regard to brain size requirements and variety of species in which play can be observed (Iwaniuk et al. 2001), there is general consensus that the animal play that most resembles human play is found in species with a long period of immaturity requiring parental care, wherein organismic self-regulation is achieved in the juvenile period and freedom from survival concerns is sustained by parental/environmental provision (the "surplus resource theory" of Burghardt [2005]). Vigorously active locomotor play (also called "rough-and-tumble play" or "play fighting") is a clearly recognizable feature in the juvenile period of almost all mammals, birds, and, according to Burghardt (2005), many other species. From an evolutionary perspective, such a ubiquitous behavior supports the notion that play serves a function in adaptation, contributing to the player's survival and/or reproductive success (Bateson and Martin 2013; Pellegrini and Smith 1998). Play is particularly challenging in this regard because it actually requires significant energy output, relies on the provision of environmental safety, diverts attention from immediate survival needs, and exposes young animals to an increased risk of predation (Bateson 2005). Evolutionary scientists and others grapple with this paradox by proposing *future advantage*; this view asserts that play provides an opportunity for the development of novel strategies and promotes a kind of flexibility that can serve adaptation in adulthood, thus conferring advantages only observable years later (Pellegrini et al. 2007; Pufall and Pufall 2008). Moreover, the inclusive imitation of adult behaviors (termed *overimitation*) is a unique aspect of human play that leads to transmission of nonessential actions in the child's re-creation of adult behavior. In human society, where cultural complexity, interpersonal skill, and technological advances proceed at dizzying speed, the overimitation typical of pretend play has been linked to both the maintenance of traditional elements and the emergence of innovations (Nielsen 2012). The evolutionary advantage may thus be "adaptive variability" (Sutton-Smith 1997, p. 221)—an outcome that is invoked by other disciplines as well, as demonstrated by the fact that flexibility is frequently cited in developmental literature (Walker and Gopnik 2013). Improved creativity and combinational flexibility, in addition to skill in extracting rules and constructing models, have been linked to play, especially social play. However, experimental proof of future benefit is sorely lacking.

Other evolutionary thinkers observe that a species' ultimate gain through play may be best described as "one benefit leads to others"

(Bateson and Martin 2013, p. 43). Creative solutions and innovation may not be the impetus for playing, but playing over development generates new problems and new approaches to old dilemmas. So, while educational intent by definition has no place in playing, play nonetheless gradually informs juveniles: they become versed in the culture of the group, discover tools and their versatility, and learn the boundaries of acceptable behavior. Another advantage conferred by play in humans may be the indirect outcome of the preference for playfulness in sexual selection, a theory proposed by Chick et al. (2012) and others and supported thus far by mate-preference data. The very fact that play appears to emerge de novo in disparate taxonomic groups suggests that it likely serves adaptation.

Because of this ubiquity of play, especially rough-and-tumble play, in mammals, Panksepp (Burgdorf and Panksepp 2001; Panksepp 2004; Panksepp et al. 1984) has suggested that the urge to play arises from shared subcortical limbic circuitries that determine affective states in all mammals and operate apart from the cortical cognitive components. A pioneer in the effort to legitimize the study of emotion within neuroscience, Panksepp (2004) proposes that play and playful emotion are likely "built into the instinctual action apparatus of the mammalian brain" (p. 54), further supporting the notion of evolutionary advantage (Mercer and Speakman 2001), despite its cost.

Play in Culture

One of the first serious scholars to address play as a topic of import, the cultural historian Huizinga (1955) described the role of play in the creation and transmission of culture and the cultural elaboration of meaning and ritual in his book *Homo Ludens: A Study of the Play-Element in Culture*. Huizinga asserted that play has been documented or inferred from artifacts of earliest human history, is an aspect of every cultural institution, and is demonstrable at every point within individual lifespans. Nonetheless, man does not play with intent; play is irreducible fun, voluntary, nonutilitarian, and pervasive. However, play generates meaning and creates importance: "In play there is something 'at play' which transcends the immediate needs of life and imparts meaning to the action" (Huizinga 1955, p. 1).

Certainly, societal attitudes toward play have varied considerably over time and have had powerful repercussions not only on its status as a topic of scientific interest but also on its expression, as adults create the milieu and the access to playtime and playthings. In humans, as in other mammals, the social conditions required for the development of the capacity to play presuppose a level of protection from survival concerns. Beyond this basic prerequisite, sociocultural factors shape and color play forms, based not only on type of economy, degree of industrialization, and technology, but also on the differential valuation of competition, aggression, creativity, ritual and mythology, and the current power hierarchy (Göncü et al. 2007). Within the larger social milieu, the subculture and socioeconomic status of the family also exert profound effects.

Parental attitudes and parental playfulness directly shape the emergence of many forms of play, especially pretend play. Through playfulness, playing is passed on from parent to child in every human culture. Indeed, playfulness and playing initiated by adults are ubiquitous features of infant care and are recognized by infants, when displayed by loving parents, as special, joyful communications; the infant's intuitive recognition of the mother's marked affect as an invitation to play is evident in the first year of life.

Just as adults transmit culture by introducing objects, games, and playfulness to children, children carry society to the next level by their imaginative vision as they ride the crest of transforming culture and demand new technology. By adolescence, "youth culture"—a heady mixture of contemporary play, music, politics, and pleasures—becomes the leading edge of social change and the driver of technological innovation.

Play in Human Development

According to psychologist Peter K. Smith (2007), the scientific study of human play has paradoxically suffered from a prevailing "play ethos"—"an uncritical and extreme assertion of the functional importance of play" (p. 33)—that has reigned since the 1920s. After being deemed beneath scientific interest in prior centuries, play was polevaulted into an arena where its merits for healthy development and improved learning were extolled without rigorous research (Lillard et al. 2013). Whereas some play forms, such as athletic games, have undisputed reverberations in the development of motor skills and strategy, pretend play's "position of prominence" in developmental theory—particularly in regard to its role in the development of cognition, affect, object relationships, language (Göncü and Gaskins 2007), creativity, and narrative capacity (Nicolopoulou and Ilgaz 2013)—in large part reflects this twentieth-century ethos rather than empirical documentation.

Much of the early twentieth-century research into pretend play (notably in the form of doll play [Sears 1947]) focused on play's reflection of the "inner person" of the child and its relationship to real experience—that is, its value as a window into the child's mind rather than as a harbinger of developmental trends or a developmental asset. Subsequent research began to tackle the task of establishing pretend play's developmental consequences in terms of specific sequelae. Two major reviews of the research, the first in 1981 by Fein and the second in 2013 by Lillard et al., document the huge challenges of definition, experimental design, and outcome measurement in this arena. Fein (1981) extracted some promising correlations from her review, particularly in regard to improved combinational flexibility, but acknowledged that the results from the majority of studies were confounded by adult "training" and no assessment of benefits beyond the immediate posttest period. Lillard et al.'s (2013) more recent review of the considerable body of current research recited a litany of methodological flaws and unconvincing findings, concluding that "existing evidence does not support strong causal claims" for any subsequent benefits (p. 1). These scholars suggest that pretend play is more likely "equifinal" and "epiphenomenal" to positive outcomes.

Critiques of Lillard et al.'s (2013) review (see Bodrova et al. 2013; Nicolopoulou and Ilgaz 2013; Walker and Gopnik 2013; Weisberg et al. 2013) reiterate the inherent challenges in studying a broadly defined, spontaneous activity with vast variations that typically occurs in the absence of adults and appears to rehearse capacities not evident for years, possibly decades. For example, to assess the role of improvised sociodramatic imaginary play, as seen during kindergarten recess, in developing theory of mind or self-regulation, one must tackle the thorny problems of how to replicate it in a laboratory setting, how to standardize the play taking place, how and when results can be measured, and where to seek correlations (Bodrova et al. 2013; Walker and Gopnik 2013). Moreover, such assessment would need to grapple with the substantial problem of pretest status and potential. As Bergen

(2013) noted in her critique of Lillard et al.'s (2013) conclusions, the overriding problem with the existing research is that the "pretend play" under investigation is more accurately termed "playful work": it is adult guided and instructed, prescripted (e.g., adult-directed enactments of familiar fairy tales and stories), performed for an audience, and lacking the crucial features that most scholars see as fundamental to play—that is, spontaneously elaborated scripts, changing themes, intense sustained internal motivation, an "as-if quality," and "in-depth metacommunicative behaviors." Moreover, Bergen (2013) observed that these studies do not address "private play," the first form of pretend play that blossoms in 3- and 4-year-olds (Bergen 2013, p. 46). Many of the critics concur that the available methodology for studying children's pretense lacks the sophistication required to look at aggregates of outcomes, multiple developmental pathways, and nonlinear dynamic interactions (Weisberg and Gopnik 2013) in order to assess such an unwieldy and pervasive aspect of childhood experience.

This debate is especially relevant to our topic, because the pretend play of early childhood is considered both a premiere therapeutic tool and a development-enhancing capacity, but this play lacks the immediately demonstrable justification of offering physical exercise, structured mental challenge, and/or direct cultivation of skills and qualities such as deductive reasoning, coordination, team spirit, sportsmanship, and perseverance. Some developmentalists suggest that seeking any function for pretend play beyond the play itself deflects attention from the fact that it is simply a "vital part of children's lives" (Bergen 2013, p. 48) that paves the young child's rocky road to adaptation to reality with precious pleasurable moments (Moran 1987). Today, when culturally sanctioned free play is threatened by the encroachment of educational agendas, there is a felt need among educators to document its value in terms of contributions to cognitive development. But even if quality of life may be of lesser status as an outcome variable, play adherents believe that pretend play's fundamental contribution is to children's subjective feeling of joy, connection to others, and creativity (Singer et al. 2009).

Moreover, most of these adherents consistently see play as facilitating development and as a crucial arena in which to practice new skills. Among these are psychoanalysts (Ablon 2001; Gilmore 2005, 2011; Meersand 2001; Solnit 1987; Solnit et al. 1993), research psychologists

(Singer and Singer 2013), cognitive psychologists (Piaget 1951, 1999; Piaget and Inhelder 1969; Vygotsky 1978), psychoanalyst teachers (Birch 1997), and child educators (Bergen 2013). Despite play's ambiguous status, these scholars and many others have generated a considerable body of literature asserting the cognitive and socioemotional value of play. Piaget's ideas about play have been credited with promoting its study, because play is crucial to his developmental schema of cognitive development. Play is contextualized in his notion of equilibrium between accommodation and assimilation: play represents "an extreme pole of assimilation of reality to the ego" (Piaget 1951/ 1999). The function of play is to protect and satisfy the "private universe of the ego" from forced accommodation (Piaget 1962, p. 168) even while play consolidates knowledge and practices skills (Carlisle 2009). Vygotsky (1967) posited the crucial role of imaginary play, especially play with others, in child development and school readiness, emphasizing that the rules of role-playing within the pretense requires self-regulation and thereby consolidates this capacity (Elias and Berk 2002). His famous statement "in play, a child becomes a head taller than himself" (Bodrova et al. 2013, p. 112) rests on his idea that "play is the source of development and creates the zone of proximal development" (Bodrova et al. 2013, p. 115). Pretend play requires that the child exceed his or her developmental level, inhibit impulses, and elaborate his or her understanding of adult roles. In the vignette at the beginning of this chapter, Jimmy's sister drew him forward into the **zone of proximal development** by offering her dollhouse and initiating him in narrative pretend play by sharing the treasured stories she had played out with her dollhouse for years. Walker and Gopnik (2013) suggest another long-term gain in their critique of Lillard et al.'s research review: pretending promotes engagement in counterfactual reasoning, which is essential to learning causal relations across domains.

Early psychoanalytic contributions to the topic of play began with Freud's (1920/1962) description of the "cultural achievement" of a 1½-year-old and his game of "fort-da" as a means of coping with separation from his mother and thereby coming to terms with reality (pp. 14–15). Waelder (1933) elaborated on Freud's observations and proposed a general "psychoanalytic theory of play," which contains the seeds for many subsequent contributions. He observed that the "cardinal functions" of play, like dreams and fantasies, are "instinctual gratification and assimilation of disagreeable experience" (p. 222). However, in contrast to dreams and fantasies, play involves objects in the world, thus straddling the boundary between fantasy and reality, which is "hazy" in childhood. Anticipating his profound insight concerning "multiple function" of mental phenomena (Waelder 1936), Waelder (1933) noted that any "single phenomenon may have various meanings, may perform various functions and cannot be explained by a single general interpretation: in short, as we say in psychoanalysis, the phenomenon has a number of determinants" (pp. 208–209). Thus, childhood play can serve the pleasure principle, yield the "functional pleasure" of performance, assimilate environmental stimuli, and dissipate traumatic experience via the repetition compulsion. The multiple functions of play include

1. Mastery.
2. Wish fulfillment (pleasure).
3. Assimilation of overpowering experience.
4. Departure from reality: it has one root in the function of fantasy.
5. Relief from superego pressures.

Peller (1954) further considered the role of play in managing anxiety, emphasizing the contribution of phase-specific conflicts arising from within in addition to environmental trauma. She described the important interface between play, psychosexual phases, and ego development, which produces a *developmental series of dominant forms*, from body play to dyadic and ultimately triadic relations. These differentiate on the basis of evolving ego capacities, phase-related conflicts and anxieties, and environmental affordances to function as the first effective mediator of synthetic function. Any iteration of play turns *passive to active* and brings a modicum of pleasure, but it is not pure instinctual gratification; it is a "step toward sublimation" (p. 180). This distinguishes play from the direct gratification of either sexual or aggressive drives; passing over the boundary to real sexual arousal or aggressive acts disrupts the state of play. Similarly, play cannot manage anxiety that exceeds its capacity to assimilate.

Winnicott's ideas, perhaps especially his concept of "transitional" space, have been highly influential in elucidating the role of play in development. Winnicott (1971) suggested that playing begins in the "potential space" between mother and infant, between psychic reality and external reality, where objects (beginning with the "transitional object") assume symbolic significance and play, creativity, and culture germinate. Throughout his clinical papers, Winnicott reiterated that the mother's playfulness is a crucial factor in establishing an arena in which both inner experience and external reality can be tempered through the emergence of symbolization and play. The research into early mother–infant exchanges conducted by Gergely et al. (1995) and elaborated on in a series of papers by Fonagy and Target (1996, 2000, 2007; Target and Fonagy 1996) underscores the importance of the primary caretaker in modulating the experience of inner and outer reality, introducing pretending via marked affect that identifies playing and toys as special, and making pretending a sanctuary. The parent's playful engagement with a very young infant supports and perpetuates the child's early play, especially pretend play, from primitive forms such as "this little piggy," "peek-a-boo," and "baby calisthenics" that the parent plays on the infant's body to the fully elaborated play of the 3- to 4-year-old. During this interval, an important shift occurs as the child of age 2–3 becomes a self-initiating player and thereby achieves independence from parental stimulus, despite the evident enhancement of the capacity by virtue of the parent's attitude of tolerance and approval (Slade 1987).

The idea of the pretending as a waystation toward reality has been addressed by an array of psychoanalytic and attachment theorists, including Fonagy and Target (1996), Gilmore (2011), Meersand (2001), Moran (1987), and Slade (1987). Moran (1987) strongly endorses parental playfulness as "a pleasure-oriented flexibility" (p. 15) that recognizes the innate pleasure orientation of the baby, deeply empathizes with his "needs and frustrations," and tries to lessen the strain of reality demands, the infant's own helplessness and incompetence, and the travails associated with these: "Playful parents find many inventive ways to lighten the demands they make on their child" (p. 16). Importantly, this play must be attuned to the state of the baby, neither drifting toward the excess of teasing and provocation nor shifting into rigidity by virtue of the parent's limited tolerance. Just as successfully playful parents use this mode to regulate their child's state, so young children, who are gradually orienting toward consensual reality, use the play arena and the "pretend mode" (increasingly initiated by the child) to let themselves down gently, as it were, thereby maintaining some degree of (pretend) omnipotence and the power to "make it come out" the way they want.

Thus, from the vantage point of psychodynamic thinking, the consistent blueprint of emerging and retreating play forms is strong evidence that in play, there is an expression of an important component of mental life that, to a greater or lesser degree, is present in every iteration, including pretend play, traumatic play, sociodramatic play, rough-and-tumble play, play fighting, and other locomotor play such as dodge ball, hopscotch, tag, and so on, into adult forms, such as baseball and Def Poetry Jams (Ablon 2001; Winnicott 1971). To some writers, adult play equivalents replace the objects of childhood with words and so are found in "puns, humor, metaphor, synonym, irony, sarcasm" (Ablon 2001, p. 346). Although childhood play is usually central to theorizing, the ideas generated in that arena have also been applied to many other situations: in particular, to transference–countertransference in the therapeutic interaction and to many endeavors involving imagination, fantasy, and creative arts. The presence of some form of play throughout life highlights its enduring importance in the mind; in the form of fiction, poetry, and fantasy, it serves to modulate and frame experience and provides an opportunity to experimentally transform it without consequences (Freud 1908/1959; Cohen and Solnit 1993). In Winnicott's (1971) metaphor, all humans, if not impeded, can realize a transitional space where creative thinking transcends current realities to find original ideas and solutions.

In regard to childhood imaginary play, the psychoanalytic literature has always privileged play as a window into the child's mind and as the resource for help in the daily management of anxiety. In addition, commentators have come to strongly endorse the development-promoting aspect of play as an overarching function. Play is the medium for such broad tasks as the integration of new ego capacities to meet developmental challenges and the development of "new ways of making meaning and new capacities to negotiate meanings with other minds" (Yanof 2012, p. 112). Its role in the latter is strongly emphasized in the work of Fonagy and Target and their colleagues (Fonagy and Target 1996, 2002; Fonagy et al. 2002; Target and Fonagy 1996), which identifies the pretend mode as the portal to the "representational aspects of thoughts" (Tessier et al. 2016) and to the growing awareness of the mutual impact of subjectivities, advancing the child toward **mentalization** and self-regulation. Pretense is an arena in which current conflicts are negotiated and future roles are tried out and practiced, contributing to the evolution of an "internal autobiographical narrative" (Tessier et al. 2016, p. 62).

THE DEVELOPMENTAL CHRONOLOGY OF PLAY FORMS

Within the various systems categorizing play, there is an implicit or explicit play chronology that has been shown to be recognizable across cultures. Piaget's (1968) developmental progression of cognitive capacities and associated play forms provided a way of categorizing play forms and facilitated the play research that has burgeoned since the 1970s (Fein 1981). The familiar sequence of *sensorimotor practice*, *pretense*, and *games with rules*, encompassing ages 1–6 years, has been further refined as each form has been characterized and understood to have its own developmental arc, often overlapping the more mature variant and remaining available in a recognizable form, at least for a period of time. As the hegemony of a given play form gives way to the next, the previous form is often retained in an attenuated version. Some variants persist indefinitely but of course evolve and mature, taking on adult meaning and sophistication. The following brief chronology of play illustrates the appearance and decline of play forms and highlights their ebb and flow.

INFANCY

Any description of play in infancy must begin with parents, because playful parents introduce playing within weeks of their child's birth and use it as an invaluable mode to child care. Adult playfulness, still an undervalued and undertheorized capacity, has suffered definitional ambiguity similar to that concerning play itself. Van Vleet and Feeney (2015) offer a broad definition of *playfulness* as "a dispositional tendency to engage in play" and thereby tether it to their preferred definition of play: "behavior or activity that is carried out *with the goal of amusement, enjoyment, and fun*." Playfulness research, like play research, is unstandardized and unwieldy. Playfulness has been studied and systematized in children from early to mid-childhood by related disciplines, especially by occupational therapists for the disabled (Brent-nall et al. 2008; Bronson and Bundy 2001; Liepold and Bundy 2000; Muys et al. 2006). Playfulness as a disposition toward spontaneous, improvisational, humorous, and adaptive activity is a huge asset for remediation and occupational or physical therapy, as it is for the enjoyment of developing play forms.

Moreover, playfulness has been recently granted important status for adults in the interpersonal sphere as serving a "signal function" in mate selection (Chick et al. 2012; Proyer and Wagner 2015) and a boon to quality of relationships (Van Vleet and Feeney 2015), ensuring its intergenerational transmission without reference to any other intrinsic evolutionary value.

Adult playfulness is important to our topic because it is essential to the infant's ultimate capacity to play. Playful parents initiate play with babies as young as 3–5 months in the same way they seek to regulate the infants' states: through the use of "marked affect" (Fonagy et al. 2007; Gergely and Watson 1996) and a particular type of motherese (Pellerin and Lecours 2015). This is the social biofeedback model, a highly complex process for self-recognition of emotion and regulation of state that is still in the process of clarification (see Pellerin and Lecours 2015). Playing and state regulation are interwoven in the parents' ministrations, because play helps a parent modulate reality for the helpless infant. There are some interesting differences, however: The playing parent does not mirror the infant's affect but rather introduces a new one intended to engage, distract, or cheer the baby. Furthermore, the parent plays with the baby, usually via baby's body, in a way that can be identified as not a real reflection of the parent's or the baby's emotions but nonetheless is recognizable to both as an indication that what is happening is special and fun; for example, "this little piggy" becomes an instantly recognized invitation to play. For an older infant, a make-believe safari (with an "elephant" ride on the parent) is a way to soften the blow of bedtime. The parent's playfulness around tasks adds pleasure to life. Similarly, the parents' playful introduction of objects endows those objects with special meaning, leading to the high valuation of toys and stuffed animals. Babies' visual and manual exploration, generated by these interactions and radiating from the body to objects in the environment, is usually considered the earliest play form.

This *exploratory play* (Morgenthaler 2006; Pellegrini and Smith 1998) is the predominant play modality of the first year of life. Piaget (1951), in his theory of cognitive development, refers to this as the *sensorimotor stage*, during which exploration facilitates knowledge of the world. This period is characterized by the familiar activities of the baby examining his or her own hand held aloft, pulling mother's hair and grabbing grandpa's glasses, and reaching to touch the light, and later rummaging in the kitchen cabinet, stacking bowls, and banging them with wooden spoons. This primarily exploratory approach to objects declines in the second year of life, as symbolic play gains momentum.

THE TODDLER

The toddler period is the preamble to pretend play. Exploration of objects declines in favor of *imitation* of adult behavior; the child now uses the bowl and spoon to feed a baby doll as a means to mimic the mother's activities This form, which is referred to as *functional play* by some writers (Luckett et al. 2007; Thiemann-Bourque et al. 2012), segues toward *object play*, because it involves using an object for its intended purpose. This intermediate form of play departs from exploration to actual use of the object, but without endowing it with properties that it does not possess.[2] From about 12 months onward, *object play* dominates and toys assume a special importance. Manipulation and *construction* occupy a considerable proportion of time the child spends with objects; some of this activity is considered *mastery play* as the junior toddler solves wooden puzzles and stacks concentric rings in the right order, gradually developing skill and frustration tolerance. Some object play, however, is moving toward pretense, as occasional objects are used to represent something else.

THE OEDIPAL-AGE CHILD

Between ages 3 and 4 years, children's play time is equally divided between *locomotor play* and *fantasy play* (also called *pretend play*, *symbolic play*, and *imaginary play*). Gender factors figure into the time

---

[2]Object play is often described in autism research, because some studies suggest that children with autism spectrum disorder use objects functionally but do not progress to using them symbolically.

spent in each, with boys exceeding girls for locomotor play and girls exceeding boys for pretense (Pellegrini and Smith 2001). Locomotor play includes rough-and-tumble play, tag, hopscotch, swinging on swings, and so on; this play form persists over the course of childhood and beyond, maturing into rope jumping and dodge ball, then double-dutch, basketball, and the vast array of other structured sports that absorb the energy and interest of young people and adults.

Fantasy or *pretend play*, the topic of Chapter 3, is of particular interest in this book because it is considered the primary modality of play therapy. It follows a universal trajectory from its appearance in the second year of life, to its peak in kindergarten (ages 5–6), its somewhat attenuated continuation during early latency, and then its gradual decline. Pretend play encompasses *object play* since it is typically linked to toys or props. It similarly incorporates *imitation*, as scenarios are enacted that involve representations of adult roles. Children in kindergarten are masters of *social play*—that is, *sociodramatic play* that involves a remarkable integration of multiple subjectivities and play agendas in a spontaneous improvisation. This category overlaps with and recruits prior modalities, dominating play in preschool and early grade school, where it can be shaped by a consensually determined "shared" fantasy or be organized into spontaneous, not yet formalized, but nonetheless rule-bound games on the playground. These outdoor play scenarios often incorporate themes derived from other sources (television, books, movies), involve elaborate thematic development extending over days or months, and have complex reverberations in the friendship hierarchy already well developed in first grade (Wohlwend 2004).

LATENCY

Piaget's cognitive progression marks age 7 as the shift to concrete operational thinking, corresponding to the child's growing capacity to perform the cognitive operations important for grade school learning; historically, this age is recognized as a turning point in the child's educability and capacity for work (Shapiro 1976). Psychoanalytic explorations of the latency period often divide it into two phases—*early latency*, from approximately age 7 to age 9, and *late latency*, from age 9 until puberty (Bornstein 1951)—based on the child's growing mastery and self-regulation, which become increasingly secure in the later half of latency with the consolidation of cognitive skills, integration of the new agency of the superego, and stabilization of defenses that regulate the impulses of the oedipal stage. Pretend play, at home and on the playground, may continue during the early phase of latency but gradually becomes displaced by the ascendance of new forms and preoccupations wherein the child's ongoing fantasy life can find both an outlet and satisfaction in reality (Sarnoff 1971). *Structured play*—various sports, board games, card games, video games, and so on—begins to take center stage. This play form demands certain gross and fine motor and cognitive skills that emerge as development proceeds. This form of playing typically involves rules that are essential to the shared goals of the game and result in the inevitability that some players must lose to allow others to win. The loosely organized culture of the playground becomes even more thoroughly sex segregated; boys' and girls' groups differ in terms of size and hierarchical organization (boys > girls) and emphasis on relationships and lingering fantasy play (girls > boys) (Friedman and Downey 2000). All of these games and play activities, from chess to soccer, from creating clubs to role-playing, entail complex psychological challenges that stabilize in the latency years.

Latency is also a time of hobbies, such as building models, making jewelry, or collecting stickers, figures, dolls, or cards linked to the narratives of the contemporary cultural scene such as movies, video games, and television shows. Hobbies serve to absorb the energy and passions of earlier childhood and are distinctly more firmly linked to reality. The freedom to depart from a realistic representation becomes increasingly curtailed as latency proceeds and the real object is valued, perhaps overvalued; for example, children who collect comic books can be overheard insisting that the recently acquired item is "worth" twice the amount paid within minutes after purchase!

LATE LATENCY AND BEYOND

The advent of electronic toys and devices has been transformative for play, and usage extends from infancy to adulthood. Electronic toys for children under age 2 are a growing industry, despite warnings from the American Academy of Pediatrics; in a demographic study from 2013 (already out of date), 38% of children under age 2 had used mobile media (Krumboltz 2013), some of which is marketed for children as young as 7 months. Infants seem to grasp the logic of their toy "remote control," "smartphone," and "tablet" and take pleasure in the readily available liveliness offered by these objects. Their parents' devices, however, are even more desirable; iPad usage among 5- to 8-year-olds was recently estimated at 52% (MDG Advertising 2016).

The debate over the impact of this rapidly expanding technology on child development is still raging, much like the debate about the technology that preceded it (i.e., television), although many scholars are adapting their thinking to contemporary realities and asking *how* (rather than *how badly*) technology is affecting and changing play, mental life, relationships, and so on (Essig 2012; Gilmore 2017; Lemma 2015). Many traditional toys and games have been absorbed into digital technology, and video games have evolved into a variety of forms and levels of complexity unimaginable at the turn of the twenty-first century. The MMORPGs (massively multiplayer online role-playing games) are highly social and allow children to talk, plan, and (usually) fight together. Other games offer modes that allow children to build and explore rather than engage in auto theft or war. The options about avatars, their characters and missions, their loyalty to the "good" side or the "bad side," the guilds they join, and the way they pursue their ends have mushroomed into a vast array of choices. Moreover, cheats and codes are accessible to resourceful players, allowing video games the same revelatory potential as the board games of old: how the game is played, how the child tolerates winning and losing, and how the child interacts with the therapist in the course of play are all understood to illuminate the child's inner life (Bellinson 2000).

Twenty-first-century play occurs in a thoroughly mediated space in which video games constitute only one part; as noted, digital devices such as smartphones and tablets are available to increasingly younger children. Today, the age of first smartphone ownership averages 10.3 years (Influence Central 2016), and kindergartners are given their own iPads in some classrooms. Despite the presumed advantage of telephone capability, smartphones are running behind tablets in popularity; both are portals to an infinite world of music, movies, television, social media, games, pornography, YouTube videos, disappearing Snapchats, tweets, and so on.

The digital devices and play portals that absorb contemporary latency-age children, in addition to their traditional games and hobbies (e.g., sports as player or spectator, word games, collecting), continue to occupy the leisure time of adolescents and young adults. Some activities transmute into adult forms that are arguably not play, such as car racing, boxing, online gambling, and pornography. Those writers who emphasize the continuation of play into adulthood refer to "symbols and myths" (Ablon 2001, p. 361) or rituals (Huizinga 1955) as adult playthings. Certainly, the notion of transitional space as a creative zone is applied equally to children and to adults. Clearly, although some of the forms of play in latency are short-lived, others persist and have the flexibility to evolve over time, thus affording pleasure in adulthood.

SUMMARY

Play is an activity enjoyed by juveniles of many species, especially mammals and birds whose play approximates some human forms. Pretense is usually considered the domain of higher primates, but some ethologists contend that forms of pretense exist throughout the animal kingdom. The self-initiated human form, more typically termed *pretend play*, *symbolic play*, or *imaginary play*, has a predictable onset, period of dominance in the child's life, and decline: its earliest forerunners are evident in the second year of life, its full blossoming occurs in the fourth, fifth, and sixth years, and its gradual diminution is clearly accomplished by preadolescence, although arguably present in sublimatory form in other creative pursuits throughout the lifespan. Play with playful adults in the first months of life is the crucial forerunner of pretend play and is considered an essential introduction to the world of make-believe.

KEY POINTS

- In humans, play begins in early infancy and evolves through a predictable sequence of forms, despite the considerable differences in their manifestations permitted and produced by a given culture.

- The extent of children's leisure time, the degree to which play is valued by society, the favored narratives, the nature of toys and technological advances, the prevalent gender stereotypes, and myriad other social factors impart character to the play of different eras and places.

- Parents have a central role in initiating the sequence of play forms, because their ministrations to their infants are intuitively playful as they try to coax them through the challenges and travails of life.

- The following sequence is consistently observed in children of all cultures:

  - *Infancy:* Parent-led playful exchanges, such as peek-a-boo, "this little piggy," tickling, and "baby calisthenics," often utilizing the baby's own body as playground

  - *Infancy and toddlerhood:* Exploratory play, in which the child examines objects, including his or her own body

  - *Toddlerhood:* Imitative play/functional play, in which the child plays with objects in ways that approximate their observed actual usages

  - *Oedipal age into latency:* Pretend play, in which the child uses toys and real objects in a representational manner and develops narrative themes played out with characters

  - *Latency:* Play involving structured games and activities, including hobbies, clubs, board games, sports, video games, crafts, and learning games

  - *Latency and beyond:* Adult forms of sports, hobbies, role-playing games, and board games

KEY TERMS

Magic circle A concept introduced by the Dutch cultural historian Huizinga (1955) to designate the physical space in which the special meanings and rules of the play reign supreme. This space could be a table top, a playground, or a virtual world; all the players implicitly or explicitly acknowledge its boundaries and agree to abide by its code.

Mentalization The developmental capacity to perceive and imagine behavior—one's own and others'—as a reflection of intentional mental states; "holding mind in mind" (Bateman and Fonagy 2012, quoted in Freeman 2016).

Playfulness   An orientation or disposition that imparts humor, lightness, and pleasure to activities. It originates in the parent–infant relationship and serves to ease the child toward an acceptance of reality, with a detour through the pretend mode.

Scaffolding   The process whereby a child, aided by an older person, is able to achieve a task or accomplish a goal at a level beyond the current level of functioning. In regard to play, this means that an older person can engage a child in play forms or versions of a given form at a level beyond the child's own capacity.

Sociodramatic play   The most advanced form of pretend play, usually seen in children in prekindergarten and kindergarten. It is distinguished by six characteristics: 1) make-believing using objects; 2) imitative role-playing in the assumption of a make-believe role; 3) make-believing about a situation, object, or action; 4) persisting or being able to continue the play in face of challenges; 5) using verbal declarations to communicate the context of play; and 6) interacting socially and verbally while playing. The last two characteristics of play, which involve interaction and communication, are critical to sociodramatic play and distinguish it from simple dramatic play. It is a play form that increases over the developmental trajectory of pretend play (Banerjee et al. 2016, p. 301; Smilansky 1968).

Zone of proximal development   A term introduced by Vygotsky (1978) to identify the distance between a child's actual developmental level and the (more advanced) one possible with guidance from an adult (Kassett et al. 2004) or any older person, such as a sibling (because older siblings are important developmental objects helping to propel a child forward).

REFERENCES

Ablon SL: Continuities of tongues: a developmental perspective on the role of play in child and adult psychoanalytic process. Journal of Clinical Psychoanalysis 10:345–365, 2001

Banerjee R, Alsalman A, Alqafari S: Supporting sociodramatic play in preschools to promote language and literacy skills of English language learners. Early Childhood Education Journal 44:299–305, 2016

Bateman AW, Fonagy P (eds): Handbook of Mentalizing in Mental Health Practice. Washington, DC, American Psychiatric Publishing, 2012

Bateson P: The role of play in the evolution of great apes and humans, in The Nature of Play: Great Apes and Humans. Edited by Pellegrini AD, Smith PK. New York, Guilford, 2005, pp 13–24

Bateson P, Martin P: Play, Playfulness, Creativity and Innovation. New York, Cambridge University Press, 2013

Bellinson J: Shut up and move: the uses of board games in child psychotherapy. J Infant Child Adolesc Psychother 1(2):23–41, 2000

Bergen D: Does pretend play matter? Searching for evidence: comment on Lillard et al. (2013). Psychol Bull 139(1):45–48, 2013 23294090

Birch M: In the land of counterpane: travels in the realm of play. Psychoanal Study Child 52:57–75, 1997 9489461

Bodrova E, Germeroth C, Leong DJ: Play and self-regulation: lessons from Vygotsky. Am J Play 6:111–123, 2013

Bornstein B: On latency. Psychoanal Study Child 6:279–285, 1951

Brentnall J, Bundy AC, Catherine F, et al: The effect of the length of observation on test of playfulness scores. OTJR: Occupation Participation Health 28(3):133–140, 2008

Bronson MR, Bundy AC: A correlational study of a test of playfulness and a test of environmental supportiveness for play. OTJR: Occupation Participation Health 21:241–259, 2001

Burgdorf J, Panksepp J: Tickling induces reward in adolescent rats. Physiol Behav 72(1–2):167–173, 2001 11239994

Burghardt GM: The Genesis of Animal Play: Testing the Limits. Cambridge, MA, MIT Press, 2005

Carlisle RP: Encyclopedia of Play in Today's Society. Thousand Oaks, CA, Sage, 2009

Chick G, Yarnal C, Purrington A: Play and mate preference: testing the signal theory of adult playfulness. Am J Play 4(4):407–440, 2012

Cohen PM, Solnit AJ: Play and therapeutic action. Psychoanal Study Child 48:49–63, 1993 7694307

Condliffe J: Time really does seem to slow down for athletes. Gizmodo, September 5, 2012. Available at: http://gizmodo.com/5940562/time-really-does-seem-to-slow-down-for-athletes. Accessed January 10, 2016.

Elias CL, Berk LE: Self-regulation in young children: is there a role for sociodramatic play? Early Child Res Q 17(2):216–238, 2002

Essig T: Psychoanalysis lost—and found—in our culture of simulation and enhancement. Psychoanal Inq 32(5):438–453, 2012

Fagen R: Animal Play Behavior. New York, Oxford University Press, 1981

Fein GG: Pretend play in childhood: an integrative review. Child Dev 52(4): 1095–1118, 1981

Fonagy P, Target M: Playing with reality, I: theory of mind and the normal development of psychic reality. Int J Psychoanal 77(Pt 2):217–233, 1996 8771375

Fonagy P, Target M: Playing with reality, III: the persistence of dual psychic reality in borderline patients. Int J Psychoanal 81(Pt 5):853–873, 2000 11109573

Fonagy P, Target M: Early intervention and the development of self-regulation. Psychoanalytic Inquiry 22:307–335, 2002

Fonagy P, Target M: The rooting of the mind in the body: new links between attachment theory and psychoanalytic thought. J Am Psychoanal Assoc 55(2):411–456, 2007 17601099

Fonagy P, Cottrell D, Phillips J, et al: What Works for Whom? A Critical Review of Treatments for Children and Adolescents, 2nd Edition. New York, Guilford, 2002

Fonagy P, Gergely G, Target M: The parent–infant dyad and the construction of the subjective self. J Child Psychol Psychiatry 48:288–328. 2007

Freeman C: What is mentalizing? An overview. Br J Psychother 32(2):189–201, 2016

Freud S: Creative writers and day-dreaming (1908), in The Standard Edition of the Complete Psychological Works of Sigmund Freud, Vol 9. Translated and edited by Strachey J. London, Hogarth, 1959, pp 141–154

Freud S: Beyond the pleasure principle (1920), in The Standard Edition of the Complete Psychological Works of Sigmund Freud, Vol 18. Translated and edited by Strachey J. London, Hogarth, 1962, pp 1–64

Friedman RC, Downey JI: The psychobiology of late childhood: significance for psychoanalytic developmental theory and clinical practice. J Am Acad Psychoanal 28(3):431–448, 2000 11109224

Gergely G, Watson JS: The social biofeedback theory of parental affect-mirroring: the development of emotional self-awareness and self-control in infancy. Int J Psychoanal 77:1181–1212, 1996 9119582

Gergely G, Nádasdy Z, Csibra G, et al: Taking the intentional stance at 12 months of age. Cognition 56(2):165–193, 1995 7554793

Gilmore K: Play in the psychoanalytic setting: ego capacity, ego state, and vehicle for intersubjective exchange. Psychoanal Study Child 60:213–238, 2005 16649681

Gilmore K: Pretend play and development in early childhood (with implications for the oedipal phase). J Am Psychoanal Assoc 59(6):1157–1182, 2011 22080503

Gilmore K: Development in the digital age. Psychoanal Study Child 70:82–90, 2017

Göncü A, Gaskins S: An integrative perspective on play and development, in Play and Development: Evolutionary, Sociocultural, and Functional Perspectives. New York, Erlbaum, 2007, pp 3–18

Göncü A, Jain J, Tuermer U: Children's play as cultural interpretation, in Play and Development: Evolutionary, Sociocultural, and Functional Perspectives. New York, Erlbaum, 2007, pp 155–178

Graham KL, Burghardt GM: Current perspectives on the biological study of play: signs of progress. Q Rev Biol 85(4):393–418, 2010 21243962

Handelman D: Anthropology of play, in The International Encyclopedia of the Social and Behavioral Sciences, Vol 17. Amsterdam, Elsevier, 2001, pp 11503–11507

Harris PL: Understanding pretense, in Children's Early Understanding of Mind: Origins and Development. Edited by Lewis C, Mitchell P. East Sussex, UK, Erlbaum, 1994, pp 235–259

Harris PL: Desires, beliefs, and language, in Theories of Theories of Mind. Edited by Carruthers P, Smith PK. Cambridge, UK, Cambridge University Press, 1996, pp 200–220

Huizinga J: Homo Ludens: A Study of the Play-Element in Culture (1938). Boston, MA, Beacon Press, 1955

Influence Central: Kids and tech: the evolution of today's digital natives, 2016. Available at: http://influence-central.com/kids-tech-the-evolution-of-todays-digital-natives. Accessed August 4, 2016.

Iwaniuk AN, Nelson JE, Pellis SM: Do big-brained animals play more? Comparative analyses of play and relative brain size in mammals. J Comp Psychol 115(1):29–41, 2001 11334216

Johnson JE, Christie JF, Yawkey D: Play and Early Childhood Development. Glenview, IL, Scott Foresman, 1987

Kassett JA, Bonanno GA, Notarius CI: Affective scaffolding: a process measure for psychotherapy with children. J Infant Child Adolesc Psychother 3(1):92–118, 2004

Krumboltz M: Study: 38% of kids under 2 use smartphones or tablets. Yahoo News, Oct 28, 2013. Available at: https://www.yahoo.com/news/blogs/sideshow/38--of-kids-under-2-use-smartphones-or-tablets--study-212548190.html. Accessed February 2016.

Lemma A: Psychoanalysis in times of technoculture: some reflections on the fate of the body in virtual space. Int J Psychoanal 96(3):569–582, 2015 26173880

Liepold EE, Bundy AC: Playfulness in children with attention deficit hyperactivity disorder. OTJR 20(1):61–79, 2000

Lillard AS, Lerner MD, Hopkins EJ, et al: The impact of pretend play on children's development: a review of the evidence. Psychol Bull 139(1):1–34, 2013 22905949

Luckett T, Bundy A, Roberts J: Do behavioural approaches teach children with autism to play or are they pretending? Autism 11(4):365–388, 2007 17656400

MDG Advertising: Kid Tech According to Apple, 2016. Available at: http://graphs.net/statistics-technology-usage-children.html. Accessed February 15, 2016.

Mechling J: Performing imaginary rhetoric. Am Q 52(2):364–370, 2000

Meersand P: Psychoanalytic aspects of play in parent-infant psychotherapy: supporting the capacity for understanding mental states. J Clin Psychoanal 10:461–480, 2001

Mercer JG, Speakman JR: Hypothalamic neuropeptide mechanisms for regulating energy balance: from rodent models to human obesity. Neurosci Biobehav Rev 25(2):101–116, 2001 11323077

Moran GS: Some functions of play and playfulness: a developmental perspective. Psychoanal Study Child 42:11–29, 1987 3438362

Morgenthaler SK: The meanings in play with objects, in Play From Birth to Twelve. Edited by Fromberg DP, Bergen D. New York, Routledge, 2006, pp 65–74

Muys V, Rodger S, Bundy AC: Assessment of playfulness in children with autistic disorder: a comparison of the children's playfulness scale and the test of playfulness. OTJR 26:159–170, 2006

Nicolopoulou A, Ilgaz H: What do we know about pretend play and narrative development? A response to Lillard, Lerner, Hopkins, Dore, Smith, and Palmquist on "The impact of pretend play on children's development: a review of the evidence." Am J Play 6(1):55–81, 2013

Nielsen M: Imitation, pretend play, and childhood: essential elements in the evolution of human culture? J Comp Psychol 126(2):170–181, 2012 21859186

Panksepp J: Textbook of Biological Psychiatry. Hoboken, NJ, Wiley, 2004

Panksepp J, Siviy S, Normansell L: The psychobiology of play: theoretical and methodological perspectives. Neurosci Biobehav Rev 8(4):465–492, 1984 6392950

Parsons M: The logic of play in psychoanalysis. Int J Psychoanal 80(Pt 5):871–884, 1999 10643568

Pellegrini AD, Bjorklund DF: The ontogeny and phylogeny of children's object and fantasy play. Hum Nat 15(1):23–43, 2004 26190292

Pellegrini AD, Smith PK: Physical activity play: the nature and function of a neglected aspect of playing. Child Dev 69(3):577–598, 1998 9680672

Pellegrini A, Smith PK: Play and development in children, in International Encyclopedia of Social and Behavioral Sciences. Edited by Smelser NJ, Bates PB. Oxford, UK, Pergamon Press, 2001. Available at: https://www.elsevier.com/books/international-encyclopedia-of-social-andam-pamp-behavioral-sciences/smelser/978-0-08-043076-8. Accessed April 11, 2017.

Pellegrini AD, Smith PK (eds): The Nature of Play: Great Apes and Humans. New York, Guilford, 2005

Pellegrini AD, Dupuis D, Smith PK: Play in evolution and development. Dev Rev 27(2):261–276, 2007

Peller LE: Libidinal phases, ego development, and play. Psychoanal Study Child 9:178–198, 1954

Pellerin N, Lecours S: Sensitization to emotions and representation formation through social biofeedback: is markedness a necessary mechanism? Psychoanal Psychol 32(1):61–93, 2015

Piaget J: The Child's Conception of the World. Lanham, MD, Littlefield Adams Quality Paperbacks, 1951

Piaget J: Play, Dreams, and Imitation in Childhood. Translated by Gattegno C, Hodgson FM. New York, WW Norton, 1962

Piaget J: Quantification, conservation, and nativism: quantitative evaluations of children aged two to three years are examined. Science 162(3857):976–981, 1968 5698850

Piaget J: The Construction of Reality in the Child. Abingdon-on-Thames, UK, Routledge, 1999

Piaget J, Inhelder B: The Psychology of the Child. New York, Basic Books, 1969

Proyer RT, Wagner L: Playfulness in adults revisited: the signal theory in German speakers. Am J Play 7(2):210–227, 2015

Pufall PB, Pufall E: The relationship between play and culture. Hum Dev 51(5–6):390–398, 2008

Sarnoff CA: Ego structure in latency. Psychoanal Q 40(3):387–414, 1971 4937100

Sears RR: Influence of methodological factors on doll play performance. Child Dev 18:190–197, 1947

Shapiro T: Latency revisited—the age 7 plus or minus 1. Psychoanal Study Child 31:79–105, 1976

Singer DG, Singer JL: Reflections on pretend play, imagination, and child development: an interview with Dorothy G. and Jerome L. Singer. Am J Play 6(1):1–14, 2013

Singer DL, Singer JL, D'Agostino H, et al: Children's pastimes and play in sixteen nations: is free play declining? Am J Play 1(3):283–312, 2009

Slade A: A longitudinal study of maternal involvement and symbolic play during the toddler period. Child Dev 58(2):367–375, 1987 2435464

Smilansky S: The Effect of Sociodramatic Play on Disadvantaged Preschool Children. New York, Wiley Press, 1968

Smith PK: Pretend play and children's cognitive and literacy development: sources of evidence and some lessons from the past, in Play and Literacy in Early Childhood: Research From Multiple Perspectives. Edited by Roskos KA, Christie JF. Mahwah, NJ, Erlbaum, 2007, pp 3–19

Solnit AJ: A psychoanalytic view of play. Psychoanal Study Child 42:205–219, 1987 3438366

Solnit AJ, Cohen DJ, Neubauer PB: The Many Meanings of Play: A Psychoanalytic Perspective. New Haven, CT, Yale University Press, 1993

Sutton-Smith B: Play as parody of emotional vulnerability, in Play and Education Theory and Practice. Edited by Lytle D. Westport, CT, Greenwood Publishing Group, 2003, pp 3–18

Sutton-Smith B: The Ambiguity of Play. Cambridge, MA, Harvard University Press, 1997

Target M, Fonagy P: Playing with reality, II: the development of psychic reality from a theoretical perspective. Int J Psychoanal 77(Pt 3):459–479, 1996 8818764

Tessier VP, Normandin L, Ensink K, et al: Fact or fiction? A longitudinal study of play and the development of reflective functioning. Bull Menninger Clin 80(1):60–79, 2016 27028339

Thiemann-Bourque KS, Brady NC, et al: Symbolic play of preschoolers with severe communication impairments with autism and other developmental delays: more similarities than differences. J Autism Dev Disord 42(5):863–873, 2012 21720725

Van Vleet M, Feeney BC: Young at heart: a perspective for advancing research on play in adulthood. Perspect Psychol Sci 10(5):639–645, 2015 26386001

Vygotsky LS: Play and its role in the mental development of the child. Soviet Psychology 5(3):6–18, 1967

Vygotsky LS: Mind in Society: The Development of Higher Psychological Processes. Cambridge, MA, Harvard University Press, 1978

Waelder R: The psychoanalytic theory of play. Psychoanal Q 2:208–224, 1933

Waelder R: The principle of multiple function. Psychoanal Q 5(1):45–62, 1936

Walker CM, Gopnik A: Pretense and possibility—a theoretical proposal about the effects of pretend play on development: comment on Lillard et al. (2013). Psychol Bull 139(1):40–44, 2013 23294089

Weisberg DS, Gopnik A: Pretense, counterfactuals, and Bayesian causal models: why what is not real really matters. Cogn Sci 37(7):1368–1381, 2013 23915198

Weisberg DS, Hirsh-Pasek K, Golinkoff RM: Embracing complexity: rethinking the relation between play and learning: comment on Lillard et al.. (2013). Psychol Bull 139(1):35–39, 2013 23294088

Winnicott DW: Playing and Reality. New York, Tavistock, 1971

Wohlwend KL: Chasing friendship acceptance, rejection, and recess play. Child Educ 81(2):77–82, 2004

Yanof JA: Treating children with affect dysregulation: discussion of Dr. Wendy Olesker's analysis of Matt. Psychoanal Study Child 66:109–121, 2012 26020994

3

Pretend Play

As a new mother, Rosie was anxious and awkward with her baby son, Sergey. In the first weeks of his life, she worried that she couldn't "interest" him in anything and he had trouble latching on and nursing. In week 4, she was bathing him in the sink and, to her great surprise, he smiled at her "out of the blue." She experienced this as a kind of epiphany that ushered in an intense feeling of attachment. She suddenly felt relaxed and even playful; she began to exercise his little arms and legs, singing "pat-a-cake" and ending the song by clapping his hands together. His enjoyment further delighted her, leading her to find more nursery rhymes, songs, and games in her collection of books about infancy; she was gratified that an Internet search led to the YouTube video "Games to Play With Baby,"[1] which provided, among other activities, "Wheels on the Bus" sung while bicycling the baby's legs. Peek-a-boo became another favorite; Rosie threw herself into the surprise moment and was rewarded by Sergey's glorious smile and, soon to follow, his crow of laughter. The receiving blanket that was typically included in these activities—as a mat, a wrap, a barrier to hide behind, and so on—was increasingly sought after by Sergey, who clutched it in nursing and at bedtime. Rosie grasped that this was Sergey's special blankie and kept close watch over its whereabouts. When Sergey was fussy, Rosie provided the blankie, and if she felt he was willing, she would offer him solace with playing out simple stories using different voices and improvised props. By the end of the first year, Sergey was particularly entranced by colorful finger puppets

[1]"Games to Play With Baby," Available at: https://www.youtube.com/watch?v=CuoD4EKkZqk. Accessed February 19, 2016.

of jungle animals, with which Rosie played out many an exciting scene. Sergey's dad joined these activities using his gruff voice to play the lion; previously scared by his dad's occasional attempts to talk "motherese," Sergey seemed thrilled by daddy playing the part of the lion (who was tamed by a parrot).

When Rosie's sister, brother-in-law, and 4-year-old twin nephews moved into her house for an extended stay while searching for their own home in the neighborhood, Sergey was delighted by his active "big" cousins; they had been regular weekend visitors, but on this visit they stayed for 2 months. As in the past, he observed their every move and gesture, but now having taken his first steps, he wanted to join in the mix. When they played with their toy lightsabers, which glowed with beautiful blue light and made sword-clashing sounds, he wanted to do that too. He grabbed a lightsaber and brandished it like a Jedi. His excited expression only briefly clouded over when his dad picked up the other one, but Sergey was soon participating in their "duel" with enthusiastic shrieks patterned after his cousins.

Star Wars characters remained a favorite for years; long before Sergey saw the movie series, he played with his father, who narrated parts of the story, and Sergey later created his own narratives and played by himself. His parents did not want him to see the latest Star Wars movie until he was "double digits" (10 years old), but he devoured illustrated guides and the animated television series. He identified with the teenage Ezra Bridger, a rebel, whose lightsaber is also a stun gun and who recognizes, at least for a time, the evils of the Empire. Sergey did not like to play out the part of the story where Ezra is drawn to the dark side, because Sergey greatly feared the Empire. He began to collect Star Wars figures and played with those too, until he decided he wanted to "make a collection" at age 8 and started placing them in a tableau on a bookshelf. As he became more interested in video games, he began to play other characters and seemed to enjoy experimenting with a range of good and evil.

In this chapter, we revisit the play form variously called *pretend*, *symbolic*, or *imaginary play* that is our primary focus in this book. We trace its origins in the earliest parent–infant exchanges; its trajectory during the years of early childhood, where it occupies about 10%–17% of a preschooler's and 33% of a kindergartner's play behaviors (Smith 2010); and its decline as a distinct play modality in late latency. More than any other play form, pretend play is credited with facilitating a remarkable transition in human development, when the child advances from toddlerhood to the point of readiness for school culture. Close observers of this period note the quantum shift in personality development that is represented, in myriad ways, in each child's version of pretend playing, in regard to narrative themes, forms, representations of others and self, and eventually in the remarkable capacity to collaborate with others. We recap the particularities and singularity of pretend play and explore the accompanying developmental moment that distinguishes it from all the other types.

In Piagetian terms, pretend play coincides with the cognitive advance from sensorimotor to preoperational thinking and is a manifestation of **semiotic function**. To the extent that this type of play, by definition, is symbolic and associated with the emergence of language (Piaget 1945/ 1962), its arrival takes the human child into an arena unique among mammals. However, some scholars rightfully point out that this characterization forecloses the recognition of pretense in other species, thereby obscuring both the evolutionary origins of symbolic activities (Mitchell 2007) and the preverbal or nonverbal evidence of pretense in human development. The definition of *pretense* independent of language hinges on a dissociation between an idea and reality: pretense "enact(s) imagination" by "intentionally allowing an idea, at least part of which an agent knows to be inaccurate about or unrelated to current reality (i.e., fictional), to guide and constrain the agent's behaviors (including mental states)" (Mitchell 2007, pp. 53–54). By this definition, pretense in nonhuman primates and mammals clearly does exist and has been described in many other species all along the evolutionary chain (Burghardt and Sutton-Smith 2006). Most commentators, however, conclude that although pretense in animals is amply demonstrated by behaviors such as "playing dead" and play fighting, it is the evolving human capacity to offer *enrichment*—the "exploitation of one piece of make-believe to create another"—that transforms pretense into pretend play (Currie 2004, p. 224). This capacity to elaborate, which of course is linked to growing semiotic function in the human child, distinguishes pretend play from the earlier and/or exclusively locomotor play forms that are shared to some degree with other immature mammals, such as rough-and-tumble, exploratory, and imitative play. Because language is further required to act as a support for later play forms that arise subsequent to imaginary play, such as the structured sports and games with rules of latency and beyond, it would appear that pretend play marks the transition to uniquely human play activities. This link to language development is clearly not coincidental, an idea we examine in detail in our discussion of the evolution of play in this chapter.

The developmental arc of pretend play has another singular feature: its emergence, dominance, and gradual disappearance follow a predictable time frame and trajectory in human cultures across the globe with the consistency of other inborn developmental milestones. As noted in Chapter 2, "Play, Playfulness, and the Sequence of Play Forms in Development," this universal finding has led some thinkers to propose "a neuropsychological timetable and biologic basis" (Harris 1994, p. 256; 1996) for pretending and has heightened the impression that pretending serves some developmental purpose. Moreover, its close connection and dependence on the emergence of the new ego capacity—semiotic function—adds it to the mix of influences in the child's acquisition of language, communication, and understanding of emotional states (Dunn 2000). New words and objects are introduced and vividly illustrated, and then can be recruited by the playing child in a remarkable burst of creative activity and invention, unparalleled in any other time of life. Equally remarkable is that the discrete entity of pretend play, replete with stories, drama, its own ego state, and its valuable social capital, usually fades away by middle school. When children are on the threshold of puberty, pretend play is relatively rare, even while its artifacts may still be present. Like Sergey in our vignette, children transform their former playthings (such as his Star Wars action figures) into collectibles and busy themselves with competitive sports, video games, and learning extracurricular skills (e.g., playing an instrument, learning hip-hop).

THE EVOLUTION OF PLAY

INFANCY AND THE ROLE OF THE PARENT

The capacity for make-believe emerges in a stepwise fashion out of the active and engaged intersubjective matrix of the mother–infant dyad. Contemporary research has cast doubt on William James's (1890) "buzzing, blooming confusion" (p. 488) as an apt descriptor of the infant experience. The infant instead comes equipped with an array of potentials and capacities that interface almost immediately with the caretaker. This interface, in turn, influences the future direction of crucial ego capacities that emerge during infancy and early childhood (Weil 1970). For example, imitation, which begins within 3 weeks after birth in regard to tongue protrusion, mouth opening, and lip protrusion (Dowling 1981; Meltzoff and Moore 1977), is understood to reflect "pre-ego psychic organization—active, coordinating, differentiating, generalizing intermodal perception, and above all, adaptive in fortifying the attachment response by the infant's caretaker" (Dowling 1981, p. 294). Imitation has also been proposed as the earliest evidence of the capacity to infer mental states, since it rests on an intuitive recognition of something "like me" in another person's expression and an innate correspondence between seeing and the subjective experience of doing (Meltzoff and Decety 2003). Similarly, the road to verbal comprehension is now understood to begin well before language production; contemporary infant researchers demonstrate convincingly that newborns have the capacity to process streams of words, break them down into discrete units, and, by the middle of the first year, recognize not only personally meaningful words, such as names of family members, but also categorical groups of words (Vivona 2012). These are only two of the array of capacities, thresholds, and proclivities that are shaped and influenced in the exchanges between baby and caregiver and whose full emergence may take years to develop. Others include anxiety potential; object relations; joint attention and social referencing; theory of mind; affective attunement, disruption, and repair (Beebe et al. 1997); language development and responsiveness; self-regulation and self-reflection (Hobson 2014); and pleasure in toys and creative access to inner life.

What does the caretaker bring to this crucial interface? The range of the mother's caretaking behaviors, her sensitivity to up- and down-regulating her baby depending on his or her state, and her pleasurable stimulation and provision of comfort are informed by her intuitive capacity for mothering and attunement, in addition to her own psychology. Winnicott's famous "good-enough mother" is no easy achievement. The mother's repertoire of engagement is almost universally informed by two features: one is *motherese*, the well-studied "infant-directed speech" or baby talk spoken by mothers the world over, and the other, intimately associated with motherese, is *playfulness*.

Motherese is present in many languages and is characterized by 1) intonational and paralinguistic phenomena (e.g., higher overall pitch);

2) words and constructions derived from the normal language but deviating from typical adult speech (e.g., the use of third-person constructions to replace first- and second-person constructions); and 3) a set of lexical items that are specific to baby talk (Saint-Georges et al. 2013). Motherese is not confined to mothers; it can be found in other caregivers, although it is demonstrably less present in fathers (Van Dam et al. 2015), who typically rely on adult-directed speech, a far less impactful discourse with infants. Motherese is credited by child specialists as promoting, via its high intensity and specific lexicon, certain vital developmental achievements: it is crucial for the communication of affects, facilitation of social interactions, attention and learning, and language acquisition (Saint-Georges et al. 2013). Indeed, some scientists believe that motherese is the midwife not only to language in individual development, but more generally to the evolution of language in our species (Falk 2009).

Playfulness, like *play*, is an unwieldy term that covers a vast range of activities; it best refers to an attitude or orientation to reality and to pleasure. Playfulness requires that the caretaker suspend adherence to reality and "make-believe" in a way that conveys "lightheartedness and an empathic understanding of what the child feels" (Moran 1987, pp. 14–15). This parental capacity is recruited to stimulate and affectively connect with the child, while simultaneously facilitating adaptation to the limits and exigencies of real life. Knowing these and knowing the vulnerability of the child, the parent blends fantasy and reality to cushion the child's journey on the difficult road ahead (Shengold 1988). Playfulness in infancy is introduced and maintained by motherese, whose repetition, syntax, and prosody are elements of the "marked affect" (Gergely and Watson 1996) that identifies a playful exchange. Although playfulness encompasses a wide range of actions and is best understood as a behavioral mode, it has been identified and studied in typical structured manifestations that are also universal despite cultural variation: baby "games" (e.g., peek-a-boo, pat-a-cake, and "this little piggy") are shaped by society but persist as recurrent tropes in parent–infant play. These early forms involve repetition, imitation, and vocalizations, delivered in the language of motherese, and typically played out on the infant's body. They become routines of interaction that are knit together from facial expressions, voice, song, and movement to create a multimodal tapestry, requiring faithful repetition of all features (gesture, expression, voice) to maintain the infant's participation (Fantasia et al. 2014). For example, omission of facial expression (as in the still-face paradigm developed by Tronick et al. [1978]) can cause a previously engaged and joyful baby to protest or unravel into disorganized movements and tears. These routines intuitively engage the baby in "play" at an appropriate developmental level and provide an experience of expectable sequences of engagement that the baby learns and relies on. Infants, from early in life, expect reciprocity and reliable sequences.

Infants immediately recognize these activities as joyful, nonutilitarian forms of engagement that are familiar but different from business as usual. The mother's exaggerated affect is not experienced as a real indication of the mother's state of mind but rather as a communication that she is playing. For example, there is evidence that infants as young as 4 months (Kleeman 1967) recognize that the parent's introduction of "peek-a-boo"—that is, the parent disappearing behind a cloth and then reappearing with a huge display of surprise—is something different from real affect and constitutes an invitation to join in mutually pleasurable fun (Gergely and Watson 1996; Gilmore 2011). This exceedingly early "make-believe," introduced by parental "action"—exaggerated emotional displays, gestures, and touch—scaffolds the child's nascent playing capacity, linguistic communication, and theory of mind (Bruner 1982; Fonagy and Fonagy 1995). It thus draws the infant forward toward a range of future developmental advances: symbolic function in the form of action and language, the capacity to process gesture and words as emotional expressions, communication patterns of give and take, and recognition of an other's subjectivity and intention. Somewhere between 9 and 12 months, infants' engagement expands to a shared point of interest, so they "flexibly and reliably look where adults are looking (gaze following),... use adults as social reference points (social referencing), and...act on objects in the way adults are acting on them (imitative learning)" (Tomasello 1999). Scholars offer a range of etiologies for this reliably recurring "9-month revolution"—whether it be due to inborn capacity, prepared learning, simulation, or the emergence of awareness of their own intention and recognition that the other is "like me." This comprehension and engagement with a third point of interest has many repercussions, including the valuation of toys introduced by a parent or sibling and the dawning of triadic relations that comes to fruition in the oedipal triangle.

Winnicott's concept of transitional phenomena, mentioned in Chapter 2, adds another dimension to these playful exchanges. Although the transitional object (Winnicott 1953) is not necessarily a toy and is infrequently used as such by the child, the establishment of the **transitional space** via playfulness creates the potential for the child's meaningful engagement in an activity that is partly grounded in reality and partly a manifestation of inner life. "The area of playing is not inner psychic reality. It is outside the individual, but it is not the external world" (Winnicott 1971, p. 51). Parental playfulness facilitates the gradual "suffusion of the external world with the internal, psychic world" (Altaian 1997, p. 726) and thereby contributes to the creation of transitional phenomena: beloved patterns of interaction, first objects, and stories (introduced by parents well before a child's full comprehension) become the creative arena that is ultimately invoked to aid the child's own management of his or her anxiety.

In the opening vignette, Sergey's rapid grasp of a culture-specific "play fight" modality illustrates the impact of slightly older children on a number of play forms. Infants with older siblings or regular playmates acquire, via imitation and scaffolding provided by the narrative power of the older children's agenda, more complex sequences of behavior, more rough-and-tumble and pretend play, and more joint pretend actions earlier (as measured at 12, 15, and 18 months) than infants lacking this important environmental nutriment (Barr and Hayne 2003). Moreover, children raised in large or extended families precociously manifest indicators of theory of mind (i.e., passing false-belief tests), another important developmental accomplishment that has been correlated with the extent of pretend play (Hughes and Dunn 1997). Notably, children spend increasing amounts of time with siblings compared with time spent with their parents: by age 1 year the time spent with siblings and parents is equivalent, but by ages 4–6, time spent with siblings is double the time spent with parents (Dunn 1983). Such extended sibling contact stimulates and instructs in the art of pretend play and in child-friendly talk of mental states, close, but still ahead of, the child's own level.

Therefore, although a child's very first (passive) experiences of pretense are typically initiated by adults, a child embedded in a family or a setting such as day care has ample opportunity to observe and delight in the play of older children and to be drawn into the make-believe games (often in the role of baby, puppy, or other diminished creature) by more skilled players. The infant's achievement of social play in which he or she is an active director and negotiator with peers is many months into the future, but sometime in the second year of life rudimentary pretend play emerges as a distinct modality, fully possessed and initiated by the toddler. Early instances of pretending, when observed in naturalistic settings, are typically performed for or with an adult, limited in complexity, and hard to distinguish from imitative behavior (Smith 2010). These simple two-part scenarios (e.g., agent–object or agent–action) benefit from a real object (e.g., a spoon or cup) to scaffold the schema (Bretherton 1984). But despite the need for real props and the close representation of real events, the little girl playing—for example, at falling asleep by re-creating the identical sequence of her own bedtime ritual and using her actual blankie—somehow makes it known to the observer (usually her parent) that the action is make-believe (Scarlett et al. 2005). Early use of objects for playing is similarly constrained by their actual function and guided by imitation; for example, the little boy grabs his parent's smartphone and scrolls the screen or "talks" into it.[2] The capacity to play entirely without objects or to mime is rarely observed before age 30 months, although partial miming, supported by the presence of a few objects, is evident much earlier, such as when a baby takes an imaginary cookie out of an empty cookie jar and offers it to an appreciative adult (Bretherton 1984). Again, the role of older children as instigators and models is considerable; they serve to draw the toddler forward toward less object-based "functional" play, and, unlike the "interested spectator" adult, they enrich the play by their own play actions, talk, and narratives (Dunn 2004). As a child's semiotic capacity and motor skills begin to blossom, his or her growing access to symbolic representation, command of narrative

---

[2]Contemporary toys reflect the electronic revolution. VTech Touch and Swipe and Fisher-Price Laugh and Learn Smart Phone are smartphone facsimiles that are available for babies as young as 5 months; however, toddlers tend to prefer the "real thing" and develop the requisite gestures quickly. (See Chapter 4, "Play in the Digital Age.")

themes, and versatile manipulation of toys and objects vastly augment pretending.

THE THIRD AND FOURTH YEARS

The remarkable developmental transformations during a child's third and fourth years amount to a quantum shift in the child's mental organization and ego capacities, ushering in a full flowering of imaginary play. These changes affect multiple arenas of personality, affect, cognition, relationships, and socioemotional range. The fact that symbolic play figures so prominently in this time period certainly supports hypotheses in regard to its developmental function (see Chapter 2). The craving for opportunities for pretend play—whether the play is solitary, is scaffolded by a parent, or occurs in the company of peers or siblings—is remarkably consistent among children by age 3 years, even before their negotiating skills permit the spontaneous peer-initiated collaborative play that characterizes 5- and 6-year-olds at school and on the playground. The following list captures the remarkable developmental advances already in evidence or nascent in this crucial developmental epoch (based on Gilmore 2011):

1. *Cognition.* In terms of Piaget's series of mental organizations, the child's thinking shifts from sensorimotor to preoperational functioning. Directly relevant to the capacity to pretend is the transition, via **decentering**, from egocentrism to the recognition of other points of view. Indeed, the discernment of make-believe as "something different" is evident in embryonic form in the infant's engagement with the playful mother's baby games, reliance on the mother's expression for reassurance, and social referencing. These achievements reflect the evolution of metarepresentational cognition, which allows the infant to grasp the mother's mental state via an activity, such as hiding or feeding a doll. Other cognitive gains, in Piaget's terms, are **decontextualization**—permitting the gradual use of objects for imaginary purposes—and **integration**—the capacity to combine pretend into sequences.

   Such cognitive developments and the emergence of the **pretend mode** contribute to the gradual transition from the cognition of psychic equivalence (Fonagy and Target 1996, 2000, 2007) to psychic reality. *Psychic equivalence* refers to the young child's equation of mental events "in terms of power, causality, and implications, to events in the physical world" (Fonagy and Target 2000, p. 854). In other words, the pretend mode facilitates the transition from infantile omnipotence to psychic reality. Of course, the achievement of consensual reality is supported by many developing systems, including perceptual and neuromuscular maturation. These achievements reflect the evolution of metarepresentational cognition, which allows the infant to grasp the mother's mental state via an activity, such as hiding or feeding a doll. *Metarepresentation* is a crucial capacity that involves both the knowing use of one thing to represent another and the recognition that another person is doing the same (i.e., that the other person is pretending). This cognitive leap "has been closely linked to the acquisition of theory of mind because when a toddler comprehends that his mother is pretending that a cup is a hat or that she is crying, he understands her relationship to this representation" (Gilmore 2011, p. 8).

2. *Semiotic function.* Semiotic function is an intrinsic feature of the cognitive advances in this age group. Beginning with the third year of life, the child's discernible capacity to use signs to symbolize things accelerates at a breathtaking pace. Freedom to use objects to represent something else in play reaches its childhood apex by age 4; as the child approaches latency, pretend play with objects is notably more constrained by their reality. Language acquisition burgeons and undergirds developing ego capacities that both enhance and further evolve during play. Verbal ability is strongly linked to children's emerging theory of mind; family conversations in which emotions are discussed—for example, in regard to siblings and book characters—predict theory-of-mind acquisition and better perspective taking, both vital for sociodramatic play (Ensink and Mayes 2010).

3. *Memory.* New memory capacity allows for greater mental representation and the evocation of relationships, narrative sequences, and events of life. Memory is the warehouse of narrative themes, object representations, and conflicts; play makes use of these supplies to create story lines, plot twists, heroes and villains, romantic figures, and happy endings. Disturbances of memory due to traumatic experience are readily apparent in play; whether such disturbances are encoded in the body (as with preverbal trauma) or warded off via

rigid defensive mechanisms, the child's play suffers disruption or remains frozen in endless loops of reenactment.

4. *Object relations.* The child's new mental capacities and emotional repertoire (see #5 below) are essential components in the marked augmentation of complexity in object relations. The designation "oedipal phase" rests on the idea that the children's relationships can encompass triangular force fields in the family or elsewhere; a child is now capable of broadening attachments to and interest in people other than the primary caretaker, of experiencing new kinds of feelings such as rivalry and guilt, and of coming to terms with the complex relationships of family life. Indeed, family life immediately multiplies the various triads, intense feelings, and dramas that all deepen and add complexity to the child's relationships. The acquisition of theory of mind, which is usually demonstrable in the false-belief test by age 4 years, is a gradual process that begins with the toddler's understanding of other people's desires at 2 years and their thoughts at 3 years. There is a rapid increment between ages 3 and 4 years in the child's understanding of the role of internal states in others' actions; this becomes an important feature of playing, not only for the successful participation in role-play but also for the comprehension of another person's declared pretending intention (Ensink and Mayes 2010).

5. *Emotion.* Among the multiple developing systems interfacing during these years, emotional repertoire shows a quantum jump in complexity and nuance. The toddler's emotional range is greatly amplified in interaction with the new importance of triadic relationships; jealousy, rivalry, hatred, desire, and the capacity for ambivalence begin to emerge, complicating emotions further by their admixture. These new feelings are oriented into vectors by the drama of family life; the infinite variations of the oedipal triangle elicit new emotions as children become acutely aware of their exclusion from the adult sexual life of parents. At the same time, they are increasingly expected to manage their feelings and to comply with parental demands.

6. *Superego.* Although multiple superego precursors predate this phase, now they begin to gradually coalesce into a more coherent system of behavioral guidelines and internalized constraints based on the child's new emotion of guilt and the wish to be good. The internaliza-

tion of parental do's and don'ts and the growing participation in extrafamilial settings help the child establish and maintain procedural guidelines. These begin to enter into pretend play scenarios and become especially prominent in the social play of the slightly older child.

7. *Self-regulation.* This crucial personality feature is in itself a complex system, reflecting improving impulse control, tolerance of frustration or "stress" management, and internalization of superego standards. Although precursors are evident from the second year, self-regulation expands considerably in the third year of life, closely associated with the development of language (Vallotton and Ayoub 2011): the child becomes capable of expressing wants and needs, can use private speech to monitor behavior, and becomes aware of the art of negotiating with peers.

8. *Gender role.* The birth of siblings and entry into preschool are external events that heighten the child's growing awareness and accrual of meaning around gender and gender difference. The relationship between designations of boy and girl and their anatomies poses ongoing challenges to the child's self-representation. The exploration of these representations often occurs in play, especially as gendered toys become increasingly common and tend to reflect cultural stereotypes.

These emerging systems constitute elements of the developmental period traditionally known as the *oedipal phase*, which transforms the toddler into a member of the "adult world…[and] moral order" (Loewald 1985, p. 439). During this phase, children are expected to manage emotions and passions, abide by rules and rituals, and gradually renounce omnipotent fantasies for the sake of learning. The emergence of oedipal dynamics in the mental life in the family setting takes shape in intense, emotionally fraught interpersonal triangles composed of a desired other, a rival, and the self, with any number of permutations: parent, parent, child; parent, sibling, child; grandparent, sibling, child; and so on. The passionate possessiveness and new recognition of other people's relationships as meaningful and important vastly enrich the child's comprehension of human interaction and attachments. Emotional complexity is greatly augmented by the capacity to experience ambivalence. The neurodevelopmental achievement of more focused genital excitement and the heightened masturbatory impulses (which peak in

5-year-olds) add an element of urgency to children's feelings at this age, often associated with a fear of damage to a newly precious part of the body. All of these developments find an outlet in the fantasies of this age group, such as in enactments based on story lines from *Star Wars*, *Frozen*, *Cinderella*, and *The Little Mermaid*, each of which contains at least some of the key features of romance, rivalry, jealousy, aggression, potential of bodily injury, and passionate love.

Pretend play is the developmental companion of the oedipal phase, providing children with a virtual world of their own design, where they can work through the yearning and desire for one parent, the rivalry and hatred toward the other, the narcissistic mortifications, the consolation of parental love, and future promises of a sexual partner of their own, by playing out their feelings and fantasies in make-believe. As noted, triadic relationships proliferate in families and then on the playground as rivalry for a favorite sibling or playmate replicates the rivalry for the desired parent, adding new complexity to play, new details to conflicts and conundrums, deepening representations of self and others, and new levels of narrative intricacy. Children's play thus evolves over this period of development, moving from the representation of real events to utilization of play sets, dolls, action figures, and the like, to early role-play with peers, siblings, and parents. Story lines are typically an admixture of contemporary cultural elements, such as animated movies, books, and fairy tales, and internal sources, including anxieties, trauma, fantasy, and dreams. This amalgam emerges in unique syntheses that highlight themes specific to each child; by crafting narratives out of stories borrowed from popular culture and internally generated wishes and fantasies, the child tackles central concerns and gains mastery (Tessier et al. 2016). Over time, these play themes may recur in different iterations or dramatically transform as the child gains new ego capacities and meets new developmental and environmental challenges.

Imaginary companions make their first appearance in children in their third and fourth year, although they can also emerge later in childhood. Despite the folklore (and early studies) that associated imaginary companions with severe psychopathology, findings from research studies over the last century have demonstrated that these associations are either absent or mild (Gleason and Hohmann 2006; Hoff 2005). Moreover, socially anxious children who develop imaginary companions are not simply manifesting a symptom but are actually coaching themselves into better real peer interactions; studies suggest that the imaginary friend may be helpful in improving peer relationships over the course of childhood (Hoff 2005). Indeed, there is even literature that documents a slight advantage for children with than for those without imaginary friends in regard to their developing social competence (Taylor and Mannering 2007), confidence, and attentional capacity (Taylor 1999). Just as there may be theoretical hypotheses but little to support an association with psychopathology, so there is also disagreement in the literature, and little empirical evidence, about correlations with precocious theory of mind or exceptional creativity. Nonetheless, there is research to support the notion that children with imaginary companions are more attentive to and conversant about mental characteristics of other people (Davis et al. 2014; Hoff 2005) and show improved "emotional understanding" (Taylor et al. 2004).

Imaginary companions represent a particular form of pretend play that is created entirely by the child "out of thin air" (i.e., the majority are not attached to an actual object) and sustained for months to years. These "friends" can serve a range of functions, including a comforting companion, dependent or protégé (more typical when the imagined character is displaced onto a real doll or stuffed animal), voice of conscience, rescuer, scapegoat, ideal self, and/or repository of unwanted and painful feelings (Hoff 2005). These companions can appear in the context of some challenge (e.g., the birth of a sibling) and clearly serve the purpose of supporting the child, in addition to providing a special arena for play; they can also appear without a clear stimulus. They have been compared to new, personified versions of transitional objects (Hoff 2005) that provide that extra momentum to the child on the path to autonomous personality functioning. Imaginary companions are famously both private and public (as in *Calvin and Hobbes*), and they often accompany younger children during family activities; those that persist into middle childhood tend be more private. When parents are introduced to the imaginary friend of their young child, they intuitively tolerate and support their child's special relationship with this new family member (Gilmore and Meersand 2014), recognizing its value for the child's inner life.

Up to 65% of children possess imaginary companions at some point in childhood; these "friends" then vanish with little fanfare, typically well before preadolescence (Gilmore and Meersand 2014); they are slightly more prevalent among girls, who tend toward the "protégé" dynamic, whereas boys are more likely to create idealized characters such as superheroes (Hoff 2005). These creatures can remain available to their creators for many years, with increasingly sophisticated and elaborate narrative arcs.

Despite the advantages afforded by the capacity to play alone and the value of the imaginary companion to sustain a child in solitude, the prevalence of such companions paradoxically highlights how much young children are oriented to play with others. Fortunately, the imaginary companion can carry the child forward toward complex and "other-oriented" play. Although interactive (as opposed to purely parallel) play with other children can be observed as early as age 2 years, the capacity to negotiate the play agenda with other children matures slowly, because it relies on the coalescence of an array of ego capacities and ego flexibility, plus the growing desire to share this modality with actual people. The imaginary companion is an intermediate step in which interpersonal negotiation is conducted with a being who is part of the self.

Over the course of the third and fourth years, explosive language development enriches the narratives and invention of children's play, creating the improvisational flow that is unique to human players. Increasingly nuanced language offers the child the capacity to elaborate role, action schema, self, other, and event representation, and to produce narrative development that sustains play sequences and deepens the portrayal of play characters with thoughts and feelings. As the child seeks to engage others in playing, language conveys that intention by the ubiquitous metacommunication "Let's pretend," immediately recognizable as an invitation to join in the "ego state of play" (Gilmore 2005): an altered state by virtue of "changes in attention, perception, mental imagery, and thought processes, and...a predominant orientation toward subjective experience and fantasy that is deliberately disengaged from consensually shared representations" (Gilmore 2011, p. 1173).

The emergence of sociodramatic play, between ages 3 and 4 years, represents further advances in the child's flexibility, relatedness, and self-regulation. In contrast to the role-playing characteristic of earlier play, sociodramatic play requires that the child take on a character role and interpret and enact the associated behaviors and mental states in complex enactments with other children. This advanced play form thus involves "participants, roles, and place" (Deunk et al. 2008); it requires the abilities to communicate, to negotiate and establish guidelines, to assume roles, and to jointly imagine the setting of the scene (the frame) while agreeing to the pretend scenario and the crucial props for the story. Children craft layer upon layer of shared pretense, thereby co-creating or re-creating a virtual world of scenes both fanciful and realistic (e.g., Arendelle from *Frozen* or a doctor's office), roles (Elsa and Anna or a mother and her sick baby), and narrative development loosely based on a movie or book or on real experiences (Deunk et al. 2008; Forys and McCune-Nicolich 1984). Although brief joint play scenarios can make their appearance as early as age 2 years, it is only the verbal child who can extend joint narratives over weeks and months, with continuing elaboration and new dramatic elements. Contemporary adolescent and adult role-play has many features in common with this advanced form of pretending, which requires a complex multiplicity of identity for the play participant (classmate, player, persona in the play) and a shared fantasy of place and narrative.

THE FIFTH AND SIXTH YEARS

Kindergartners are usually expert sociodramatic players; historically, their classrooms had make-believe stations expressly for the purpose of such playing, and teachers used guided sociodramatic play to recruit intrinsic motivation for curricular goals. This type of play is different from the spontaneous play in the dress-up corner; it is likely an example of playfulness in the teacher's approach to learning a task. Because adding a pleasure quotient is obviously a successful technique with children from early infancy, it would seem self-evident that playful learning for young school-age children is likely to be met with greater success. However, with a heightened emphasis on early academic achievement in American classrooms, many educators and scholars feel that sociodramatic play, whether it is guided by the teacher's agenda or it emerges spontaneously in allotted "choice" time, has declined, and the opportunities it affords for learning in various arenas, including language, early literacy, motor skills, socioemotional skills, creativity, and various specific cognitive arenas such as mathematics, are thereby diminished (Bergen 2002; Lynch 2015). Teachers, under pressure to produce demonstrable academic gains, tend to focus on other teaching methods; in a recent survey, Lynch (2015) noted that a significant number of teachers did not know how to incorporate play into the curriculum.

Some advocates of the importance of unstructured time to play in the classroom and elsewhere believe that the equivocal research about the development-promoting value of play misses several key points: play is important in and of itself for the child's quality of life and individual psychology; play is a "right" and an intrinsic part of life for a child; and much of play is private by nature and therefore impossible to study (Bergen 2013). The urge to pretend play continues in this age group and, if excluded from the classroom, this play finds its way into other activities. For example, at recess and during free time in the classroom, kindergartners and first graders are typically engaged in activities around which pretending may be a shared or individual orientation; for example, they may create narratives around block constructions or in chasing games, sometimes borrowing familiar plot lines from television shows or movies. Children in this age group still gravitate toward pretending while engaged in solitary activities (e.g., in play with dolls or action figures) and seek opportunities in playdates to engage in both dramatic play (role-playing) and play with objects. As in the school setting, these iterations of role-play are typically based on favorite television shows, books, or movies, in addition to situations from daily life.

LATENCY AND BEYOND

Although pretend play can be readily observed in middle childhood, it occupies a less central place in a child's life and typically declines in the years leading up to puberty. Play preferences trend toward more structured games, art projects, building sets, and sports (Hughes 2010). Latency-stage children may continue to engage in pretense with favorite dolls and action figures and even in group scenarios, but the cognitive transformation occurring in this age group increasingly orients them to consensual reality. Nonetheless, many children retain some elements of pretending in their lives—in private play, creative writing, and humor, or as an enhancement of daily activities; for example, boys may inject fantasy elements into competitive sports, perhaps imagining the oedipal victory of "getting the desirable girl" as the prize for the winner (Altaian 1997; Clowes 1996; Sarnoff 1971). Moreover, early video game play may reinstate the opportunities for a version of fantasy play, shaped by the narrative premises and the vastly increased choices of avatar features in contemporary games. The video game genre offers a rapidly expanding range of game subjects, types of play, atmospherics, and avatars, as well as growing opportunities for socialization in game play, especially **MMORPGs** (massively multiplayer online role-playing games), such that each child's imagination can find a niche and a vehicle for fantasy.

Because the treatment situation is often experienced as an invitation to play, it can extend pretend play deep into latency or even adolescence in a safe and supportive environment without risk of exposure or embarrassment (Meersand 2009). A given child's propensity to pretend play cannot be immediately assumed to reflect immaturity or resistance to growing up, although it may serve to illustrate conflict around such desires in the treatment setting. In addition, it is not unusual for a latency child to bring handheld electronic games to sessions; the management of such increasingly common situations (with younger and younger children) is the topic of Chapter 4, "Play in the Digital Age."

Pretending, for some children, is a treasured mental state that provides a range of pleasures; developmental scholars suggest that with the decline of pretending, the older child finds a transitional outlet in daydreaming (Solnit 1998). There are many partial outlets for pretending in later childhood and adolescence, but these begin to border on other forms of creative expression and imagination; creative writing, improvisational drama, and guided story enactments in school are genres unto themselves, genres that resemble play but that are not the complete experience because one feature or another is missing.

In addition, live-action role-playing games, as exemplified by the tabletop game *Dungeons and Dragons* (D&D), Renaissance faires, and costume play (cosplay), approximate mature forms of imaginary play. The play associated with these activities is remarkably low tech and interpersonal, conducted at convention centers, outdoor parks, or local comic book stores. Their popularity persists despite their influence on or derivation from electronic gaming or other screen-related activities.

Often credited as the grandfather of fantasy video games, the unfairly maligned D&D involves live players (or player-characters [PCs]) who gather together, often on a regular basis, to play out ongoing narratives. D&D was developed in the late 1960s and became commercially available by 1974. Its first iteration was a tabletop game requiring one player in the role of Dungeon Master, other PCs, a rule book, and dice (Dormans 2006). Although each player chooses and to some extent crafts his or her own character from an array of given possibilities, the Dungeon Master is the primary source of the imaginary scenarios. The Dungeon Master dictates the events, the rulebook creates the blueprint for and the constraints on the game's action, and the various dice introduce the element of randomness or chance (Waskul and Lust 2004). As D&D grew in popularity in the 1980s, some gamers took it into live-action role-playing games where players enacted the stylized Medieval-influenced narrative with costumes and props. The Dungeon Master remains the creator of the imaginary realm, but there is room for improvisation for every player, with tension and uncertainty sustained by the roll of the dice. Deviations from the script create excitement and take the players into fantastical situations that are unpredictable and partly scripted but also partly created de novo (Shank 2015). Infinite possibilities are present because D&D's "metarule" is that there are no rules requiring that the players follow the rules (Waskul and Lust 2004).

A PC has features similar to a child engaged in sociodramatic imaginary play with other children or adults. Each PC carries elements of the persona (the character), the player (the player's attitude toward and conduct in the play), and the person (the nonplaying personality) (Waskul and Lust 2004); this multiplicity of identities is typically present in make-believe, as children move in and out of the pretend mode. The potential for a blurring of boundaries may be greater with older children because of their action orientation and mature bodies; no doubt this contributed to the "moral panic" around D&D's alleged promotion of real violence (Haberman 2016). There is no doubt that this type of live-action role-playing game, which has spawned a number of themed narrative role-play games, such as Dragon Quest, Spycraft, and Star Wars, usually relies on explicit violence as a key narrative element, but it is typically stylized violence and represents a violation of known rules, which then reequilibrate. Many elements of D&D were incorporated in contemporary MMORPGs.

Renaissance faires, also called Medieval Fairs, Renaissance Festivals, Knights Tournaments, and the like, are recurring events, most popular in the United States but also found in Europe and Australia, that began to appear in the 1960s. The early prototype of these annual festivals was developed by Phyllis Patterson in Laurel Canyon, California. An educator and children's theatre instructor, she borrowed elements from Commedia dell'arte and 60s counterculture to create an enacted, costumed, parodic event with a political "edge" (Rubin 2012). The original faires were deliberate anti-establishment affairs; while they have become increasingly commercial and lavish, they retain an admixture of defiant, queer,[3] and heroic elements that make them especially appealing to emerging adults. These weekend events encourage participants to create extravagant costumes, engage in historical enactments such as jousting tournaments and historical romances, adopt historical idioms in speech, and perform ancient music on period instruments. Participants also draw the nonparticipants into the play, creating spontaneous (but not entirely unplanned) "immersion theater" (Rubin 2012, p. 114) that amounts to an adult form of improvised play. They also accommodate popular narratives—from fairy tales to videogame plots; the faire-grounds become fictional landscapes that can be "saturated with meaning" that will vary according to the faire-goers.

Another late-adolescent and adult genre of pretending is *cosplay*, which originated in Japan in the 1980s. Players dress as characters from the contemporary scene, anime (animated stories), manga (comics), and pop culture. Although costume/persona display (with pictures and social media posts) is often an aim in and of itself, some participants engage in fantasy interactions at the "carnivalesque space" of cosplay conventions (Lamerichs 2014), often spilling over to the surrounding area. This form of role-play is focused on bodily transformation into the character, achieved by elaborate costuming, cross-dressing, and subversive (caricaturing) appropriation of popular characters from anime, pop music, video games, and cultural sources, including queer politics. Narrative development is not a major focus.

---

[3]Originally a derogatory term for gay men, queer has come to signify a political or theoretical stance that rejects normative thinking in regard to gender and sexuality. Many queer theorists refuse to define the term because a definition immediately co-opts its inherent subversiveness.

SUMMARY

The developmental trajectory of pretend play begins in infancy and can extend, in certain forms, into adulthood. Its heyday is in early childhood, starting in the third year of life with simple pretend acts, usually based on real experience, like rocking a baby-doll or feeding a cookie (real or imagined) to a grown-up. As semiotic function advances and language capacity accelerates between ages three and four, the full flowering of pretend play occurs. This is the period of the most unfettered and fanciful play sequences, ones that utilize objects without regard to their intended purpose to create narratives entirely outside of lived experience. The timing of this progression can be observed in all human cultures, leading some to suggest its foundation in universal neurophysiological development. Play continues to evolve, becoming increasingly social and simultaneously more concrete until it begins to fade in importance in latency (Gilmore 2011). However, the developmental function of pretend play—despite its consistent trajectory and its apparent role in identity formation, interpersonal relations, role exploration, the management of conflict and anxiety—has not been empirically demonstrated. Many theorists consider this a problem of experimental design and the challenge of elucidating the developmental value of a spontaneous, often private, and mostly ephemeral activity that bears fruit many years later in life.

KEY POINTS

- Make-believe play begins in playful interaction with a parent, usually the mother, who uses marked affect and motherese to engage the infant in a playful exchange, typically with the baby's own body as playground. While other adults, notably the father, can also participate in very early play, the special combination of motherese and extravagant emotional display, in this culture mostly confined to women, seems to be crucial. The mother's marked affect and prosody facilitate the infant's recognition that the unfolding spectacle—the exaggerated facial expression, sing-song baby-talk, and affectionate physical contact—has no "real" purpose. Even 3-month-old babies respond accordingly, with excitement and pleasure; they "know" that their mother is playing.

- Exploratory, imitative, and object play—forms that precede the appearance of child-initiated pretending—are often incorporated into the earliest pretend play of the child late in the second year of life; short sequences of "playing bedtime" or "feeding the baby" or "giving mommy a cookie" are typical examples. Adults or older children can facilitate these forays by encouraging narrative development.

- Play is hugely advanced by the emergence of symbolic function in general. Metarepresentation is a key element in pretending, and the child who is 3–6 years old is more at home with creative metarepresentation than later in childhood, when consensual reality has taken hold. Language is essential for establishing play parameters and for narrative development.

- Play similarly benefits from the newly enlarged relational capacity and affective complexity of 4- and 5-year-olds.

- The function of make-believe has proved especially difficult to research (Lillard et al. 2013) because most of make-believe is spontaneous and/or private; attempts to study it have been inconclusive, in large part because the research designs are flawed. Theorists and educators offer a range of proposals regarding play: play is a right of childhood and intrinsic to its proper experience; play promotes theory of mind; play promotes counterfactual reasoning, important for understanding causality (Walker and Gopnik 2013); play promotes literacy; and play promotes prosocial behaviors.

KEY TERMS

Decentering, decontextualization, integration   Piagetian terms referring to aspects of cognitive development. **Decentering** refers to the process of achieving equilibrium between assimilation and accommodation, which allows children to understand perspectives different from their own. **Decontextualization** allows objects to be used for imaginary purposes and thus freed from their real context. **Integration** refers to the assimilation of external elements into evolving mental structures.

MMORPG   Massively multiplayer online role-playing game. These games involve social interaction in collaborative virtual environments that are "persistent worlds" (i.e., they are not dependent on the presence of users). They are played by literally millions of players daily. *World of Warcraft* hit its peak in 2010 with 12 million subscribers; today it is at 5.5 million subscribers and is still considered among the top 10 MMORPGs (Conditt 2016).

Pretend mode   A concept introduced by Fonagy et al. (2004) that designates the role of imagination as the child moves from a "psychic equivalence mode" (where thoughts are felt to mirror reality) to consensual reality. The pretend mode allows the child to "partially … free representations from their referents and allow these freed representations to be modified" (p. 261). Children can pretend and elaborate stories, self-representations, and situations "in their heads" and understand that they are imagining something that does not and must not be confused with the real. This mode follows the course of pretend play, emerges at 2½–3 years, and declines in importance as a bridge to reality as the child moves into latency.

Scaffolding   A term associated with Vygotsky's (1978) theorizing about the *zone of proximal development* (ZPD). He pointed out that adults or older children interact with younger ones at a slightly higher level of development than they possess, drawing them forward toward the achievement of next steps. They thereby scaffold the younger child: "with adult intervention over a series of interactions, a child is able to solve a problem, carry out a task or achieve a goal that would be beyond the child's unassisted efforts. In other words, the adult provides an implicit scaffold that helps the child move to a higher level within the ZPD" (Kassett et al. 2004, p. 94).

Semiotic function   The human capacity to use signs to represent objects, ideas, or other aspects of reality in the service of communication in social interactions. Verbal language is the primary example of semiotic function, but the concept has been applied by many disciplines to their object of study, from films to cosmology (Johnson 2015).

Transitional space   The "space" between me and not-me in which transitional objects and other transitional phenomena can develop. It is the "realm of illusion." "This intermediate area of experience, unchallenged in respect of its belonging to inner or external (shared) reality, constitutes the greater part of the infant's experience, and throughout life is retained in the intense experiencing that belongs to the arts and to religion and to imaginative living, and to creative scientific work" (Winnicott 1953, p. 97).

REFERENCES

Altaian N: The case of Ronald: oedipal issues in the treatment of a seven-year-old boy. Psychoanal Dialogues 7(6):725–739, 1997

Barr R, Hayne H: It's not what you know, it's who you know: older siblings facilitate imitation during infancy. Int J Early Years Educ 11(1):7–21, 2003

Beebe B, Lachmann F, Jaffe J: Mother-infant interaction structures and pre-symbolic self- and object representations. Psychoanal Dialogues 7(2):133–182, 1997

Bergen D: The role of early pretend play in children's cognitive development. Early Childhood Res Practice 4(1):2–13, 2002

Bergen D: Does pretend play matter? Searching for evidence: comment on Lillard et al. (2013). Psychol Bull 139(1):45–48, 2013 23294090

Bretherton I: Representing the social world in symbolic play: reality and fantasy, in Symbolic Play: The Development of Social Understanding. Edited by Bretherton I. Orlando, FL, Academic Press, 1984, pp 3–49

Bruner J: The organization of action and the nature of adult-infant transaction, in The Analysis of Action. Edited by von Cranach M, Harre R. New York, Cambridge University Press, 1982, pp 313–327

Burghardt GM, Sutton-Smith B: The Genesis of Animal Play: Testing the Limits. Cambridge MA, MIT Press, 2006

Clowes EK: Oedipal themes in latency: analysis of the "farmer's daughter" joke. Psychoanal Study Child 51:436–454, 1996 9029970

Conditt J: "World of Warcraft" keeps growing with "Legion" in August. Engadget, April 19, 2016. Available at: https://www.engadget.com/2016/04/19/world-of-warcraft-legion-release-date/. Accessed October 1, 2016.

Currie G: Arts and Minds. Oxford, UK, Clarendon Press, 2004

Davis PE, Meins E, Fernyhough C: Children with imaginary companions focus on mental characteristics when describing their real-life friends. Infant Child Dev 23(6):622–633, 2014 25685093

Deunk M, Berenst J, De Glopper K: The development of early sociodramatic play. Discourse Stud 10(5):615–633, 2008

Dormans J: On the role of the die: a brief ludologic study of pen-and-paper ro-
leplaying games and their rules. Game Studies 6(1), 2006. Available at:
http://gamestudies.org/0601/articles/dormans. Accessed March 12, 2016.

Dowling S: Abstract report from the literature on neonatology. Psychoanal
Q 50:290–295, 1981

Dunn J: Sibling relationships in early childhood. Child Dev 54:787–811,
1983

Dunn J: Mind-reading, emotion understanding, and relationships. Int J Behav
Dev 24:142–144, 2000

Dunn J: Children's Friendships: The Beginnings of Intimacy. Oxford, UK,
Blackwell, 2004

Ensink K, Mayes L: The development of mentalisation in children from a
theory of mind perspective. Psychoanal Inq 30(4):301–337, 2010

Falk D: Finding Our Tongues: Mothers, Infants and the Origins of Language.
New York, Basic Books, 2009

Fantasia V, Fasulo A, Costall A, López B: Changing the game: exploring infants' participation in early play routines. Front Psychol 5:522, 2014
24936192

Fonagy I, Fonagy P: Communication with pretend actions in language, literature and psychoanalysis. Psychoanalysis and Contemporary Thought
18:363–418, 1995

Fonagy P, Target M: Playing with reality, I: theory of mind and the normal development of psychic reality. Int J Psychoanal 77(Pt 2):217–233, 1996
8771375

Fonagy P, Target M: Playing with reality, III: the persistence of dual psychic
reality in borderline patients. Int J Psychoanal 81(Pt 5):853–873, 2000
11109573

Fonagy P, Target M: The rooting of the mind in the body: new links between
attachment theory and psychoanalytic thought. J Am Psychoanal Assoc
55(2):411–456, 2007 17601099

Fonagy P, Gergely G, Jurist EL, Target M: Affect Regulation, Mentalization
and the Development of the Self. New York, Other Press, 2004

Forys S, McCune-Nicolich L: Shared pretend: sociodramatic play at 3 years
of age, in Symbolic Play: The Development of Social Understanding.
Edited by Bretherton I. Orlando, FL, Academic Press, 1984, pp 159–191

Gergely G, Watson JS: The social biofeedback theory of parental affect-
mirroring: the development of emotional self-awareness and self-control
in infancy. Int J Psychoanal 77(Pt 6):1181–1212, 1996 9119582

Gilmore K: Play in the psychoanalytic setting: ego capacity, ego state, and
vehicle for intersubjective exchange. Psychoanal Study Child 60:213–
238, 2005 16649681

Gilmore K: Pretend play and development in early childhood (with implications for the oedipal phase). J Am Psychoanal Assoc 59(6):1157–1182, 2011 22080503

Gilmore K, Meersand P: Normal Child and Adolescent Development: A Psychodynamic Primer. Washington, DC, American Psychiatric Publishing, 2014

Gleason TR, Hohmann LM: Concepts of real and imaginary friendship in early childhood. Soc Dev 15(1):128–144, 2006

Haberman C: When Dungeons and Dragons set off a "moral panic." Retro report. The New York Times, April 17, 2016. Available at: http://www.nytimes.com/2016/04/18/us/when-dungeons-dragons-set-off-a-moral-panic.html?_r=0. Accessed August 15, 2016.

Harris PL: Understanding pretense, in Children's Early Understanding of Mind: Origins and Development. Edited by Lewis C, Mitchell P. East Sussex, UK, Erlbaum, 1994, pp 235–259

Harris PL: Desires, beliefs, and language, in Theories of Theories of Mind. Edited by Carruthers P, Smith PK. Cambridge, UK, Cambridge University Press, 1996, pp 200–222

Hobson R: The making of mind. Psychoanal Inq 34(8):817–830, 2014

Hoff EV: Imaginary companions, creativity, and self-image in middle childhood. Creat Res J 17(2–3):167–180, 2005

Hughes C, Dunn J: "Pretend you didn't know": preschoolers' talk about mental states in pretend play. Cogn Dev 12(4):477–497, 1997

Hughes FP: Children, Play and Development, 4th Edition. Thousand Oaks, CA, Sage, 2010

James W: Principles of Psychology. New York, Henry Holt, 1890

Johnson KB: Semiotics, in International Encyclopedia of the Social and Behavioral Sciences, 2nd Edition. Edited by Wright JD. New York, Elsevier, 2015, pp 592–597

Kassett JA, Bonanno GA, Notarius CI: Affective scaffolding: a process measure for psychotherapy with children. J Infant Child Adolesc Psychother 3(1):92–118, 2004

Kleeman JA: The peek-a-boo game, I: its origins, meanings, and related phenomena in the first year. Psychoanal Study Child 22:239–273, 1967 5590067

Lamerichs N: Embodied fantasy: the affective space of anime conventions, in The Ashgate Research Companion to Fan Cultures. Edited by Duits L, Zwaan K, Reijnders S. New York, Routledge, 2014, pp 263–274

Lillard AS, Lerner MD, Hopkins EJ, et al: The impact of pretend play on children's development: a review of the evidence. Psychol Bull 139(1):1–34, 2013 22905949

Loewald HW: Oedipus complex and development of self. Psychoanal Q 54(3):435–443, 1985 4023124

Lynch M: More play please: the perspective of kindergarten teachers on play in the classroom. Am J Play 7(3):347–370, 2015

Meersand P: Play and the older child: developmental and clinical opportunities. Psychoanal Study Child 64:112–130, 2009 20578436

Meltzoff AN, Decety J: What imitation tells us about social cognition: a rapprochement between developmental psychology and cognitive neuroscience. Philos Trans R Soc Lond B Biol Sci 358(1431):491–500, 2003 12689375

Meltzoff AN, Moore MK: Imitation of facial and manual gestures by human neonates. Science 198(4312):75–78, 1977 17741897

Mitchell RW: Pretense in animals: the continuing relevance of children's pretense, in Play and Development: Evolutionary, Sociocultural, and Functional Perspectives. Edited by Göncü A, Gaskins S. New York, Erlbaum, 2007, pp 51–75

Moran GS: Some functions of play and playfulness: a developmental perspective. Psychoanal Study Child 42:14–15, 1987 3438362

Piaget J: Play, Dreams and Imitation in Childhood (1945). New York, WW Norton, 1962

Rubin RL: Well Met: Renaissance Faires and the American Counterculture. New York, New York University Press, 2012

Saint-Georges C, Chetouani M, Cassel R, et al: Motherese in interaction: at the cross-road of emotion and cognition? (A systematic review). PLoS One 8(10):e78103, 2013 24205112

Sarnoff CA: Ego structure in latency. Psychoanal Q 40(3):387–414, 1971 4937100

Scarlett WG, Naudeau S, Salonius-Pasternak D, et al: Children's Play. Thousand Oaks, CA, Sage, 2005

Shank N: Productive violence and poststructural play in the Dungeons and Dragons narrative. J Pop Cult 48(1):184–197, 2015

Shengold L: Some notes on play and playfulness. Bulletin of the Anna Freud Centre 11:146–151, 1988

Smith CL: Multiple determinants of parenting: predicting individual differences in maternal parenting behaviors with toddlers. Parent Sci Pract 10(1):1–17, 2010

Solnit AJ: Beyond play and playfulness. Psychoanal Study Child 53:102–110, 1998 9990826

Taylor M: Imaginary Companions and the Children Who Create Them. New York, Oxford University Press, 1999

Taylor M, Mannering AM: Of Hobbes and Harvey: the imaginary companions created by children and adults, in Play and Development: Evolutionary, Sociocultural, and Functional Perspectives. Edited by Göncü A, Gaskins S. New York, Erlbaum, 2007, pp 227–246

Taylor M, Carlson SM, Maring BL, et al: The characteristics and correlates of fantasy in school-age children: imaginary companions, impersonation, and social understanding. Dev Psychol 40(6):1173–1187, 2004 15535765

Tessier VP, Normandin L, Ensink K, et al: Fact or fiction? A longitudinal study of play and the development of reflective functioning. Bull Menninger Clin 80(1):60–79, 2016 27028339

Tomasello M: Social cognition before the revolution, in Early Social Cognition: Understanding Others in the First Months of Life. Edited by Rochat P. Mahwah, NJ, Erlbaum, 1999, pp 301–314

Tronick E, Als H, Adamson L, et al: The infant's response to entrapment between contradictory messages in face-to-face interaction. J Am Acad Child Psychiatry 17(1):1–13, 1978 632477

Vallotton C, Ayoub C: Use your words: the role of language in the development of toddlers' self-regulation. Early Child Res Q 26(2):169–181, 2011 21969766

Van Dam M, De Palma P, Strong WE: Father's use of fundamental frequency in motherese. Journal of the Acoustical Society of America 137(4):2267, 2015. Available at: http://asa.scitation.org/doi/abs/10.1121/1.4920275. Accessed March 2, 2016.

Vivona JM: Is there a nonverbal period of development? J Am Psychoanal Assoc 60(2):231–265, discussion 305–310, 2012 22467444

Vygotsky LS: The Mind in Society: The Development of Higher Psychological Processes. Cambridge, MA, Harvard University Press, 1978

Walker CM, Gopnik A: Pretense and possibility—a theoretical proposal about the effects of pretend play on development: comment on Lillard et al. (2013). Psychol Bull 139(1):40–44, 2013 23294089

Waskul D, Lust M: Role-playing and playing roles: the person, player, and the persona in fantasy role-playing. Symbolic Interact 27(3):333–356, 2004

Weil AP: The basic core. Psychoanal Study Child 25:442–460, 1970 5532125

Winnicott DW: Transitional objects and transitional phenomena: a study of the first not-me possession. Int J Psychoanal 34(2):89–97, 1953 13061115

Winnicott DW: Playing and Reality. London, Tavistock, 1971

4

Play in the Digital Age

Jeff began therapy with Dr. Howard at age 8 due to social anxiety and mood disturbance. He had three siblings, an 18-year-old brother and 14-year-old twin sisters, and his parents were wealthy professionals who employed a large staff of nannies, tutors, assistants, drivers, and security guards. Jeff was a phobic, lonely boy who relied on his live-in tutor and nanny and shied away from activities with other children. He had had a severe bout of hypochondriacal anxiety in second grade after a painful gastrointestinal illness; for 3 months, he was fearful of touching anything at school and would avoid the toilets by retaining for the entire school day. This was viewed as a transient reaction, and no psychiatric treatment was considered. However, a waxing-and-waning school resistance persisted such that he missed many days in the spring. In his current third-grade year, his poor attendance persisted and he appeared very disengaged at school, did not record his assignments or participate in class, and was listless at home. The only pleasure he pursued was playing video games; he was an avid Minecraft enthusiast and spent almost all of his after-school time playing the game, exploring the online community of devotees, and seeking to establish a relationship with a wildly popular older boy who performed and discussed strategies in YouTube videos. His preoccupation with Minecraft had escalated to the point that he resisted participation in any family activities, tutoring sessions, and scheduled family trips. His parents expressed their concerns to his pediatrician and raised the possibility that he was "addicted" to the game. The pediatrician recommended consulting with Dr. Howard, a 37-year-old media-savvy child psychiatrist who had written a number of essays on video games (including Minecraft) and video-game addiction.

Jeff was dropped off at his first appointment by a driver, so it was left to Dr. Howard to introduce himself. Dr. Howard was struck by Jeff's

thin, pale, and rather disconsolate appearance; an atmosphere of loneliness followed him like a cloud when he came into the office. Jeff chose
to sit in the chair beside the desk and did not look around the room.
Dr. Howard acknowledged Jeff's reluctance and guessed that he was
worried that this meeting was about his gaming. Jeff angrily described
his parents' new rules: Minecraft play was limited to the weekends and
"not only that, but I can only play for 2 hours total! Did you tell them
that's what they should do?" Dr. Howard was sincerely puzzled, because he had done no such thing and was concerned that such a "coincidence" would brand him as "the enemy." While admitting that Jeff's
parents had talked to him about their concern regarding Jeff's gaming, he told Jeff that he was pretty sure that he hadn't recommended
any new rules but that he understood why Jeff must think he was behind it. Dr. Howard noted that he was a kind of student of video games
and tried to learn about them and understand which one became
someone's favorite and why. This comment transformed the atmosphere. Jeff began to describe his participation in a multiplayer realm
(by invitation) in the Survival Mode of Minecraft, his comradery with
the other players, and their joint projects and combined defenses
against the deadly mobs who arise at night. He extolled the brilliance
of the YouTube "star" who shared his ideas and responded to comments and questions. Glancing at Dr. Howard's PC, Jeff offered to show
him a short clip. Dr. Howard agreed and added that he actually wanted
to understand more about Jeff and his love of Minecraft; he would
clear it with Jeff's parents, but he thought it might be helpful to play
Minecraft together, understanding that it would be separate from his
multiplayer realm, just between them. He told Jeff that he had some
experience with Minecraft and liked it too.

Electronic play can provide an adequate platform for psychodynamic
treatment. Dr. Howard conducted play therapy with Jeff almost exclusively through Minecraft for the first 18 months of treatment. Even in
this first meeting, it was clear to Dr. Howard that Jeff was managing
his isolation, loneliness, and desire for an older boy as mentor by his
involvement in the game. Dr. Howard's willingness to permit the play
directly in the treatment was facilitated by a number of factors: he
knew the game well and felt confident he could manage whatever might
come up in the actual game play; he felt strongly that Jeff was using
the game for a range of psychological reasons, many of which would
be productive to explore without prejudice; and he was concerned that
the parents' abrupt prohibition would derail the treatment from the out-

set. Furthermore, Dr. Howard was convinced that Jeff's life was in Minecraft and that the best way to open the door would be to play the game
with him.

OVERVIEW: ELECTRONICS, DIGITAL MEDIA, AND PLAY

Any perspective on young children and their development in the
twenty-first century must reckon with the fact that they are digital
natives, born and raised in seamlessly mediated environments. This reality has special significance in early twenty-first-century developmental science because many of the researchers and scholars studying young
people have grown up in an analog world and, as digital "immigrants"
(Zevenbergen 2007) or "settlers" (Palfrey and Gasser 2008), they are
fundamentally different from their subjects. They can easily be faulted
for not appreciating the developmental experience of anyone born after
1980, in particular the children of the 2000s and 2010s who were themselves raised by digital natives. Although therapists like Dr. Howard will
increasingly populate the ranks of child clinicians, training in play theory and technique is only beginning to address this kind of play.

Most experts agree that these children, the digital natives, see and experience the world differently from their parents and teachers (Zevenbergen 2007). From birth, today's infants are exposed to a steady stream
of stimuli emanating from **technoculture**: background television, baby-
oriented videos, apps for kids ages 2–4 on smartphones and tablets, and
online communities such as Penguin Club open to 6-year-olds, to
name just a few. Today's young children are "born digital" and raised in
a media-saturated world in which "humans and computers interact in
hundreds of ways daily, often unobtrusively; technology-mediated
experiences are simply everywhere and everywhere taken for granted"
(de Zengotita 2005, quoted in Essig 2012, p. 440). Perhaps inevitably,
the disconnect between generations has triggered grave concerns about
the impact of technology on development, as represented in the reports
from pediatric, educational, and developmental literature. However,
following Flanagan's (2014) admonition that "we must make sense of
our own times" (p. 29), there is an expanding literature that aims at understanding the interplay of children and contemporary culture with a
more dispassionate eye and finds therein benefits, opportunities, and,
perhaps most important, preparation for a posthuman future in which
human life and machines are indistinguishable. Inevitably, the funda-

mental features of children change with the culture, because childhood is a social construct that has varied dramatically over history. As play therapists, we must play with children as they present themselves to us, with the same cultural sensitivity we strive for when treating children from foreign cultures or local subcultures.

A BRIEF HISTORY OF TECHNOLOGY AND CHILD DEVELOPMENT

Beginning with the advent of television more than 60 years ago, the question of deleterious and/or beneficial effects of technoculture on growing children has been researched and debated. From the point of view of child development—for example, in regard to learning, attention, brain development, emotional regulation, and aggression—even the most evenhanded research reviews describe a complex mosaic of benefits and risks. Considered from the vantage point of future citizenship in a digital world, media literacy is clearly necessary; early exposure to technology plays a role in fostering both comprehension and facility, such that very young children have command of the devices, avenues of access, and communication potential that far exceeds that of their parents. The tendency of today's more senior commentators to be negative about digital impact on various aspects of child development—on creative play, empathy, mentalization, socialization, interpersonal communication, attention, and so on—is nothing new; indeed, each technological advance has been greeted with concern by the older generation. Perhaps because many believe that technoculture has radically reconfigured our society—including its centuries-old traditions, professions, and value systems—the disconnect between generations and the critique of new technology have reached new levels.

More specifically in regard to play, the impact of electronic media on typical developmental progression and the mind of the child is a topic of urgent concern to play advocates who maintain the importance of play for human development (Singer and Singer 2007). Many believe that the future of play is at risk in the context of cultural transformation to a technologically driven society, and as play goes, so goes childhood (Strasburger 2017). Of course, electronic media are both product and shaper of contemporary culture as it undergoes a remarkably rapid transformation to a fully digital society and posthuman ethos. Some, perhaps more optimistic, commentators suggest that the children of today, while playing with contemporary playthings, are inducted into the technoculture, develop expertise, and stimulate its further development, without significant loss to creativity or imagination (Gelfond and Salonius-Pasternak 2005; Zevenbergen 2007). They can then advance to playing and developing **serious games** that purposefully promote an array of skills crucial for adaptation to the twenty-first century: "communication, collaboration, social and cultural skills, creativity, critical thinking, problem-solving, productivity in a globalized world, learning to learn skills, self-direction, planning, flexibility, risk taking, conflict management and a sense of initiative and entrepreneurship" (Romero et al. 2015, p. 149). Dismay about or rejection of this aspect of youth culture is out of step with the world in which we live.

In this chapter, we consider these changes as they relate to play and also address the potential of electronic devices—toys, games, and computers—for play therapy. Important considerations include whether these devices should be allowed into the consultation room and whether electronic play on screens and mobile devices bars access to inner life, squelches creativity, and leads to robotic minds.

TELEVISION

We first revisit the debate about television, the first screen technology to invade the American household and the potential portal to later use of electronic toys, video games, and computer games (Vandewater et al. 2005). Television and its remarkable spread into American homes, with ownership jumping from 7% to 83% between 1950 and 1957 (Wartella et al. 2010) and to 96% in 2016 (Nielsen 2009), has stirred controversy that continues today. In and of itself, television does not constitute playing, but television is of interest in this discussion because it has been criticized as an *interference to play* and also because it is typically children's first introduction to screens, both historically and in the course of a child's life.

The exponential surge in television ownership in the 1950s and the likelihood of children under age 2 years being exposed to television increased steadily over time, as homes with more televisions than people became the norm (Nielsen 2009). In regard to programming specifically for children, *Sesame Street* began broadcasting in 1969, but it was not until 1997, with the production of *Baby Einstein*, that television videos were created with the explicit intention of engaging a baby viewer (Wartella et al. 2010). Shortly thereafter, the American Academy of Pediatrics Committee on Public Education (1999) issued an advisory, warning parents against screen exposure before age 2. In this regard, it is noteworthy that the pediatric literature consistently documents negative outcomes of baby television watching (Landhuis et al. 2007; Radesky et al. 2014; Zimmerman and Christakis 2005), whereas developmental research is not nearly so negative and may even demonstrate positive effects (Courage and Howe 2010; Wartella et al. 2010). Nonetheless, the *Baby Genius* video series targeting children under age 2 has been convincingly proven to not produce educational benefits. In fact, there is substantial evidence that infants under age 18 months are not really capable of processing screen media. Television or video viewing has an independent developmental course with its own demands on mental processing; very young children lack the perceptual, cognitive, and social maturity to decode it (Anderson and Hanson 2010; Singer and Singer 2005). This is one contribution to the well-documented **video deficit**, a term referencing the finding that infants learn better from people than from videos—for example, in the acquisition of skills such as object retrieval and imitation. The video deficit is typically corrected by age 5 (Anderson and Hanson 2010). Highly interactive videos and parental participation can compensate for the deficit, even in younger children, but such conditions essentially confirm the importance of human input.

The concerns about brain development for the age 0–3 screen-exposed population in regard to attentional processes, language learning, and so on, while amply represented in the literature, are based on correlations rather than causal evidence (Courage and Setliff 2010). The frequently cited association of early television viewing and attention-deficit/hyperactivity disorder in later childhood (Christakis et al. 2004) has not been supported by many subsequent studies and information about infant attention that refutes the connection. Many studies highlight the mediation of other factors, including inborn neurobiological factors and genetic predisposition unrelated to environmental input. In contrast, violent television content has been robustly linked to attentional problems (Courage and Setliff 2010) and, in combination with other violent media exposure, has been postulated to have an impact on neural maturation (Hummer 2015), but this requires further neuroimaging research. Studies exploring television's role in language development vary, depending on the program and its embedded language-learning methodology; interactive prompts or parental coviewing are helpful, especially to children with larger vocabularies to begin with. Programs with sustained storybook formats are superior to those with series of vignettes and babyish characters whose vocabularies are limited (Linebarger and Walker 2005). Children from impoverished backgrounds do seem to gain in literacy and vocabulary from explicitly language-learning-focused television.

Television's postulated deleterious impact on play of all types, from practicing in infancy to pretend play to outdoor locomotor activities, is usually attributed to promotion of passivity, diminution of dedicated play time, and the level of distraction from play when television is in the background. In regard to passivity, many researchers differentiate the intellectual from physical inactivity because of the significant mental capacities required by television viewing. A close examination of television watching by infants suggests that comprehension of "television space" follows its own developmental trajectory that evolves over childhood with a steep learning curve in the first years of life. For television space to be visually understood by young children, they must master and integrate a visual/spatial/auditory experience with limited interactive potential, which is further complicated by rapid transitions based on point of view, camera angles, and shifting location. The neurocognitive capacities to synthesize the imagery and simultaneous auditory input only emerge and become fully operational toward the end of the third year of life (Anderson and Hanson 2010). Television cannot, therefore, be considered a purely passive activity in regard to its comprehension and is seen favorably as a step in the development of media literacy. However, watching television is clearly not a physical activity; television sets in the bedroom and time spent viewing television have been shown to be risk factors for obesity and cardiometabolic disease in children (Staiano et al. 2013). Reports vary about the impact of television watching on outdoor play (Anderson and Hanson 2010; Natsiopoulou and Bletsou 2011): paradoxically, in television-heavy households (where television is on all the time), television time is not associated with diminished outdoor time or indoor toy play. The more significant differences between children from these households and those from light-television homes is that the former are delayed and less adept at reading and more dedicated to other electronic media later in childhood (Vandewater et al. 2005). Some researchers suggest that play is more interrupted and less absorbing when accompanied by background television (Masur et al. 2015; Singer and Singer 2007).

ELECTRONIC TOYS AND GAMES

PARENTS' TOYS

Mastering television is a step in the development of media literacy, but television is no longer the only screen opportunity for children under age 2 years. Another potent and ubiquitous source of screen exposure is the smartphone, a device that is owned by close to 80% of 30- to 49-year-olds (Smith 2015), roughly the age group that includes parents of young children. The pursuit of screens starts very early; parents' phones are alluring and are often offered to occupy young children. Literature examining the impact of smartphones on children's development reflects radical cultural differences in attitudes and approaches. In South Korea, where smartphone "addiction" is felt to have a specific deleterious effect on frontal lobe development, the addiction rate for preschool children was 4.3% in a 2012 national survey (Park and Park 2014, p. 147). Smartphone apps targeting preschoolers are on the rise; these apps dedicated to kids are downloaded by parents for the express purpose of turning this presumably adult object into a child-oriented toy. Indeed, the still small collection of smartphone studies in the United States also documents very early use of and facility with smartphones; moreover, new apps for kids appear regularly, such as Monkey Preschool Lunchbox, Peek-a-Boo, and Angry Birds. The smartphone is touted as a highly successful babysitter, such that the online newsletter *Techadvisor* promotes its use with the following advice: "And the hardest thing of all is to entertain and educate, whilst grabbing back a bit of time for yourself. I have good news for you reader: your smartphone and tablet are your friends. Kids love playing good apps" (Egan 2016).

ELECTRONIC TOYS MADE FOR YOUNG CHILDREN

Although screens form a continuous thread in children's experience of the digital world, there are other genres of electronic toys—such as electronically motored figures from beloved television shows and movies, which can dance and sing; remote-controlled vehicles and robots; talking or otherwise interactive devices ranging from cash registers to spy-gear night goggles—that are oriented toward different age groups. Controversy about these toys continues, likened to the "moral panic" that greets every iteration of "children's popular culture" (Marsh 2005, p. 133); this, of course, is an echo of the controversy about television. Some educators, pediatricians, and play experts raise the alarm about the harmful effect of electronic toys on imaginary play (Levin and Rosenquest 2001), whereas others suggest that 1) toys always reflect the prevailing culture and commercial interests, 2) mastery of electronic devices is a vital learning experience for today's children, and 3) children will use any toy for personal expression, no matter how pre-scripted (Marsh 2005).

The empirical verdict is still out, however; research is typically more focused on the learning value of these toys, to the neglect of the play quotient, since the latter is notoriously difficult to measure and apparently not considered a marketing tool. Electronic toys for very young children are almost without exception advertised as educational, but there is little proof of conventional or developmental learning, such as improving vocabulary or theory of mind (Siraj-Blatchford and Siraj-Blatchford 2002). As an example, one study demonstrates a decline in communicative interaction when parents use an electronic toy to play with children ages 10–16 months, as compared to reading or playing with a nonelectronic toy (Sosa 2016). Another study of 24-month-olds playing with shape sorters shows that although parents produce comparable numbers of words using traditional and electronic versions, there is less unique language with the latter: "parents may take a back seat to electronic toys" (Zosh et al. 2015, p. 141). The conclusion is that electronic toys apparently do not foster the richness of discourse that a nonelectronic toy can. Similarly, a study using videoconferencing as a tool for 4-year-olds to enhance theory-of-mind acquisition (in a research design that is minimally techie at best) demonstrated its failure to do so in any precocious way (Siraj-Blatchford and Siraj-Blatchford 2002). Another study tested the hypothesis that novel technology could accelerate theory-of-mind acquisition in 4-year-olds by placing two video screens in their classroom and conducting **false-belief tests**. Videoconferencing allowed the children to witness the deception on screen. While the exposure helped children develop familiarity with video equipment, it had no effect on the pace of their theory-of-mind acquisition (Siraj-Blatchford and Siraj-Blatchford 2002). It appears that the presence and quality of input by the parent, caretaker, or, in theory-of-mind studies, a peer whose theory of mind is already developed, are the keys to achieving learning objectives that are not enhanced by the technology alone.

As in studies of television viewing, researchers examining electronic toys for the very young highlight the steep learning curve that must be scaled before infants are able to fully appreciate digital toys. For the manufacturer-recommended age range of 6 months to 3 years, toys such as the Fisher-Price Laugh and Learn series or Bright Beats Dance and Move BeatBo (a colorful robot with music, lights, and dance moves, reported in 2016 to be Infant/Toddler Toy of the Year by the Toy Industry Foundation) are introduced long before a young child recognizes their representational nature. Moreover, even at the age at which a child begins to develop the symbolic capacity to grasp that a toy cellphone represents a real smartphone, the child is frequently more captivated by the songs, lights, and commentary emitted by the toy at the expense of elaborated play with the toy as a prop. In fact, although the toy captures the child's attention, it mostly elicits exploratory play and can provoke laughter and/or dancing (Bergen et al. 2010; Younger and Johnson 2004). As children develop the capacity for symbolic play, this type of toy is far less malleable than an inanimate or nonelectronic object that bends more neutrally to their playing agenda. Indeed, research confirms that electronic toys are sufficiently busy—with noise, lights, speech, and movement—to stimulate interest and exploration, but too specific to encourage creative elaboration (Bergen et al. 2010).

It may be, however, that exploration of electronically activated devices is in itself a crucial stepping stone to media literacy and promotes a new kind of creative thinking. It is important to keep in mind the wide twenty-first-century digital gap between scientists, educators, and parents on the one hand and very young children on the other. Young people, from preschoolers to law students, are so fully immersed in digital culture that most models of childhood applied to them are outdated and irrelevant; not only is educational methodology lagging but so are notions of creativity and imagination (Strasburger 2012).

Forward-looking thinkers have begun to critique the mainstream literature for its patent nostalgia for the childhood of yesteryear. Indeed, any study showing detrimental impact of electronic activities can be matched by one showing positive effects (Pujol et al. 2016). Contemporary children's interaction with electronic toys provides them with fun, challenges, and learning and play opportunities *about the world in which they live*. It has been persuasively argued that what children are gaining are the skills to master, manage, play with, and manipulate technology and that this opens a wide vista of potential playgrounds in virtual reality (Gelfond and Salonius-Pasternak 2005), where most play is likely to be found in the twenty-first century. Furthermore, this familiarity migrates to facility with screens in general—the premiere portal into the new reality.

SCREENS

Screens are a feature of many early childhood electronic toys, including toy cellphones, tablets, and laptops, each ostensibly offering a learning experience with built-in interactive rewards for the playing child. In our experience, as soon as children have the set of skills and capacities to really comprehend the representational nature of the toy screens they are given, they gravitate toward the "adult" versions of these devices; these are the alluring items that successfully compete for their parents' attention and are loaded with apps and animated movies for kids, beginning with those for ages 0–3 years (iPadFamily.com.au 2016a), which are usually simple narratives with some interactive add-ons.

Almost all the apps for young children promise an "educational" purpose combined with fun and entertainment: for example, the Toca Store app makes the following claims: "this educational app promotes creativity, imagination, choice, decision making, service, empathy, counting and negotiation all within the context of fun!…This is perfect for role-playing between friends, siblings, parent and child…. Teaching business skills, from an early age!" (iPadFamily.com.au 2016d). Another app, Cookie Doodle, allows children to assemble, mix, and bake ingredients for virtual cookies that they can decorate, serve, and even eat. The latter (virtual) experience is accompanied by eating sounds and a disappearing cookie (iPadFamily.com.au 2016c). This may be an eerily virtual experience of a highly embodied activity, but whether it is any better or worse than the pretend "cookie" offered to a parent who "munches" enthusiastically is unclear. Some observers decry the absence of "embodied cognition"—that is, thought in action or enactive thinking (Bergen et al. 2016, pp. 15–18), noting that such play lacks physicality, the palpable objects and the bodily action of a child playing in a play kitchen, but instead offers visual imagery and sound, previously left to the "imagination." The role of body in play is significantly reduced—a deficit that is clearly amplified by the screen apps for young children (Mangen 2010). Even with current and anticipated haptic technology, those who see the centrality of the hand (Wilson 1999) and of sensory experience that follows a predictable sequence in the real world are concerned by the condensing of all these varied physical events to "point and click." The increasingly "naturalized" relationship to mouse and keyboard and the refinement of haptic controls suggest that these will be the predominant sensorimotor experiences of young children. Despite inevitable losses in the direct, palpable, and predictable series of events—that is, action and reaction—it is increasingly clear that digital skills are the crucial vehicle for engaging with the contemporary world. Digital natives' dexterity in this domain, which often astonishes their parents, amply demonstrates this new skill.

Kid-oriented apps are proliferating rapidly. There are, for example, apps that play free animated films, apps that offer educational games, and apps that promote commercial products such as tie-ins to current popular movies. All of these entertain children and are frequently offered and accepted more readily than traditional toys. For older children, there are apps designed to facilitate their own movie making, animation, fashion design, and character creating; these apps bridge the transition from symbolic play to latency play and foster continued creative invention and narrative (iPadFamily.com.au 2016b).

Developmental educators and play advocates concerned with early childhood see contemporary threats to play from a number of quarters: premature academic pressure, parental anxiety and restrictions on unsupervised outdoor play, digital media, and unfettered access to a universe that is still opaque to adults. Traditional educators are hard put to consider ways that electronic toys and games can be used to advantage for the young child. Certainly, parental presence and high level of parental verbal activity may enhance the vocabulary gains afforded by electronic toys, but this is furthering the toys' "educational" purpose rather than their play potential (Gelfond and Salonius-Pasternak 2005). Even educational value can be challenging to extract from programs aimed at young children. Given that play is considered an essential developmental capacity and a "right," the electronic evolution of toys and games and the advent of digital devices have elicited some dismay among play advocates (Singer and Singer 2007). In contrast, a growing number of commentators believe that these electronic toys and digital media successfully use entertainment and play to provide practice in the fundamental language of the future, build media literacy, expand awareness of technological potential, and offer opportunities for adventure, social interaction, and mastery (Goetz 2017; Thomas and Brown 2007).

OLDER CHILDREN AND PLAY ON SCREENS

The culture of latency (ages 6 to 10–11) has undergone significant changes in the last half century. Digital technology is a central part of its transformation and is deeply woven into the lives of school-age children who have essentially been "digitalized" since birth. Access to smartphones, electronic toys, computers, and tablets (sometimes provided in school) has been a highly valued part of their academic and pleasure pursuits. Parents, many of whom are less technologically adept than their school-age children, are concerned over their children's facility with electronic devices and Internet access and fear that their children's online travels are potentially dangerous and difficult to monitor.[1] The peer culture endorses and rewards knowledge of various video games, YouTube videos, and other Internet opportunities. These activities can dominate school-yard conversations and are the focus of play dates, both in virtual space (online in massively multiplayer online role-playing games [**MMORPGs**]) and in real space, where people play together using multiple controls. Parents are especially concerned that the open portal to the Internet in multiplayer games is bidirectional, exposing children to possible predators and to commercial incursions. There is ample literature documenting the dangers of early social media usage, excessive gaming, and unchaperoned Internet searches.

---

[1]Some cultural observers believe that the tension between contemporary adolescents ("screenagers") and their parents is a direct result of the generational gap in the use of electronic media (Gergen 2015); fortunately, such reasoning holds the promise of gradual improvement as that gap narrows.

Video games in particular have been a focus of research, much of it flawed in design and strongly influenced by preconceived attitudes toward this rapidly mushrooming industry and leisure time activity (Latham et al. 2013; Shams et al. 2015), recently estimated to occupy about 10,000 hours by the time the player is age 21 (Kühn et al. 2014a, 2014b). Some research regarding the impact of games has been critical, highlighting their tendency to replace real relationships (Snodgrass et al. 2011), to model violence and promote insensitivity to it (Funk 2005), and to foster addictive usage (Dini 2009; Gelfond and Salonius-Pasternak 2005; Lopez-Fernandez 2015; Taylor 2008). However, in contrast to these findings, there is a growing body of literature that challenges the games' links to real violence and aggression (Ferguson and Olson 2013) and instead demonstrates improvement in a variety of cognitive functions and brain structure and activation patterns; even studies that confirm the potential for aggressive arousal find that prosocial games can similarly influence players toward positive social changes (Greitemeyer and Mügge 2014). This information appears to have affected some game makers. For example, Minecraft (Jeff's favorite in the vignette at the beginning of this chapter) offers a range of "modes" that permit regulation of aggressive content: hardcore survival, survival, creative, adventure, and spectator.

In terms of cognition, several recent reviews of research (Bavelier and Green 2016; Latham et al. 2013; Shams et al. 2015) have documented findings showing that video games enhance cognitive abilities, such as increased working memory, processing speed, attention/attentional biases, reduction of positive schizophrenic symptoms, and improved self-control and coping strategies (Shams et al. 2015, p. 71). These changes have been corroborated in imaging studies demonstrating increased gray matter volume and plasticity of white matter. Specific application of video games (i.e., serious games) in the treatment of designated child populations, such as those who are medically ill, who have learning disability or autism, or who are traumatized or maltreated, has been highly effective, and video games have been successfully used for purposes of medical education, pain management, and rehabilitation (Eichenbaum et al. 2014; Li et al. 2011; Parry et al. 2012; Taylor 2008). Scientists interested in this arena have begun to collaborate with the game industry to develop specific games for specific therapeutic purposes and clinical populations (Fernández-Aranda et al. 2012; Gelfond and Salonius-Pasternak 2005).

Some commentators suggest that video game playing can foster creativity and imagination (Thomas and Brown 2007). In an attempt to reframe the conversation about video games, researchers reconfigured their questions to consider children's positive motivations to play and children's role in demanding advances in technology. Those studies looking at the experience of the player challenge the stereotype of the socially isolated maladjusted child with a tendency toward aggressive fantasy (Ferguson and Olson 2013) and emphasize the importance of socialization with friends, catharsis, and fantasy in video game play. The association with game play and psychopathology has been consistently disproven (Ferguson and Olson 2013).

In the spirit of meeting the child where he or she is, many psychodynamic clinicians have recognized the value of treating the child through the vehicles that give him or her pleasure and self-expression. Children of every era play with toys that are cultural artifacts and represent the sensibility and values of contemporary society. Today children grow up in a mediated world with radically altered dimensions of space and time, expanded by an array of absorbing virtual worlds full of historical, fantastical, and futuristic elements; instant access to friends and strangers all over the globe; information without the barriers of "age-appropriateness" and time-consuming research; and other people's fantasy as in wildly popular fan-fiction and "alternative universes" (players' own spin-offs of existing games that are shared in blogging sites). In that spirit, a more sanguine perspective on video games has growing momentum and presence in the literature. Clinicians are more eager to tackle the world in which their patients live (Dini 2012) and, as a consequence, there is a greater appreciation of the specific therapeutic play affordances of video games despite their pitfalls. In the opening vignette, Jeff's relatively young therapist had himself played Minecraft through college and had even written a paper about its adolescent themes. Undoubtedly, this transition to a cadre of digital therapists is already beginning.

ELECTRONICS IN THE TREATMENT SETTING

In the past decade or so, the reports of video games used in clinical settings have predominantly focused on their targeted use in certain disorders or certain situations (e.g., preparation for surgery [Rassin et al. 2004]). The idea of actual collaboration between game designers and health care professionals to address specific therapeutic needs is frequently mentioned in contemporary literature. However, the use of video games or other games requiring screens is still rarely described in the dynamic play therapy setting, where play is deliberately unguided and interpreted as a reflection of the child's mental life (but see Bertolini and Nissim 2002; Bonovitz 2004; Ceranoglu 2010; Dauphin 2013; Dini 2012; Zelnick 2005).

In fact, some of the still sparse literature as well as anecdotal reports suggest that electronics and computers are often viewed as intrusions and are deliberately excluded from psychodynamic treatment settings due to a range of factors: they continue to be viewed by parents as deleterious and, as in the vignette about Jeff, may figure significantly in the parents' presenting complaints; they have been associated with violence, desensitization to violence, and the trend toward childhood obesity; they are fast paced and diminish face-to-face interaction; and they tend to discourage conversation, reduce abstract representations, and provide prefabricated imagery that substitutes for the elaboration of idiosyncratic fantasy (Bellinson 2000; Ceranoglu 2010; Weisel 2015; Zelnick 2005). The penultimate objection is countered to some extent by the obvious reminder that the classic (adult) psychoanalytic situation is characterized by lack of eye contact (Zelnick 2005) and that in traditional play therapy with children there is also relatively little eye contact, for example, during drawing and other crafts, board games, and narrative play with action figures or dolls where the "eye contact" is between the (toy) characters in the play. No doubt, some children continue to play with and enjoy classic toys (Whelan 2017; Zelnick 2005), but many contemporary children's real interests, conflicts, and impulses are no longer captured by Barbie dolls, Legos, board games, or action figures that were popular in the previous century. Electronic games and media are the children's toys of today (Davis 2011). Traditional figures and games are no more neutral or fundamental than a robotic toy or video game; every toy or game reflects its time and culture.

One serious objection to the presence of technology in play therapy concerns pathological usage in "addicted" individuals. Despite its lack of diagnostic legitimacy in DSM-5 (American Psychiatric Association 2013), *media addiction* is a term used and recognized in the literature, implying out-of-control gaming or social media use, to the neglect of real-life tasks and obligations, leading to withdrawal, loss of relationships, and decline in self-care, and often associated with significant mental illness (Baer et al. 2012). In an in-depth report of two cases, Weisel (2015) illustrates the powerfully impenetrable ego state of the addicted player. She justifies her eventual prohibition of the game's actual presence in her office because it was impossible for her to follow its action and, as elsewhere in their lives, the patients' overwhelming preoccupation obliterated the possibility of a meaningful dialogue. Nonetheless, the video games remained a central part of the conversation and eventually offered opportunities for meaning making. Prohibition of game play in some cases arises from therapeutic necessity and most certainly does not banish the involvement and thinking about games from the work.

Therapists' reluctance may also be based on relative unfamiliarity with contemporary games and technology in general, due in part to the unusually rapid cultural transformation and technological advances that have occurred since 1980. As Dauphin (2013) notes, the older generation of child clinicians have only recently faced the challenge of working with children raised from birth in a digital world, possessed of skills and facility to master a technological culture totally unfamiliar to their seniors. The reversal of the power differential may contribute to clinicians' resistance. This generational divide, however, is likely to naturally self-correct over a brief period of time, because at the time of our writing in 2016 the typical gamer is 35 years old and gamers are almost equally divided between men and women (Pew Research Center 2015; Statista.com 2016). Nonetheless, the problem of psychotherapist education persists; to the extent that play therapy is part of training, some older clinicians are unable to teach the therapeutic uses of electronic media and may discourage their younger colleagues from incorporating such media. Teachers of play therapy must know something about video games, Facebook, Instagram, and Snapchat to speak to the innovative ways in which electronics can be folded into interpretations of transference, ego defenses, and unconscious fantasy. As technology advances and children's leisure activities become swallowed up by digital media, the mental health professionals trained to help children risk obsolescence if they ignore cultural realities (Dauphin 2013; Dini 2012; Essig 2012). Clinicians who work with children are obligated to familiarize themselves with the world in which their patients live. Although statistics fluctuate, the consensus is that *normal* teenagers spend up to 9 hours per day using media, and children ages 8–12 years spend 6 hours per day in similar pursuits (Pew Research Center 2015). This means that media literacy is becoming a requirement for child work, and this is a challenging task for older therapists with less technology experience (Dini 2012). Short of immersing themselves in the millions of games currently available, clinicians may have to learn more about their patients' preferred games; there is no better way than asking for explanations and watching play. Even though statistical analyses suggest that the majority of parents play video games with their kids, the children brought to treatment for this problem are seen as "addicted" and unmanageable, like Jeff, or as, at the very least, overinvolved in games at the expense of friends, family, and school work, and, in our clinical experience, the adults around them have rarely been willing or able to truly enjoy their favorites. Many children want a parent to "watch me!" in this arena just as much as they do in the traditional performative sports, recitals, school play, or talent show.

Therapy with a computer or gaming console in the playroom is relatively uncharted territory, but there are a number of thoughtful contributions showing that video games in the treatment setting can be rich sources of information about a given patient's conscious and unconscious fantasy, much like other cultural products made for children in prior generations. Despite their relative paucity, clinical descriptions of the use of video games in play therapy (or for that matter, in adult treatment [see Dini 2012]) illustrate how therapists can harvest meaning of the same complexity from video games as from doll-house play, checkers, drawing, or any other play behavior (Bellinson 2005; Bertolini and Nissim 2002; Ceranoglu 2010; Dini 2012; Fernández-Aranda et al. 2012; Gelfond and Salonius-Pasternak 2005). Even in Weisel's case, where the therapist felt the need to banish the game from the office because it directly interfered with the therapeutic conversation, the meanings of gaming in terms of both content and impact on the patient's life continued to be a rich source of information (Weisel 2015). Other media have also found their way into offices. Smartphones, social media, music videos, chatrooms, blogs, and YouTube videos are often a focus of children's emotional life; a therapist who expresses interest and "wants to see" has an advantage over one who waits silently and implicitly disapproves.

Of course, interpretive work involving electronic usage must be introduced with the same tact as interpretations of any form of play.

Pathologizing electronic play can only create mistrust. Dr. Howard was cautious not to rush into interpretations that would immediately link Jeff's loneliness at home and school to his excessive involvement with the Minecraft community. This connection could only be broached when Jeff complained about his parents' travel or some kind of rejection at school and then interrupted further discussion by turning to Minecraft. In Jeff's case, Dr. Howard felt strongly that excluding video games from the office was not "neutral" and would put him squarely in the camp of the critical parents. To the digitally savvy, video games are in many respects no different from play of any type: prefabricated fantasy, readily available in books and movies, is typically borrowed by the playing child and has always been interpretable. These games allow children to manifest their interests and play pursuits as they actually are. In their early iterations, video games were felt to be inflexible, rigidly scripted, and cheat-proof (Bellinson 2000), but young therapists, more adept at assimilating the rapid pace of technological advance, see increasing opportunity for patients' expression of conflictual material and conscious and unconscious aspects of self-representation in their choices of their avatars' appearance, gear, weaponry, ethnicity, and so on. Children can now express their idiosyncratic and unique selves through the myriad decision points involved in game play: choice of system, game, modality (e.g., exploration vs. fighting the enemy), avatar's class (e.g., wizard or warrior), gender, features, attire, and "side" to be on; use of readily available cheats and shortcuts; and adhesiveness to this form of play. The preferred game, the avatar adopted, the social aspects of the game world, and the way the game is played, including or excluding the therapist, are all grist for the mill. As with any defense or presentation of fantasy material, snap interpretations are usually not helpful; the clinician needs to wait until the moment that such commentary seems natural and "part of the play."

THE 21st CENTURY CHILD PATIENT AND THE CHALLENGES FOR PLAY THERAPY

In the more than half century of their existence, video games have evolved into remarkably complex, visually striking, and sophisticated portals to alternate worlds. Their special appeal to children today has been attributed to their "graphics and realism," their multiple levels of increasing challenge, their interpersonal interactive potential with peers and other players (Gelfond and Salonius-Pasternak 2005), their rich utilization and seamless blend of real and virtual worlds, and their infinite variety and customizable features. Rather than feeling limited and coerced by a rigid predetermined scenario, children take pleasure in the release from the usual constraints, rules, even laws of physics; the loss of childhood freedoms due to legally enforced restrictions on outdoor activities[2] in the real world is compensated by the license to wander through increasingly elaborate and explorable virtual ones. Games liberate children from the demands and constraints of "real life"—limits on their geographic, physical, and nonconforming impulses—but they do come with their own sets of values, rules, interpersonal potential, economy, heroes, villains, and so on, which provide the therapist with opportunities to understand how the child navigates his or her chosen experience.

Childhood gaming, as well as other daily uses of computers and electronic toys, has skyrocketed and dominates leisure time. This applies to very young as well as grade school children. Many master touch-screen technology as junior toddlers, long before they can tie their shoes: "44% of 2- and 3-year-olds can play a basic online computer game, and one quarter can use a cell phone to make a call" (Geist 2014, p. 58). Given the ubiquity of digital technology and its reach into the lives of children from preschool onward, it is likely that children in therapy will have already had extensive experience with digital media and its unique affordances. Some games are simply "electronified"; for example, puzzle and word games on devices and the computer are similar to their former incarnation although sometimes with a new twist—like the possibility of playing all day long with someone in a foreign country (as with Words With Friends).

Technology and electronic games introduce new challenges to the play therapist's work in the following ways:

1. Any video game play involves access to a computer, handheld device, or game console. Use of an office computer can be potentially problematic because it contains confidential information and be-

---

[2]As in the 2015 case involving the Meitiv parents, who allowed their three children to roam their Maryland neighborhood (Wright et al. 2015).

cause downloading games requires a great deal of memory. The disadvantage of playing or observing play on a handheld device is self-evident: the tiny screen and single player format eliminates the therapist's role as co-player or opponent and impedes understanding of the game's content and meaning. If clinicians do provide a computer or game console, children may be artificially drawn toward game play because they want to please the therapist or feel gratified by an opportunity denied or restricted at home. As with any provision in therapy, whether it be the newest playset, action figure, or gaming console, clinicians have to be attentive to multiple levels of response, complicating interactions with their young patients while simultaneously offering a window to their passionate pursuits.

2. The vast diversity of electronic games and children's relative freedom to self-select particular challenges and environments, rules, and personas provide specificity in the expression of each child's inner life. A potential problem is that most play therapists are not conversant with the huge number of games available (Dini 2012). Nonetheless, if these games are not allowed into the consulting room, the therapist is excluded from a space in which the patient may spend hours every day. This is a serious loss of information for treatment, because each child tends to gravitate toward his or her own preferred virtual and mixed worlds, choosing among tens of millions of games. Verbal description of an environment in which visual experience is preeminent can be difficult for a child or adolescent and inadequate for a therapist's understanding. Hours spent in game play are hours lived in different spaces, increasingly augmented by haptic chairs, gloves, and other paraphernalia, where the child can address his or her conflicts, disappointments, and yearnings with greater agency than in real life. Therapists need to encourage patients to introduce and explain their favored games. Gaming is often a source of considerable strife at home, and children may be wary, defiant, and/or defensive about the possibility of further censure. It is not unusual for children to encapsulate themselves in playing video games, disavowing their need for unavailable parents by deep absorption in multiplayer or even single-player games. Games may have become a recurrent trigger for conflict with parents. Mobile systems can become constant companions, serving the child's defenses of avoidance and retreat. Indeed, this is a

typical way that games arrive in the consultation room; they serve to exclude the therapist as totally superfluous to an autonomous and compelling activity. Thus, the child and therapist's first interaction concerning games can reproduce the interpersonal conflicts occurring at home, ideally providing a window into the child's history, interpersonal relatedness, and willingness to trust; these features may ultimately be far more important than the game's content (Bellinson 2005).

3. Mixed-reality play, such as in Pokémon GO, unites a smartphone app with real geography and allows communities to engage in team play. This type of game provides a social context that has potential to extend the peer group in real life, distinguishing it from the multiplayer games that allow for virtual teams and communities. Like other outdoor play in groups, a game of this type poses challenges because play in therapy is often limited to indoor play and not (typically) usefully invaded by playmates. Children often resist playing multiplayer games in the therapist's company because they want to avoid an adult invasion of established (online) peer relationships that are distinguished by their lack of supervision and freedom. Giving the therapist an opportunity to just peruse the virtual world of a favorite game may be a first step toward allowing access and meaningful communication.

4. The incarnation of "second-order selves" through avatars in games is a unique and informative feature of electronic games (Gergen 2015, p. 62). Games and Web sites vary in terms of the flexibility offered for self-representation; choices are of course meaningfully related to children's central conflicts arising from unconscious, conscious, social, and familial sources. A child's adoption of an avatar can correct or reveal aspects of the self that may be much less accessible or impossible to portray in other play forms. Self-representation offers a rich vein of conscious and unconscious meaning and also provides an invaluable measure of growth in treatment. As with any other self-representation in any other play form (e.g., the identification with a particular character in doll or action figure play), the therapist's interpretation of its usual multiplicity of meanings requires opportunity, deep familiarity with the patient's dynamics or circumstances, and a tactful way to say it "in the game," as in "your guy is a real loner who seems kind of worried about being controlled

by the other guild members" or "she is an amazingly powerful sorceress but she seems really afraid of everyone."

5. Competition in electronic gaming has elements that differ from those in nonelectronic games. The relationship to winning and losing may seem somewhat attenuated in video games, because there is perpetual potential to renew oneself and take on the challenge once again. Also, levels reached or challenges conquered confer superiority and renown to a given player. Many game sites rank players both by level and the time it took them to succeed; these leader boards provide constant competitive challenges, feelings of accomplishment and inferiority, and idols to emulate or surpass. Even for beginners, there are opportunities to strive competitively where losing can be quickly reversed and where winning can accrue a following of admiring peers, all with little real consequence. Especially with the evolution of gaming as a spectator sport, excellent gamers gain widespread acclaim. Children's idols and tolerance of competition are meaningful for treatment. Their preoccupation with status is readily revealed in the management or disregard for the statistics and numerical accounts of expertise.

6. Despite what may appear to be pre-scripted and unvarying progression, games are increasingly customizable and variable by virtue of the player's choices. Moreover, there are ways to "game" the game, typically by using readily available cheats (Dini 2012). The child's relationship to rules and constraints is often more readily revealed in video games for which a vast array of tricks and codes can be retrieved from other players, YouTube, and various Internet sites, all without consequence.

7. In MMORPGs, access to fellow gamers who can play with or against the player is an expanding component of gaming. This socialization is usually geographically unbounded and develops naturally in the context of the game structure; battles, building projects, and criminal activities can lead to teams, gangs, and rivalries. The Internet experience of globalization permeates these types of video games and allows children to connect to others in many other countries. It also generates a vast library of videos demonstrating skills, offering instruction, and enabling customization of some video games, created by gamers of all ages. Games with millions of dedicated players promote their products with online tournaments, prize

money, and global renown. Children can be awed observers or avid participants depending on what games they have access to and how far they can penetrate the Internet.

Contemporary case reports consistently show the therapeutic use of video games as introduced by the child; therapist-introduced gaming has not been widely utilized in open-ended psychotherapy situations (but see Gardner 1993). The availability of a gaming console in the therapy room is rarely referred to (but see Dini 2012), although a computer is a standard part of the therapist's office equipment. The advantage of adequate equipment with larger screens as opposed to handheld devices is that they eliminate the functional exclusion of the clinician; however, exclusion has multiple forms, and even a handheld device can serve to advance the therapeutic work (Bellinson 2005). Case reports showing the use of video games in dynamic psychotherapy demonstrate their value in elucidating the relationship with the therapist, the child's avoidance of challenges (Dini 2012), the child's impulse to betray the other player (Zelnick 2005), and an infinite number of other personality traits.

OTHER SCREENS/MEDIA IN THE OFFICE

An occasional paper (e.g., Sugarman 2017; Zelnick 2005) addresses the presence of social media in treatment settings. Children often have their own smartphones by late latency, and their opportunities to communicate with peers, whether familiar or unfamiliar/masked/anonymous, have expanded with Web sites such as Tumblr and Instagram and on communication channels such as Snapchat, instant messaging, WhatsApp, and Skype. If a child brings these resources into the consulting room, via smartphones or access to the clinician's computer, the therapist obtains a vivid display of the child's style of socialization, sophistication, and online behavior. Although screens and media are not precisely "play," their presence in the therapist's office has been likened to the presence of "transitional objects" (Sugarman 2017) and can be understood as a special form of communication from children to their therapists, even though the objects might seem to exclude the therapists or make them passive onlookers.

SUMMARY

The debate about the impact of screen technology on child development is ongoing, but play therapists are increasingly required to keep pace with their patients in regard to media literacy and familiarity with the icons of child culture. Clinicians' familiarity and skill at navigating the world of video games, social media, and the Internet in general are vital links to the mental lives of children in the twenty-first century, in addition to older millennials whose social world occurs as much online as in real life.

KEY POINTS

- Social media and video games are a fundamental part of experience in the twenty-first century. For millennial children, the virtual–real world continuum is the world they know. Their sensibilities, leisure activities, social lives, and professional aspirations are created from complex and seamlessly connected real-life and virtual environments. Most children today are more media literate than their parents; if the pace of technology continues unabated, it will always be up to young patients to educate therapists about the raw material with which they construct their fantasy life.

- Therapists need to remain open to learning how children represent their experience, in normative as well as psychopathological ways. Overinterpretation of children's involvement with technology is not helpful and may actually create distance between patients and therapists.

- Play occurs in whatever playground contemporary culture provides. If child patients resist playing with the toys of yesteryear and prefer contemporary ones, they are in sync with their time. Because children inevitably express their inner life through the iconic elements—heroes, narratives, media, and modalities—that their culture provides, it is the obligation of child clinicians to keep pace with their patients in order to understand them.

- Despite ongoing cultural transformation, current-day children develop by progressing through a recognizable sequence of emerging ego capacities and environmental expectations. No doubt this may change over time, as society and child development are increasingly saturated in technology. Clinicians must change too and must learn the contemporary language of childhood.

KEY TERMS

False-belief test   Test used to assess the child's achievement of theory of mind by examining whether the child can understand that another individual will not "know" something has been displaced unless he or she witnesses the move. Children under age 4 do not typically possess the capacity to recognize that others can maintain false beliefs (i.e., can have a different subjectivity).

MMORPG   Massively multiplayer online role-playing game. These games involve social interaction in collaborative virtual environments that are "persistent worlds" (i.e., they are not dependent on the presence of users). They are played by literally millions of players daily. World of Warcraft hit its peak in 2010 with 12 million subscribers; today it is at 5.5 subscribers and is still considered among the top 10 MMORPGs (Conditt 2016).

Serious games   Games that are created with a specific educational or remedial purpose, not for the sake of entertainment alone. They can look and play like any other game but are designed to promote skill learning.

Technoculture   The cultural condition produced by the interaction between, and politics of, technology and society. It is a term invented and used in academic writings.

Video deficit   The demonstrated learning difference for infants under age 30 months when taught by video or closely matched live presentation. The infants are less able to reproduce the action after a delay if instructed by video rather than live instruction unless the video presentation is repeated at least six times (Anderson and Kirkorian 2015).

REFERENCES

American Academy of Pediatrics Committee on Public Education: Media education. Pediatrics 104(2 Pt 1):341–343, 1999 10429023

American Psychiatric Association: Diagnostic and Statistical Manual of Mental Disorders, 5th Edition. Arlington, VA, American Psychiatric Association, 2013

Anderson DR, Hanson KG: From blooming, buzzing confusion to media literacy: the early development of television viewing. Dev Rev 30(2):239–255, 2010

Anderson DR, Kirkorian HL: Media and cognitive development, in Handbook of Child Psychology and Developmental Science, Vol 2, Cognitive Processes. Edited by Liben LS, Muller U. Hoboken, NJ, Wiley, 2015, pp. 949–994

Baer S, Saran K, Green DA, et al: Electronic media use and addiction among youth in psychiatric clinic versus school populations. Can J Psychiatry 57(12):728–735, 2012 23228231

Bavelier D, Green CS: The brain-boosting power of video games. Sci Am 315(1):26–31, 2016 27348376

Bellinson J: Shut up and move: the use of board games in child psychotherapy. J Infant Child Adolesc Psychother 1(2):23–41, 2000

Bellinson J: I beat the level: children's use of Gameboy as therapeutic communication. J Infant Child Adolesc Psychother 4(2):198–208, 2005

Bergen D, Hutchinson K, Nolan JT, et al: Effects of infant-parent play with a technology-enhanced toy: affordance-related actions and communicative interactions. J Res Child Educ 24(1):1–17, 2010

Bergen D, Davis DR, Abbitt JT: Technology Play and Brain Development. New York, Routledge, 2016

Bertolini R, Nissim S: Video games and children's imaginations. J Child Psychother 28(3):305–325, 2002

Bonovitz C: Unconscious communication and the transmission of trauma. J Infant Child Adolesc Psychother 3(1):1–27, 2004

Ceranoglu TA: Video games in psychotherapy. Rev Gen Psychol 14:141–146, 2010

Christakis DA, Zimmerman FJ, DiGiuseppe DL, et al: Early television exposure and subsequent attentional problems in children. Pediatrics 113(4):708–713, 2004 15060216

Conditt J: "World of Warcraft" keeps growing with "Legion" in August. Engadget, April 19, 2016. Available at: https://www.engadget.com/2016/04/19/world-of-warcraft-legion-release-date/. Accessed October 1, 2016.

Courage M, Howe M: To watch or not to watch: infants and toddlers in a brave new electronic world. Dev Rev 30(2):101–115, 2010

Courage M, Setliff A: When babies watch television: attention-getting, attention holding, and the implications for learning from video material. Dev Rev 30(2):220–238, 2010

Dauphin B: Therapists' resistance to understanding the importance of technology for child and adolescent psychotherapy. J Infant Child Adolesc Psychother 12(1):45–50, 2013

Davis A: What about digital toys? Looking into the idea of using digital media in play. Play Therapy, December 2011. Available at: http://www.mlppubsonline.com/article/What_About_The_Digital_Toys%3F_Looking_Into_ The_Idea_Of_Using_Digital_Media_In_Play_Therapy_Sessions!/887087/88264/article.html. Accessed July 17, 2016.

Dini K: Internet interaction: the effects on patients' lives and analytic process. Panel report. J Am Psychoanal Assoc 57(4):979–988, 2009 19724073

Dini K: On video games, culture, and therapy. Psychoanal Inq 32(5):496–505, 2012

Egan M: Best kids apps 2016/2017: best free and cheap apps for kids, toddlers, and teens. PC Advisor, 2016. Available at: http://www.pcadvisor.co.uk/test-centre/software/best-kids-apps-2016-best-apps-for-children-3647437. Accessed October 1, 2016.

Eichenbaum A, Bavelier D, Green CS: Video games: play that can do serious good. Am J Play 7(1):50–72, 2014

Essig T: Psychoanalysis lost—and found—in our culture of simulation and enhancement. Psychoanal Inq 32(5):438–453, 2012

Ferguson C, Olson C: Friends, fun, frustration and fantasy: child motivations for video game play. Motiv Emot 37(1):154–164, 2013

Fernández-Aranda F, Jiménez-Murcia S, Santamaría JJ, et al: Video games as a complementary therapy tool in mental disorders: PlayMancer, a European multicentre study. J Ment Health 21(4):364–374, 2012 22548300

Flanagan V: Technology and identity in young adult fiction: the posthuman subject. London, UK, Palgrave Macmillan, 2014

Funk JB: Children's exposure to violent video games and desensitization to violence. Child Adolesc Psychiatr Clin N Am 14(3):387–404, vii–viii, 2005 15936665

Gardner J: Nintendo games, in Play Therapy Techniques, 2nd Edition. Edited by Schaefer CE, Candelosi DM. Northvale, NJ, Jason Aronson, 1993, pp 357–364

Geist E: Using tablet computers with toddlers and young preschoolers. Young Child 69(1):58–63, 2014

Gelfond HS, Salonius-Pasternak DE: The play's the thing: a clinical-developmental perspective on video games. Child Adolesc Psychiatr Clin N Am 14(3):491–508, ix, 2005 15936670

Gergen K: Playland: technology, self, and cultural transformation, in Playful Identities: The Ludification of Digital Media Cultures. Edited by Frissen V, Lammes S, de Lange M, et al. Amsterdam, Amsterdam University Press, 2015, pp 55–74

Goetz C: Securing home base: separation-individuation, attachment theory, and the "virtual worlds" paradigm in videogames. Psychoanal Study Child 70:101–116, 2017

Greitemeyer T, Mügge DO: Video games do affect social outcomes: a meta-analytic review of the effects of violent and prosocial video game play. Pers Soc Psychol Bull 40(5):578–589, 2014 24458215

Hummer TA: Media violence effects on brain development: what neuroimaging has revealed and what lies ahead. Am Behav Sci 59(14):1790–1806, 2015

iPadFamily.com.au: Best iPad Apps for Children Age 0–3, 2016a. Available at: http://www.ipadfamily.com.au/apps-for-kids-age-0-3. Accessed June 23, 2016.

iPadFamily.com.au: Best iPad Apps for Children Age 6 to 9 Reviewed, 2016b. Available at: http://www.ipadfamily.com.au/apps-for-kids-age-6-9. Accessed June 23, 2016.

iPadFamily.com.au: Review: Cookie Doodle HD, 2016c. Available at: http://www.ipadfamily.com.au/ipad-app-reviews/cookie-doodle-for-ipad. Accessed June 23, 2016.

iPadFamily.com.au: Review: Toca Store, 2016d. Available at: http://www.ipadfamily.com.au/ipad-app-reviews/toca-store. Accessed June 23, 2016.

Kühn S, Gleich T, Lorenz RC, et al: Playing Super Mario induces structural brain plasticity: gray matter changes resulting from training with a commercial video game. Mol Psychiatry 19(2):265–271, 2014a 24166407

Kühn S, Lorenz R, Banaschewski T, et al: Positive association of video game playing with left frontal cortical thickness in adolescents. PLoS One 9(3):e91506, 2014b 24633348

Landhuis CE, Poulton R, Welch D, et al: Does childhood television viewing lead to attention problems in adolescence? Results from a prospective longitudinal study. Pediatrics 120(3):532–537, 2007 17766526

Latham AJ, Patston LL, Tippett LJ: Just how expert are "expert" video-game players? Assessing the experience and expertise of video-game players across "action" video-game genres. Front Psychol 4:941, 2013 24379796

Levin DE, Rosenquest B: The increasing role of electronic toys in the lives of infants and toddlers: should we be concerned? Contemp Issues Early Child 2(2):242–247, 2001

Li RW, Ngo C, Nguyen J, et al: Video-game play induces plasticity in the visual system of adults with amblyopia. PLoS Biol 9(8):e1001135, 2011 21912514

Linebarger DL, Walker D: Infants' and toddlers' television viewing and language outcomes. Am Behav Sci 48(5):624–645, 2005

Lopez-Fernandez O: How has Internet addiction research evolved since the advent of Internet gaming disorder? An overview of cyberaddictions from a psychological perspective. Curr Addict Rep 2(3):263–271, 2015

Mangen A: Point and click: theoretical and phenomenological reflections on the digitization of early childhood education. Contemp Issues Early Child 11(4):415–431, 2010

Marsh J: Popular Culture, New Media and Digital Literacy in Early Childhood. New York, Routledge Palmer, 2005

Masur EF, Flynn V, Olson J: The presence of background television during young children's play in American homes. J Child Media 9:349–367, 2015

Natsiopoulou T, Bletsou M: Greek preschoolers' use of electronic media and their preferences for media or books. International Journal of Caring Sciences 4(2):97–104, 2011

Nielsen: More than half the homes in U.S. have three or more TVs. Media and Entertainment page, July 20, 2009. Available at: http://www.nielsen.com/us/en/insights/news/2015/nielsen-estimates-116-4-million-tv-homes-in-the-us-for-the-2015-16-tv-season.html. Accessed May 10, 2016.

Palfrey J, Gasser U: Born Digital: Understanding the First Generation of Digital Natives. New York, Basic Books, 2008

Park C, Park YR: The conceptual model on smartphone addiction among early childhood. International Journal of Social Science and Humanity 4(2):147–150, 2014

Parry IS, Bagley A, Kawada J, et al: Commercially available interactive video games in burn rehabilitation: therapeutic potential. Burns 38(4):493–500, 2012 22385641

Pew Research Center: 5. Children's extracurricular activities, in Parenting in America. December 17, 2015. Available at: http://www.pewsocial-trends.org/2015/12/17/5-childrens-extracurricular-activities/. Accessed July 18, 2016.

Pujol J, Fenoll R, Forns J, et al: Video gaming in school children: How much is enough? Ann Neurol 80(3):424–433, 2016 27463843

Radesky JS, Silverstein M, Zuckerman B, et al: Infant self-regulation and early childhood media exposure. Pediatrics 133(5):e1172–e1178, 2014 24733868

Rassin, M, Gutman, Y, Silner D: Developing a computer game to prepare children for surgery. AORN J 80(6):1095–1096, 1099–1102, 2004 15641663

Romero M, Usart M, Ott M: Can serious games contribute to developing and sustaining 21st century skills? Games and Culture 10(2):148–177, 2015

Shams TA, Foussias G, Zawadzki JA, et al: The effects of video games on cognition and brain structure: potential implications for neuropsychiatric disorders. Curr Psychiatry Rep 17(9):71, 2015 26216589

Singer DG, Singer JL: Imagination and Play in the Electronic Age. Cambridge, MA, Harvard University Press, 2007

Singer JL, Singer DG: Preschoolers' imaginative play as precursor of narrative consciousness. Imagin Cogn Pers 25(2):97–117, 2005

Siraj-Blatchford J, Siraj-Blatchford I: Developmentally appropriate technology in early childhood: "video conferencing." Contemporary Issues in Early Childhood 3:216–225, 2002

Smith A: Chapter one: a portrait of smartphone ownership. Pew Research Center, April 1, 2015. Available at: http://www.pewinternet.org/2015/04/01/chapter-one-a-portrait-of-smartphone-ownership. Accessed September 15, 2016.

Snodgrass JG, Lacy MG, Denagh HF, et al: Enhancing one life rather than living two: playing MMOs with offline friends. Comput Human Behav 27(3):1211–1222, 2011

Sosa AV: Association of the type of toy used during play with the quantity and quality of parent-infant communication. JAMA Pediatr 170(2):132–137, 2016 26720437

Staiano AE, Harrington DM, Broyles ST, et al: Television, adiposity, and cardiometabolic risk in children and adolescents. Am J Prev Med 44(1):40–47, 2013 23253648

Statista.com: Age breakdown of video game players in the United States in 2016, Statista.com, 2016. Available at: https://www.statista.com/statistics/189582/age-of-us-video-game-players-since-2010/. Accessed July 18, 2016.

Strasburger VC: School daze: why are teachers and schools missing the boat on media? Pediatr Clin North Am 59(3):705–715, ix, 2012 22643175

Strasburger V: The death of childhood. Psychoanal Study Child 70:91–100, 2017

Sugarman A: The transitional phenomena functions of smartphones for adolescents. Psychoanal Study Child 70:135–150, 2017

Taylor L: Positive features of video games, in Handbook of Children, Culture, and Violence. Edited by Dowd NE, Singer DG, Wilson RF. Thousand Oaks, CA, Sage, 2008, pp 247–266

Thomas D, Brown JS: The play of imagination: extending the literary mind. Games and Culture 2(2):140–172, 2007

Vandewater EA, Bickham DS, Lee JH: When the television is always on: heavy television exposure and young children's development. Am Behav Sci 48(5):562–577, 2005

Wartella E, Richert R, Robb M: Babies, television and videos: how did we get here? Dev Rev 30(2):116–127, 2010

Weisel A: Virtual reality and the psyche. Some psychoanalytic approaches to media addiction. J Anal Psychol 60:198–219, 2015 25808470

Whelan R: Technological advances in play therapy: tradition versus innovation. Dissertation, The Chicago School of Professional Psychology, ProQuest Dissertations & Theses, 2017 10106004

Wilson FR: The Hand: How Its Use Shapes the Brain, Language, and Human Culture. New York, Vintage Books, 1999

Wright D, Smith C, Effron L: Free-range parenting debate: should kids be allowed to roam unsupervised? ABC News Online, January 30, 2015. Available at: http://abcnews.go.com/Lifestyle/free-range-parenting-debate-kids-allowed-roam-unsupervised/story?id=28594061. Accessed July 20, 2016.

Younger BA, Johnson KE: Infants' comprehension of toy replicas as symbols for real objects. Cognit Psychol 48(2):207–242, 2004 14732411

Zevenbergen R: Digital natives come to preschool: implications for early childhood practice. Contemporary Issues in Early Childhood 8(1):19–29, 2007

Zelnick L: The computer as an object of play in child treatment. J Infant Child Adolesc Psychother 4(2):209–217, 2005

Zimmerman FJ, Christakis DA: Children's television viewing and cognitive outcomes: a longitudinal analysis of national data. Arch Pediatr Adolesc Med 159(7):619–625, 2005 15996993

Zosh JM, Verdine BN, Filipowicz A, et al: Talking shape: parental language with electronic versus traditional shape sorters. Mind, Brain, and Education 9(3):136–144, 2015

5

Basic Psychodynamic Concepts and Their Use in Play Therapy

Seven-year-old Alex was brought to Dr. Chen, a child psychiatrist, because of increasingly disruptive behavior: his parents reported his taunting of his younger sister, and first-grade teachers complained about his aggression toward peers. Alex's early academic skills appeared very solid, but in-class assignments and homework often led him to tears and protests. Both parents and teachers had begun to realize that their mildly punitive responses (loss of recess time, removal of his technology) did little to improve the child's cooperation or motivation.

Alex appeared polite and subdued upon meeting Dr. Chen. He spent numerous sessions diligently constructing Lego vehicles and buildings, often seeking her suggestions for planning out a toy village. He explained that the vehicles formed a "Jedi-led special ops defense force" equipped with secret intricate parts for launching projectiles, dropping bombs, and repelling enemy fire. The village comprised fortlike structures for the townspeople, who were under attack from Darth Vader's minions; all that stood between the inhabitants and total annihilation, Alex declared soberly, was the strength and courage of the Jedi warriors. During these initial hours, Dr. Chen functioned mostly as a curious observer who asked questions about the various characters and their conflicts. Alex responded pleasantly but disinterestedly, reserving a more impatient attitude for her queries about the history of the current war: "It's just always been this way; it doesn't matter how it started."

Following a particularly problematic school day, during which Alex's mother called and reported to Dr. Chen that he was denied recess for pushing a classmate, a more aggressive demeanor emerged in Alex. He focused on one Jedi leader whose mission included "infiltrating enemy lines"; confusingly, this took the form of blasting and breaking the townspeople's homes after spying on them through their windows. Dr. Chen commented on the Jedi's power and gleeful attitude, and vocalized the confusion of the townspeople, who had previously relied on their Jedi protectors. Alex remarked, "My guy gets out of control sometimes. He's probably just mad at his friends. Only the top Jedi trainer can stop him going rogue." She observed that there was no sign of this ultimate authority figure, and Alex grimly agreed, adding that no one had seen him for a long time.

Next, Alex enlisted the therapist as a warrior-in-training, directing her in an increasingly imperious manner to construct an armed Lego vehicle. He soon grew dissatisfied with Dr. Chen's efforts, complaining that she had created inferior fighting equipment. With mounting dissatisfaction, he briefly departed from the play to insist that she procure better building pieces for her playroom before their next visit. Dr. Chen spontaneously exclaimed, "I really feel like one of your minions right now!" Alex paused and responded, "It's usually grown-ups ordering *me* around." As the game continued, his character grew wilder, bashing the villagers as well as their homes, scattering small figures and building pieces all over the office. He insisted that the therapist, through her play character, mimic his activities. After a momentary hesitation, Dr. Chen complied; Alex immediately expressed disgruntlement, whining, "I knew it, you only wanna do girlie games." She replied, "I did hold back for a second, there. It made you think I don't like playing with boys as much as girls." As the session came to an end, Alex grew even surlier, refusing to clean up. Dr. Chen retrieved his storage bin, stating, "This was a pretty exciting game, but we have to stop. Should we put the rest of the buildings in here for next time?" "Yes, but you do it yourself!" and he ran out of the room.

OVERVIEW OF PSYCHODYNAMIC CONCEPTS

The spontaneous nature of the play, Dr. Chen's attention to Alex's affective experience and to the meanings of his narratives and behaviors, and her attempts to verbalize aspects of their interaction mark this vignette as an example of psychodynamic play therapy. Early in the treatment, child and therapist begin to develop their relationship by entering a mutual playing state; their joint participation in imaginary play creates a safe, intermediary space within which the treatment can begin to unfold. Following a brief period of guardedness and reserve, important aspects of Alex's inner life—conscious attitudes and beliefs, as well as unconscious fears, fantasies, conflicts, and defenses—are gradually revealed through his reactions to Dr. Chen as well as in the contents of his play. He eventually demonstrates that he worries about power and control, fears helplessness and bodily injury, struggles to manage aggressive feelings, wishes to surround himself in protective armor, and equates tough attitudes with boyishness. Working mostly but not exclusively within the play itself, Dr. Chen finds ways to talk to Alex about his use of grandiosity as a defense against feeling scared, vulnerable, and out of control. Her knowledge of his developmental capacities and sensitivities allows her to address potentially uncomfortable issues without causing him to feel exposed and criticized. For example, she verbalizes his fear that girls are preferred to boys, but she does not link this to known sibling rivalry in his real life. Moreover, despite imagery that derives from body-based phallic and anal issues (erected fortresses, launched missiles, exploded bombs) and references to oedipal-phase curiosities ("spying" and "infiltrating"), Dr. Chen makes no attempt to comment on earlier phases of Alex's development.

As is typical of young children, Alex demonstrates a distinct disinterest in the past and a limited capacity to engage in insight-oriented exchanges that link current behaviors with personal history ("It's just always been this way; it doesn't matter how it started"); nonetheless, his proffered explanation for the Jedi's actions—"He's probably just mad at his friends"—hints at current feelings about self and peers. The creation of coherent autobiographical narratives, often referred to as "reconstruction" in psychoanalysis, is not necessarily a central feature of play therapy. Indeed, the forward push of development powerfully shapes the nature of child treatments, necessitating the therapist's sensitive and judicious use of such clinical procedures as looking backward and linking here-and-now experience with the past. In Chapter 6 ("Therapeutic Action and the Multiple Functions of Play Therapy"), we provide a more detailed discussion of the way in which play therapists approach sensitive contents, respecting the child's need for self-protection and balancing interventions that are aimed at resolving earlier conflicts with those that seek to facilitate developmental progress.

Alex observes Dr. Chen's behavior closely; he comments on the unique aspects of their interactions ("It's usually grown-ups ordering me around") and immediately senses her brief hesitation to enact aggressive pretense. Moreover, Alex's interpretation of her reluctance, his conviction that she prefers "girlie" games, and his accompanying anger reveal crucial information about **transference**; his interpersonal wishes, impulses, perceptions, and fantasies originate within familial relationships but powerfully shape his experience of the therapist (Abrams et al. 1999). Dr. Chen allows Alex to perceive her behavior in his own way; she does not seek to rebuff or correct his sense of their interactions. When her own spontaneous behavior elicits a strong response from Alex, she acknowledges his reality-based observation ("I did hold back for a second, there") and suggests a meaningful way for them to think about his response ("It made you think I don't like playing with boys as much as girls"). At different points in this vignette, the therapist embodies multiple and shifting roles: she is inquisitive onlooker, reflective commentator, and active playing partner, as well as an adult who helps contain and manage the child's impulses and wishes, safeguarding the boundaries of the therapy.

It is not only Alex's inner life that is revealed as he and his therapist interact and mutually enliven the play. The clinician's **countertransference** reactions are an inherent, inevitable, and valuable component of play therapy; evoked emotional responses in the therapist reflect her unique personality but also represent a trove of information about the child's past and present attachments, modes of relating, and self-protective mechanisms. In play treatments, young children's inner conflicts and worries are often transformed into actions that may quickly escalate, potentially eliciting uncomfortable responses in clinicians. In this case, Alex's demand that Dr. Chen bash and plunder pretend town dwellers, creating a mess of her playroom in the process, unmasks her private inhibitions and reveals unintended discomfort with his imaginary scenarios; while momentarily uncomfortable to the therapist, this interaction ultimately deepens the therapy and leads to fresh insight about the child's sense of self.

THE CHILD–THERAPIST RELATIONSHIP IN PLAY THERAPY

The patient–clinician relationship represents a key mutative agent for intrapsychic change, including new modes of relating, transformed perceptions of self and others, and strengthened ego capacities. In child treatments, this relationship is particularly complex because the therapist must manage multiple assignments as a recipient of transference, a coparticipant in a **real relationship**, and an adult who is recruited as a **new object**; these represent roles that may be seen as serving the child's past, present, and future, respectively (Abrams and Solnit 1998; Freud 1965). In addition, the clinician functions as a **developmental object**, scaffolding the child's vulnerable capacities for emotional self-regulation (Sugarman 2003a, 2009b). Although we discuss these designations individually for purposes of clarity, they are always intertwined and often appear inseparable in the child's actions, play, and accompanying verbalizations. Indeed, for both children and adults, there is continual interplay between the patient's reality-based and more personalized perceptions of the therapist (Greenson 1967; Loewald 1960); even such basic, "real" behaviors as the clinician's greetings and endings, interested attitude, and nonjudgmental responsiveness are interpreted in subjective ways. Inevitably, therapists' appearances, nonverbal behaviors, and office setups communicate personal attitudes and preferences (Galatzer-Levy 2008).

Certain realities of child therapy are undeniable. Children's perceptions of the clinician's greater physical size and skill, or of the disparity between adult authority and relative child powerlessness, reflect reality-based conditions; they cannot be viewed purely as artifacts of fantasy and distortion, although such elements further influence children's perceptions in unique and subjective ways. In adult treatments, the concrete reality-based distinctions between therapist and patient are less stark; however, meaningful hierarchical differences in power nonetheless exist. For example, an adult patient might experience a feeling of helplessness or inadequacy in relation to the clinician, based partly on transference distortions (e.g., a long-standing tendency to view others as controlling, demanding authorities) but also on the therapist's real status as relatively more informed about psychological matters, as the caretaker of the patient, and as the one who determines key aspects of the work, such as payment.

THE ROLE OF TRANSFERENCE IN CHILD PSYCHOTHERAPY

Contemporary definitions of *transference* in the therapeutic relationship refer to the total process of the patient's unfolding conscious and unconscious reactions to the therapist and the treatment. A central feature of transference involves use of the therapist for revival of conflicts and relational paradigms that predate the treatment, having originated with the parents; indeed, most psychodynamic clinicians, even if they do not privilege early experience in their clinical work, make the assumption that the here-and-now relationship between therapist and patient contains important clues to past traumas, conflicts, and modes of relating (Govrin 2006). Although the clinician working with adults is largely concerned with the patient's internalized representation of early bonds, child therapists are additionally working with their patients' intense ongoing need for and attachment to the real parents. Historically, these complications led to major controversies in the way child analysts viewed the nature of transference: Melanie Klein (1927) believed that very young children could develop transference analogous to that of adults, but Anna Freud (1965) took the position that the child's naïve cognition, limited ego strength, and ongoing dependency on the parents had an impact on the depth and scope of the transference relationship, rendering it distinct from that which emerges during adult therapy.

Drawing from the work of numerous psychoanalytic theorists who have shaped contemporary attitudes, we take the position that transference is a central aspect of child treatment while simultaneously acknowledging the ongoing primacy of the parent–child relationship, the impact of the child's maturation on perceptions of the therapist, and the variety of the therapist's functions; these clinician functions, which include less fantasy-based, more direct developmental assistance to the child and a working relationship with the parents, are also pivotal in shaping the therapeutic bond and the clinical outcome (Chused 1988; Fraiberg 1951; Neubauer 2001; Sandler et al. 1980; Sugarman 2003a; Yanof 1996a, 1996b). Children feel deeply about their therapists, but the quality of the relationship reflects their mental development: self–other differentiation, theory of mind, and affect tolerance are among the maturational achievements that powerfully affect the nature of the therapeutic bond and the extent to which it can be explored meaningfully in play treatments (Fraiberg 1951). Young children do not necessarily grasp the "as-if" quality of the transference relationship, instead often experiencing it in an immediate and literal fashion. Children, like adults, vary widely in their motivation and tolerance for self-examination, but no child can recognize the influence of the past on the present or realize that the therapist is the recipient of wishes that derive from the parent–child relationship, before the necessary underlying capacities for such emotional knowing are available.

NEW AND DEVELOPMENTAL OBJECTS IN CHILD TREATMENT

The child–therapist relationship is fueled not only by the dyad's separate and unique histories, personalities, and mutual here-and-now play interactions, but also by the very process of development itself; the child's entry into periods of mental reorganization requires that the therapist inhabit changing roles, offer opportunities for varying identifications, and serve novel meanings (Sugarman 2003a, 2009a; Yanof 1996a, 1996b). Such new object functions help move development forward. During certain phases, for example, children may relate to the therapist as an oedipal rival, a figure to whom the child can attach in order to lessen dependency on parents, or a mentor and teacher (Abrams 2003). Although the phenomenon of the new object relationship is a component of adult treatment as well, it is more prevalent and vivid in child therapy because of the ongoing normative need for new identifications in order to fulfill developmental tasks (Chused 1988). Indeed, treatment can free the child for wider use of others as new objects, allowing for essential growth opportunities that might previously have been hampered; children who cannot tolerate peer competition or who rigidly oppose adult authority may be helped to gain greater freedom and autonomy and move into the important spheres of teacher/mentor connections and friendships via identifications with the clinician's affect tolerance, nonjudgmental attitudes, and reflective stance. The two-person nature of play therapy, in which child and therapist jointly create and negotiate affectively charged narratives and meanings, facilitates capacities that are needed for a wide range of future relationships (Lyons-Ruth 2006).

Additionally, the child therapist functions as a "developmental object," providing needed ego support when the child's self-regulatory capacities are not sufficient for tolerating the structure of treatment (e.g., parameters having to do with session times, the therapist's office space, acceptable behaviors) or the affects that emerge during play. The therapist's provision of direct support, such as actively setting limits and containing affects, is sometimes referred to as *developmental help or assistance* (Neubauer 2001; Sugarman 2003a, 2009b). The therapist's developmental and new object functions are interconnected in work with young children, who use their identifications with the clinician's observant, reflective, and attuned stance both to shore up existing vulnerabilities and to facilitate the emergence of novel capacities.

In the opening vignette, Alex relates to Dr. Chen in multiple ways: he recruits her as a teacher, seeking her advice for planning his Lego village; he enacts a familiar and rigidified mode of relating, in which others are blamed as the source of his internal dissatisfactions; he projects onto her his disowned inadequacies, accusing her of operating with substandard equipment; he re-creates with her a specific facet of his parental relationships, wherein he interprets her hesitation to play as gender-based rejection; and he relies on her help with self-regulation when he becomes overstimulated and has trouble transitioning out of the session.

THERAPEUTIC ALLIANCE

Another important aspect of the child–clinician relationship is the **therapeutic alliance**, which involves the child's basic trust in the therapist's essential benevolence and helpfulness. This component of the therapeutic bond allows the child to sustain motivation and willingness to work with the clinician despite the inevitable anxieties and discomforts of treatment. Indeed, the quality of the alliance is most apparent during times when the child is distressed by uncomfortable affects that emerge due to some aspect of therapy (the contents of play, the intensity of the transference) and when rejection or avoidance of the situation would likely bring immediate relief (Novick 1970). A therapeutic (or working) alliance is distinct from passive compliance; in the latter, the child merely submits to the clinician's interventions. A true alliance requires that the child actively maintain participation in the treatment, identifying with the therapist's observing and reflecting behaviors, even during moments of adverse emotional arousal (Kabcenell 1993; Novick 1970). In the treatment of young children, the therapist's participation in play is key to facilitating a sense of cooperation, mutuality, and shared exploration. While interacting through the safe displacement of a play scenario, young children are better able to communicate distress and tolerate affects that might feel overwhelming in a more direct, less metaphorical mode of treatment (Sugarman 2008).

Because children's capacities for autonomous emotional regulation, deferred gratification, and self-observation are limited, the working alliance extends to the parents. The majority of young children do not seek therapy of their own accord; although some possess conscious awareness of personal difficulties and desire relief, most are brought to treatment only because parents or teachers perceive the children's emotional states and behaviors as problematic. Parents are crucial to the treatment relationship in that they must ensure the continuity of the sessions through their tacit support and their willingness to cope with any temporary discomforts, including the child's vehement protests, for future developmental gains. In Chapter 10, "Working With Parents Over the Course of Treatment," we focus on ways to establish a positive working relationship with parents.

COUNTERTRANSFERENCE IN PLAY THERAPY

Contemporary definitions of *countertransference*, like those of *transference*, have shifted toward a broader conceptualization that includes the total of the therapist's subjective reactions to the child and to the clinical situation. Countertransference arises in the interface between the therapist's individual qualities (history and experience, current concerns, personality dynamics) and the myriad, potentially evocative aspects of treatment. In play therapy, the latter may include the child's appearance, temperament, and behavior; the nature of the transference relationship; the mutual interactions and play creations of the therapy time; and manifestations of the child's developmental phase. The continuous interaction of the therapist's and patient's unique minds and subjectivities represents an inevitable process that operates both in and outside of the clinician's consciousness, enriches the treatment, and yields crucial information that may not be accessible through more direct channels (Chused 1991; Eagle 2000; Jacobs 1999; Schafer 2000).

Often, a clinician's dawning awareness of countertransference emerges via self-observation of subtle shifts in feelings and attitudes, or realization of participation in unconsciously motivated patient–therapist interactions, known as **enactments**. These symbolically meaningful behaviors are differentiated from countertransference in that enactments involve manifest therapist–patient interactions rather than the clinician's internal response. Often, enactments arise as children seek to actualize latent fantasies in the treatment situation, eliciting both countertransference feelings and behavioral responses that initially go unrealized by the therapist. For example, a child behaves in an increasingly provocative manner, consistent with an unconscious wish for adult punishment. The therapist, pressured by a mounting inner sense of burden and irritation, misreads his watch by 5 minutes and abruptly informs the child that it is time to clean up as the session is nearly over. After the child leaves, the therapist is quite surprised to look at his watch and realize that he ended the session too early.

In the fast-paced, stimulating environment of play therapy, enactments represent the ongoing and ubiquitous process of patient–therapist unconscious communication. Indeed, their presence is essential to all psychodynamic treatments, both child and adult, wherein the therapist must sustain adequate emotional openness to receive the patient's myriad verbal and nonverbal signals. Inevitably, such continuous affective reciprocity (and mutual action and play, in the case of child treatments) stimulates the therapist's personal conflicts and leads to unconsciously driven responses. When the therapist is attuned to personal behavior and reflects on the sources, in the patient but also in the self, enactments provide unique opportunities for learning about patients' interpersonal dynamics that are relived in the treatment situation (Chused 1991).

Of course, the pervasive nature of action in child treatments sometimes precludes the therapist's immediate self-observation and self-analysis. In the vignette at the beginning of this chapter, Dr. Chen becomes aware of an uncharacteristically inhibited response only when Alex protests her behavior. Then she realizes that the child's play directive—his insistence that she mimic his openly gleeful and sadistic annihilation of "townspeople"—has elicited her internal discomfort. Dr. Chen's further reflections, once the session is over, might reveal a deep superego prohibition, such as fear of her own aggression. Within the session, a series of interpersonal events—Alex's complaint about her reluctance and his accusation that "you only wanna do girlie games"; Dr. Chen's realization of unusual hesitation and her verbal acknowledgment; and her vocalization of the boy's interpretation—serve to open up new material and deepen the treatment. Dr. Chen experiences a clearer sense of Alex's fear of being out of control, his worries about his own destructive potential, and his unconscious wish for adult prohibition and protection, whereas Alex realizes that his emotional responses are accepted in therapy and begins to hear how his reactions reflect deep-seated expectations and fears.

The child clinician is buffeted by a unique set of emotional factors, leading to countertransference reactions that are distinct from those evoked during adult treatments. Child therapists often interact with people in addition to the child, leading some writers to propose definitions of countertransference that include responses to parents, other family members, and even agencies involved in the child's care (Gabel and Bemporad 1994). Parental attitudes and behaviors may provoke intense responses in the therapist, sometimes leading to rescue fantasies and overidentification with the child. Moreover, children's normative developmental struggles and their active recruitment of the clinician as a new object further engender affective reactions; these often include revival of the therapist's unresolved feelings and early conflicts (Bonovitz 2009). Examples include an overly fastidious response to a young child's messy anal trends; punitive feelings in the presence of a latency-phase youngster's projection of unwanted guilt-based conflicts; or negative reactions toward an oedipal-phase child's intense curiosity. The action-based nature of play therapy, the young child's vivid presentation of frankly sexual and aggressive material, and the inevitable moments of physical contact between child and therapist create unique personal pressures for the clinician. Common countertransference reactions include a subtle desire to steer play away from uncomfortable contents, an urge to reject distasteful play roles, and a wish to impose logic and rationality on chaotic or confusing play narratives.

CONFLICT, DEFENSE, AFFECTS, AND EVOLVING EGO CAPACITIES

Conflict and defense represent ubiquitous mental processes that powerfully shape the child's emerging personality. Recognizing inner tensions and self-protective mechanisms in therapy, via the child's actions, play, affective expression, and interpersonal responses, is key to understanding and treating disruptions in development. Often, the clinical presentation involves external struggles between the child and the central attachment or authority figures (e.g., the vignette about Alex describes his increasingly defiant disregard of adults' parameters).

However, psychodynamic play therapy focuses not only on interpersonal conflicts but also on the inevitable intrapsychic tensions that accompany maturation. As ego and superego capacities evolve, the child's wishes and impulses encounter mounting opposition from inner guilt and self-evaluation, leading to intense anxiety and affective discomfort. Indeed, the developmental process itself introduces conflict and disequilibrium, such as when the relative quiescence of the latency phase is disrupted by the preadolescent's increasing sense of bodily change and internal pressure. Such interior tensions burden children's limited capacity for affect tolerance and self-regulation, sometimes leading to rigid or maladaptive modes of self-defense.

CONFLICT AND DEFENSE IN THE FIRST YEARS OF LIFE

Potential sources of conflict proliferate throughout childhood, developing alongside the child's growing ego capacities and expanding repertoire of defense mechanisms (Cramer 2006). Both conflict and defense are observable from the earliest months of life; initially, both are closely tied to the baby's basic needs (i.e., managing affective experience and maintaining proximity to the parent). Occasional inevitable discomforts, such as momentary social overstimulation, are handled via body-based self-protections; these include an effective but limited range of capacities, such as gaze aversion. Transient stressors, within the context of a secure parent–child attachment wherein the infant's affective states are mirrored and modulated, are unlikely to impede a developing sense of emotional reciprocity. When the parent–infant relationship fails more globally, however, the child is forced into a more rigid and enduring defensive stance. Faced with a parent who cannot tolerate affective expression, a baby must resolve competing desires; the innate need for maternal closeness and felt security vies with emotional knowledge that the parent responds unfavorably to affective signals. As a result, babies may engage in more persistent self-protective maneuvers, such as avoidance or freezing behaviors during times of emotional arousal; indeed, they may downregulate or heighten their overall affective expression, ultimately behaving in ways that suit parental struggles to manage affect and defend against personal vulnerability (Fraiberg 1982; Lyons-Ruth 1991; Main 2000). In essence, children in such situations identify with parental defenses and sacrifice aspects of their own natural emotionality (Winnicott 1960).

The child's awareness of parental attitudes intensifies during the toddler years; when the parents' aims, such as toilet training, oppose the child's urges and wishes, the toddler begins to experience conflict between autonomous strivings and desire for adult approval. Environmental expectations increase exponentially beyond age 3 years (the preschooler is required to share possessions and cope with brief periods of separation from parents; the latency-age child needs to master a dizzying array of skills, function autonomously for many hours at a time, and follow classroom rules), creating myriad opportunities for inner tension and frustration. Scrutiny by parents and other authorities, combined with the child's emerging capacity for guilt and self-appraisal, creates multiple sources of potential anxiety and a need to develop protections from threats to self-esteem.

Simultaneously, the child's ability to tolerate frustration, manage social complexity, defer gratification, and employ a range of defensive resources evolves; indeed, Anna Freud (1963) observed that by early latency the child possesses access to many of the defense mechanisms (e.g., sublimation, regression, reaction formation, fantasy formation) that adults employ to manage internal pressures. Expansion of the available defensive systems and social-emotional outlets, including shared fantasy play, softens the immediacy of painful affects and conflicts. As the child grows in competence and skill, diverse outlets (intellectual, creative, social, and athletic pursuits) further transform aggressive or competitive urges while offering new opportunities for a sense of competence and achievement.

Nonetheless, imbalances between the child's capacity for emotional self-regulation and the pressures of environmental expectations are common. The child clinician is likely to acquire copious experience with common manifestations of such developmental discrepancies; typical scenarios involve young latency-phase children whose modes of coping with increased social and academic demands may include transient losses of self-control, increased passivity or aggression, and avoidance of newfound responsibilities. Externalization of inner conflicts is highly characteristic of this age group, whose newly formed superegos tend toward rigidity and severity (Furman 1980). In the vignette at the beginning of this chapter, Alex responds to his internal discomforts via disruptive and oppositional behaviors, ultimately eliciting his parents' and teachers' castigations; successful attainment of adults' punishments allows him to eschew the far more painful prospect of internal guilt and self-recrimination.

Although the presence of conflict in mental life is inevitable, the child therapist must be alert to other sources of developmental disruption (Gilmore 2005; Pine 1994). Knowledge about children's endowments, including any neurologically based learning challenges, as well as their exposure to early trauma or deprivation, is essential to a full understanding of the clinical picture. For example, a child's failure to demonstrate imaginary play may reflect a confluence of influences, including inhibitions and conflicts around self-expression and fantasy, but might also signal constitutional vulnerabilities, such as attentional limitations, or attachment-based deprivations in the early years of life. Similarly, a child who repeatedly mishears the clinician's comments may very well be engaging in defensive maneuvers because the remarks generate internal discomfort, but this is only a partial understanding if the child suffers from a receptive language deficit. See Chapters 7, "Play and Developmental Psychopathology, Deprivation, or Disability," and 13, "Play Therapy, Variations in Child Development, and More Serious Psychopathology," for further discussions about assessing and working with various learning, emotional, and behavioral conditions that disrupt children's ego development and pose challenges to their relational capacities.

DEFENSES IN PLAY THERAPY

A major goal of psychodynamic treatment is to soften defenses that lock children into maladaptive modes of relating and restrict their engagement in various parts of life. Although the child's unique endowment, environment, and experiences yield highly individualized presentations, familiar defensive trends of childhood include the following: aggressive and oppositional behaviors or grandiose attitudes, which belie underlying fears and vulnerabilities; a tendency to seek external conflicts and consequences, which allows the child to eschew internal self-reproaches; a pattern of anxious, avoidant behaviors, which protect the child from challenging social and academic situations; overreliance on the parent, which helps to manage intense emotional experience; or insistence on mildly compulsive actions to (magically) undo angry thoughts and hostile wishes. These and many other rigid patterns interfere with the child's ability to establish social connections, function autonomously, and flexibly negotiate complex developmental tasks.

Achieving change in children with entrenched, habitual defensive modes requires that the clinician engage in a gradual, sensitive exploration of the ways in which children protect themselves from intensely uncomfortable feelings. Indeed, the vulnerable nature of young children's defenses, the fragility of their self-regulatory resources, and their dread of overwhelming affects pose special challenges for the clinician (Bornstein 1951; Hoffman 2007; Yanof 1996a, 1996b). The child's newly developed systems of self-control are easily disrupted, and the therapist's comments may feel threatening, exposing, and invasive. In Chapter 6, "Therapeutic Action and the Multiple Functions of Play Therapy," we discuss more fully the ways in which clinicians use play and judicious verbalizations to raise the child's conscious awareness of defensive patterns and enhance tolerance of affective states.

The metaphoric nature of play fosters a uniquely safe environment within which child and clinician can explore fears and wishes via their displacement onto play narratives, without directly attributing meanings to the child. However, many children soon realize that play with a therapist is a special situation through which hidden aspects of the self are examined and revealed. Moreover, even seemingly neutral questions or observations by the clinician may elicit the child's distress; at times, the child's own narrative may fall threateningly close to anxiety-laden contents, leading to disruption of play. **Resistance** is the process by which children and adults recruit defenses in order to oppose psychological change, maintain an internal status quo, and interfere with the ongoing process of treatment (Miller 1993); indeed, the process of therapy can be conceptualized as the ongoing tension between the competing forces for revelation and those of resistance that seek to maintain the child's current internal situation (Mahon 2000). At times, the developmental process itself can create normative resistances, such as the latency-age child's natural dread of feeling overcome by recently repressed oedipal wishes; such fears are easily elicited by interventions that too quickly reveal hidden affects or expose impulses and may intensify the child's opposition to therapy. Often, children's resistances are vivid and action-based, such as declining to enter or running out of the playroom, refusing to speak, crying, covering ears when the therapist comments, crumpling up drawings, disrupting a particular play scenario, yelling "shut up," and even striking out at the clinician.

ROLE OF INSIGHT AND INTERPRETATION IN PLAY THERAPY

In psychodynamic therapy, **interpretation** is the term reserved for verbal interventions that seek to raise patients' awareness of unconscious processes and thereby enhance their emotional self-knowledge. The therapist's interpretive comments are delivered over time, in a series of steps designed to orient the individual toward the meanings of certain behavioral and interpersonal patterns; gradually, such surface-to-depth work reveals disavowed affects and defensive trends, as well as enduring wishes and fantasies that might originate in earlier phases of development. When the clinician employs such verbalizations tactfully in child therapy, with consideration of the child's developmental capacities and vulnerabilities, they can facilitate self-observation and reflection, ultimately expanding the child's ego control over previously repudiated affects and impulses (Glenn 1992; Hoffman 2007; Mahon 2000; Sugarman 2003b). However, the clinician's use of insight-oriented interventions is modified with prelatency and latency children, whose capacity for self-examination is limited and who are likely to feel overwhelmed by direct comments and the uncomfortable emotions they elicit.

Traditionally, psychoanalytic definitions of *insight* involve emotional as well as intellectual self-knowing, with particular emphasis on elucidation of unconscious contents and motivations. The following ego capacities are prerequisites for insight-oriented work: comprehension of the connections between external actions and inner states, and between past experience and the self in the present; sustained self-observation; and tolerance for the affects that are evoked during the self-reflective process (Kennedy 1979; Mayes and Cohen 1996; Schmukler 1999). Consolidation and integration of these various functions are achieved gradually during childhood; emergence of mental state knowledge during the oedipal phase marks a fundamental achievement, facilitating self-understanding and emotional self-regulation, and assuaging the child's desire for immediate affective discharge (Fonagy and Target 1996). However, certain developmental tendencies and normative defensive reactions run counter to the therapeutic goal of self-discovery;

these include the latency child's inevitable intolerance for uncomfortable affects, predilection for externalizing inner tensions and blaming personal problems on others, and distinct preference for concrete, practical solutions to problems of all kind (Kennedy 1979; Schmukler 1999). Complaints about the unfairness of adult expectations and reports of peers' transgressions are likely responses to the therapist's direct attempts at eliciting the child's self-reflection and sense of personal responsibility. Moreover, despite their increased capacity to reflect on their own mental states and grasp multiple perspectives, latency-age children may struggle to comprehend complex emotional phenomena, such as the notion that opposing feelings (i.e., conflict) may reside in the same individual (Jemerin 2004).

In addition, the forward pull of development and children's present and future, rather than past, orientation run counter to certain therapeutic efforts; interventions that seek to link an individual's current conflicts and defenses to historical material, sometimes referred to as *reconstructions*, represent an important component of adult psychodynamic treatments but are employed far more judiciously by the child clinician (Abrams et al. 1999). The opening vignette in this chapter illustrates some of the challenges posed by a child's developmental status: when Dr. Chen attempts to reference a connection between past and present, via her questions about the play characters' current conflicts and potential links to former events, Alex manifests impatience and disinterest. Working within the here-and-now, or connecting a current affective reaction to events in the immediate rather than distant past, is often of greater value to the child than is invoking a dimly recalled autobiographical event; emphasis on the remote past involves highly abstract verbal interventions that may serve the clinician's need for organization and coherence but that run the risk of eliciting from the child either disengagement or cognitive rather than experiential self-understanding (Chused 1988).

In the treatment of prelatency children, whose capacities for self-reflection and affect tolerance are very limited, the therapist's facilitation of insight is often achieved primarily via comments made *within the play itself*. Indeed, the therapist must deliver more direct remarks to and about the child with care, to avoid disrupting the flow of the child's imaginative fantasy, engendering unnecessary self-consciousness and feelings of exposure, or inhibiting overall self-expression (Birch 1997;

Mayes and Cohen 1996). A number of writers suggest that the therapeutic play process, uniquely suited to young children's cognitive and emotional equipment, allows for the fluid displacement of central wishes, fantasies, and conflicts onto pretend scenarios wherein the child may achieve greater awareness of internal states without the act of conscious self-reflection (Birch 1997; Cohen and Solnit 1993; Neubauer 1994; Yanof 1996a, 1996b). The playing state promotes children's consideration of multiple viewpoints and relational paradigms, allows for experimentation with varying affective states, and fosters the child's realization of the mind as a representation of ideas and emotions; these functions may lay the groundwork for insight by aiding in the integration of complex experience, the differentiation of one's own and others' emotional reactions, and the tolerance of uncomfortable feelings (Cohen and Solnit 1993; Fonagy and Target 1996; Vygotsky 1978). Sugarman 2003b, 2009a) proposes that the notion of insight, when applied to prelatency children, is best viewed as a process of "insight-fulness" whereby the therapist facilitates curiosity and self-reflection rather than the discovery of specific unconscious repudiated mental contents.

SUMMARY

Psychodynamic play therapy incorporates fundamental concepts from psychoanalysis, such as transference, countertransference, conflict, and defense. Application of these ideas is adjusted to accommodate children's emerging ego capacities, ongoing attachment to their parents, need for identifications with adult figures in order to complete developmental tasks, and play and action-based modes of communication. The therapist is particularly attuned to the child's affective states, fantasies about self and others, use of self-protective mechanisms to avoid intense and unwanted emotions and impulses, and interpersonal patterns. Play, rather than direct verbal comments about the child, is the primary vehicle intervention that seeks to expand the child's capacity for self-observation, affect regulation, and insight.

KEY POINTS

- The child–therapist relationship involves multiple, inseparable elements such as transference, the working alliance, and the therapist's roles as a new and developmental object. Current notions of transference encompass the sum of the child's feelings about and reactions to both the real and imagined aspects of the clinician.

- Countertransference is an inherent, often unconscious aspect of play therapy involving the therapist's reactions to the child's real qualities, transference manifestations, and developmental phase as well as to the mutual interactions of the therapy. Awareness of countertransference reactions and enactments (unconsciously driven, symbolically meaningful child–therapist interactions) yields a trove of information about the child's fears, fantasies, and relational patterns that may not be available through more direct channels.

- Defense and conflict are ubiquitous, normative mental processes that are present from birth; they develop and expand along with the child's ego functions, including awareness of environmental attitudes and expectations, and capacity for self-appraisal and guilt. Play therapy seeks to soften those rigid, maladaptive patterns of defense that interfere with developmental progression. However, because of children's shaky sense of self-control and their limited tolerance for uncomfortable affects, the clinician must use a gradual, sensitive approach to interpreting their inner struggles. The child's resistance to treatment may be increased if the therapist's premature comments engender a sense of exposure.

- Insight-oriented work, which involves an expansion of cognitive-emotional self-knowledge, is a cornerstone of psychodynamic treatment. The child therapist, however, must adjust modes of intervention to accommodate children's evolving capacities for self-observation and affect tolerance.

KEY TERMS

Countertransference   The sum of the therapist's reactions to the patient and to their mutual interactions.

Developmental object   The therapist's role as a provider of developmental assistance, such as limit setting, affect labeling, and containment of the child's impulses.

Enactments   Symbolic patient–therapist interactions wherein their mutual unconscious conflicts and fantasies are actualized in the treatment.

Interpretation   A set of verbal, insight-oriented comments that seek to raise the patient's awareness of unconscious forces.

New object   The therapist's functions as a potential figure for identifications that serve the child's developmental progression, such as use of the clinician's affect tolerance and reflective stance to scaffold emerging capacities.

Real relationship   Aspects of the therapeutic relationship that are relatively unaffected by distortion and are based on the therapist's reality-based behavior, such as greetings, here-and-now reactions, and attitudes.

Resistance   The patient's self-protective tendencies that may at times oppose the therapeutic process in order to maintain a psychological status quo.

Therapeutic alliance   The part of the patient–clinician relationship that involves the patient's motivation and willingness to engage in treatment, even during times of distress and discomfort.

Transference   The sum of the patient's reactions to the therapist, including the revival of past wishes and urges.

REFERENCES

Abrams S: Looking forwards and backwards. Psychoanal Study Child 58(1): 172–186, 2003

Abrams S, Solnit AJ: Coordinating developmental and psychoanalytic processes: conceptualizing technique. J Am Psychoanal Assoc 46(1):85–103, 1998 9565900

Abrams S, Neubauer PB, Solnit AJ: Coordinating the developmental and psychoanalytic processes: three case reports. Introduction (Discussion). Psychoanal Study Child 54:19–24, discussion 87–90, 1999 10748626

Birch M: In the land of counterpane: travels in the realm of play. Psychoanal Study Child 52:57–75, 1997 9489461

Bonovitz C: Countertransference in child psychoanalytic psychotherapy: the emergence of the analyst's childhood. Psychoanal Psychol 26(3):235–245, 2009

Bornstein B: On latency. Psychoanal Study Child 6:279–285, 1951

Chused JF: The transference neurosis in child analysis. Psychoanal Study Child 43:51–81, 1988 3227088

Chused JF: The evocative power of enactments. J Am Psychoanal Assoc 39(3):615–639, 1991 1719055

Cohen PM, Solnit AJ: Play and therapeutic action. Psychoanal Study Child 48:49–63, 1993 7694307

Cramer P: Protecting the Self: Defense Mechanisms in Action. New York, Guilford, 2006

Eagle MN: A critical evaluation of current conceptions of transference and countertransference. Psychoanal Psychol 17(1):24–37, 2000

Fonagy P, Target M: Playing with reality, I: theory of mind and the normal development of psychic reality. Int J Psychoanal 77(Pt 2):217–233, 1996 8771375

Fraiberg S: Clinical notes on the nature of transference in child analysis. Psychoanal Study Child 6:286–306, 1951

Fraiberg S: Pathological defenses in infancy. Psychoanal Q 51(4):612–635, 1982 6758010

Freud A: The concept of developmental lines. Psychoanal Study Child 18:245–265, 1963 14147280

Freud A: Normality and Pathology in Childhood. New York, International Universities Press, 1965

Furman E: Transference and externalization in latency. Psychoanal Study Child 35:267–284, 1980 7433582

Gabel S, Bemporad J: An expanded concept of countertransference. J Am Acad Child Adolesc Psychiatry 33(1):140–141, 1994 8138511

Galatzer-Levy RM: The nuts and bolts of child psychoanalysis. Annu Psychoanal 36:189–202, 2008

Gilmore K: Play in the psychoanalytic setting: ego capacity, ego state, and vehicle for intersubjective exchange. Psychoanal Study Child 60:213–238, 2005 16649681

Glenn J: Child Analysis and Therapy. Northvale, NJ, Jason Aronson, 1992

Govrin A: The dilemma of contemporary psychoanalysis: toward a "knowing" post-postmodernism. J Am Psychoanal Assoc 54(2):507–535, 2006 16773820

Greenson R: The Technique and Practice of Psychoanalysis. New York, International Universities Press, 1967

Hoffman L: Do children get better when we interpret their defenses against painful feelings? Psychoanal Study Child 62:291–313, 2007 18524096

Jacobs TJ: Countertransference past and present: a review of the concept. Int J Psychoanal 80(Pt 3):575–594, 1999 10407752

Jemerin JM: Latency and the capacity to reflect on mental states. Psychoanal Study Child 59:211–239, 2004 16240613

Kabcenell RJ: Some aspects of the "treatment alliance" in child analysis. Journal of Clinical Psychoanalysis 2(1):27–41, 1993

Kennedy H: The role of insight in child analysis: a developmental viewpoint. J Am Psychoanal Assoc 27(suppl):9–28, 1979 263976

Klein M: Symposium on child-analysis. Int J Psychoanal 8:339–370, 1927

Loewald HW: On the therapeutic action of psycho-analysis. Int J Psychoanal 41:16–33, 1960 14417912

Lyons-Ruth K: Rapprochement or approchement: Mahler's theory reconsidered from the vantage point of recent research in early attachment relationships. Psychoanal Psychol 8(1):1–23, 1991

Lyons-Ruth K: Play, precariousness and the negotiation of shared meaning: a developmental research perspective on child psychotherapy. J Infant Child Adolesc Psychother 5(2):142–159, 2006

Mahon E: A "good hour" in child analysis and adult analysis. Psychoanal Study Child 55:124–142, 2000 11338985

Main M: The organized categories of infant, child, and adult attachment: flexible vs. inflexible attention under attachment-related stress. J Am Psychoanal Assoc 48(4):1055–1096, discussion 1175–1187, 2000 11212183

Mayes LC, Cohen DJ: Children's developing theory of mind. J Am Psychoanal Assoc 44(1):117–142, 1996 8717481

Miller JM: Resistance in child psychoanalysis. Journal of Child Psychotherapy 19(1):33–45, 1993

Neubauer PB: The role of displacement in psychoanalysis. Psychoanal Study Child 49:107–119, 1994 7809278

Neubauer PB: Some observations about changes in technique in child analysis. Psychoanal Study Child 56:16–26, 2001 12102011

Novick J: The vicissitudes of the "working alliance" in the analysis of a latency girl. Psychoanal Study Child 25:231–256, 1970 4100204

Pine F: Some impressions regarding conflict, defect, and deficit. Psychoanal Study Child 49:222–240, 1994 7809286

Sandler J, Kennedy H, Tyson RL: The Technique of Child Analysis. Cambridge, MA, Harvard University Press, 1980

Schafer R: Reflections on "thinking in the presence of the other." Int J Psychoanal 81(Pt 1):85–96, 2000 10816846

Schmukler AG: Use of insight in child analysis. Psychoanal Study Child 54:339–355, 1999 10748639

Sugarman A: Dimensions of the child analyst's role as a developmental object: affect regulation and limit setting. Psychoanal Study Child 58:189–213, 2003a 14982021

Sugarman A: A new model for conceptualizing insightfulness in the psychoanalysis of young children. Psychoanal Q 72(2):325–355, 2003b 12718248

Sugarman A: The use of play to promote insightfulness in the analysis of children suffering from cumulative trauma. Psychoanal Q 77(3):799–833, 2008 18686791

Sugarman A: Child versus adult psychoanalysis: two processes or one? Int J Psychoanal 90(6):1255–1276, 2009a 20002815

Sugarman A: The contribution of the analyst's actions to mutative action: a developmental perspective. Psychoanal Study Child 64:247–272, 2009b 20578441

Vygotsky LS: Mind in Society. Cambridge, MA, Harvard University Press, 1978

Winnicott DW: The theory of the parent-infant relationship. Int J Psychoanal 41:585–595, 1960 13785877

Yanof J: Language, communication and transference in child analysis, I: selective mutism: the medium is the message. J Am Psychoanal Assoc 44(1):79–100, 1996a 8717479

Yanof J: Language, communication, and transference in child analysis, II: is child analysis really analysis? J Am Psychoanal Assoc 44(1):100–116, 1996b 8717480

6

Therapeutic Action and the Multiple Functions of Play Therapy

Kate's parents brought her to Dr. Enright, a pediatric social worker, seeking help with the 5-year-old's prolonged struggles over bowel training. Kate's refusals and tears, when she was pressed toward continence, had followed a brief period of successful potty usage between ages 2½ and 3 years; the onset of subsequent battles had coincided with the birth of a brother. Despite her previously cheerful and affectionate demeanor, Kate had begun to direct angry outbursts at her now 2-year-old sibling, whose frequent tantrums dominated family life. Her parents ruefully observed that everyone, including Kate, had adopted the habit of treading carefully and catering to the toddler's demands to avert his protracted outbursts; now, however, Kate seemed more likely to provoke him via teasing and physical aggression. Equally concerning to her parents were Kate's periods of passivity in which she appeared to withdraw from her usual play activities. The parents, busy professionals, tended to communicate with Dr. Enright in brief news updates, via e-mail or phone, but it had not been easy to find time for full sessions wherein deeper discussions could develop.

In their first session together, Kate greeted Dr. Enright somewhat shyly but followed her into the playroom with her babysitter's encouragement; she immediately gravitated toward the dollhouse and was happy to include Dr. Enright in her play. "Pretend I'm the mommy and you're the daddy and I have a lot of babies," Kate suggested, beginning to fill the house with small figures; when this supply was exhausted, she added a collection of tiny animals until every room was filled with crying "babies," all demanding to be fed. "I've never seen so

147

many babies!" exclaimed Dr. Enright. Kate nodded eagerly and squeezed a few additional small creatures into the overflowing spaces. Standing back to survey the house, she appeared satisfied. "How did you get so many babies?" the therapist inquired, careful to follow Kate's initial comments in which the babies were stated to belong to the mother alone. "I ate a lot of food and got a very big tummy (gesturing toward her own abdomen and tracing a huge imaginary protuberance), and a lot of babies started coming out!" Kate then encouraged the therapist to join her in a cacophony of crying and whining that represented the babies' collective pleas. After several minutes of joint noise making, Kate placed her hands over her ears and yelled, "We have to shut them up! They're too loud!" Dr. Enright agreed that the babies were extremely demanding and disruptive, and appeared to be taking over the home. "Of course they are," replied Kate, "because they want all the food! Nobody else will get anything!" "What about the older children in the house?" asked Dr. Enright. "No, because all the milk and the cupcakes are being eaten by those babies!" For a few moments, they jointly opined about the unfairness of this; Dr. Enright suggested various affects that the older children might experience, such as anger and disappointment. Kate expanded this, asserting that they don't even like the babies anymore. For a brief second, Kate stood still and her facial expression shifted to something sad or worried; the moment passed quickly, and she then returned to play. Dr. Enright commented quietly, as they returned to the game, "You looked uncomfortable there for a bit." Ignoring this comment, and gesturing for Dr. Enright's participation, Kate demonstrated how the many babies would gobble play food and then fill their diapers with vast quantities of poop. As the play continued, Kate further elaborated the selfishness and greed of the infants: their incessant demands turned from food to toys to maternal attention. The culminating scene depicted a frazzled mother doll running about in a series of futile efforts, none of which silenced the constant stream of wailing. Indeed, it was soon revealed that the mother was so busy that the older children had been forgotten at school.

Two days later, Kate returned for her next session. Her babysitter brought her directly after kindergarten, and she and Kate read books and colored together for about a half hour as they waited for her time with Dr. Enright to begin. Kate greeted the therapist enthusiastically and entered the playroom, commenting, "I thought you forgot about me today. I had to wait for so long." Dr. Enright registered a sense of pressure and unfairness; she experienced a strong urge to protest that the session was beginning on time and to point out that Kate had arrived quite early. Instead, she agreed that it was hard to wait, especially when one was not sure that the person you were waiting for remembered you. Kate did not respond; she had already begun to resume the play from the previous session and impatiently handed Dr. Enright some dolls so that they could re-create the scene in which the babies dominated the dollhouse. Dr. Enright followed along, feeling somewhat frustrated; she believed that the prior moment between them was important, but there was no time to revisit it or even to reflect on its meanings.

Kate added a new element to the play scenario. She shifted to another area of the playroom that she designated "the schoolyard"; here, she and Dr. Enright embodied the two kindergartners in the large family whose parents had failed to collect them at the end of the school day. "Where are Mommy and Daddy?" asked Dr. Enright, to which Kate responded in a sad voice, "Daddy is at work and Mommy is feeding the babies. What should we do? We're all alone!" Pausing for a minute, Kate brightened and said, "Wait, I know, I'm the oldest girl and I know the way to Daddy's office! We'll go and surprise him!" A triumphant arrival at the father's workplace brought the session to an end. As she carefully placed the father and older girl dolls into a bin, Kate looked directly at Dr. Enright and stated proudly, "I actually know how to get to Daddy's office."

OVERVIEW OF THERAPEUTIC ACTION

Therapeutic action refers to those aspects of treatment that are hypothesized to foster psychological change and ultimately improve people's lives. Psychoanalysts' views of these mutative agents are diverse, inextricably linked to their theories about the goals of treatment and the relative weight they assign to various intrapsychic and interpersonal processes. Verbal interpretations, the clinician's consistent availability and empathic attunement, and various conscious and more implicit aspects of patient–therapist interactions are variously privileged as contributing to the individual's personal growth. Within psychodynamic theory, desirable changes include increased insight and self-reflection, affect tolerance, softening of rigid relational and defensive patterns, expanded capacities for intersubjective sharing and communication, and a more coherent sense of self (Ablon 2005; Friedman 2007; Michels 2007). Most contemporary writers conceive of the therapeutic process as multifaceted rather than unidimensional, highly reflective of both patients' and therapists' unique individual qualities and powerfully shaped by the dyad's collaborative style. Inevitably, any discussion of therapeutic action includes the complex interplay of the clinician's theories, a repertoire of techniques and less consciously derived interventions, the evolving patient–therapist relationship, their verbal and nonverbal here-and-now interactions, and the structure and consistency of the treatment.

What constitutes therapeutic action in the treatment of young children, and how does play therapy help restore the forward progression of development? Although each child–therapist dyad brings unique qualities to the treatment and shapes the progress of therapy in highly subjective ways, the following potentially mutative components are central to the therapeutic process:

- The achievement of a child–therapist mutual playing state wherein affects, meanings, and narratives are shared and co-created
- The clinician's use of joint pretense for naming affects, connecting inner states to behavior, elucidating transference, and clarifying defensive patterns
- As treatment progresses and opportunities arise, the therapist's more direct comments about the child's wishes, anxieties, and defense mechanisms as these are revealed in the context of their unfolding interactional patterns
- The clinician's provision of a **new object relationship** in which the child develops and internalizes emerging capacities for self-knowledge and self-reflection, affect tolerance, and emotional self-regulation
- The therapist's work with parents to establish greater awareness of the child's individuality

In this chapter, we discuss multiple aspects of the play therapy process and examine how they help mobilize inherent growth-promoting forces, foster the integration of disavowed aspects of self-experience, and ultimately facilitate the child's access to less rigid, more adaptive ways of relating and functioning (Abrams 2008).

As depicted in the opening vignette, Kate is a child who requires little help entering a mutual playing state; she immediately engages in pretense and is happy to include the therapist in her imaginary world. This child spontaneously and fluidly adopts and assigns roles, and generates and embellishes narratives. Dr. Enright accepts Kate's designation of the "daddy" role; she moves the narrative along a meaningful path, asking, "How did you get so many babies?" without transgressing the boundaries of the play scenario (i.e., she does not verbalize the obvious links between Kate's reality and the fantasy depicted in the treatment). Kate reveals her "theory" of human reproduction, in which the various orifices of the body are conflated; like many oedipal-age children, Kate envisions that eating and defecation are closely linked to childbirth. Dr. Enright's later query, "What about the older children in the house?" is pointed, in that she creates an opening for Kate to express intense sibling feelings, but it is offered in the form of a question that Kate can freely integrate or ignore. In this way, the greediness of babies—and their potential to edge out their older siblings—is organically linked to the play narrative rather than to Kate herself, and causes the child no discomfort or self-consciousness. In addition, we learn of Kate's wishful fantasy in which the babies belong to mother alone, leaving father safely out of the loop and potentially available for a dyadic connection, perhaps in the form of a surprise visit from his clever older daughter.

Through mutually created play, Kate reveals key aspects of her symptomatic problems and stalled developmental progression (defecation is scary: it involves babies and hateful feelings toward them; moreover, the achievement of toilet training signals growing up, which portends abandonment by mother). Dr. Enright's approach to the play characters suggests acceptance of and interest in strong affects; once these are expressed via displacement in pretense, Kate can freely communicate, explore, and better understand emotional states of mind. Ultimately, this little girl discovers a creative solution to certain dilemmas and oedipal dramas: via pretending, Kate transforms the passive experience of neglect and abandonment via her own ingenuity, and an adventurous and brave little girl saves the day. Such satisfying imaginary resolutions to painful and potentially mortifying real-life feelings—exclusion from the parental couple and the sense of losing to a sibling rival—are powerful tools that the young child uses to gain mastery over intense feelings and to strengthen tolerance for inner conflict.

At the end of the vignette, there is a hint of Kate's potential to respond to more direct work outside of the play scenario: she indicates her identification with the older sister doll, while glancing meaningfully at Dr. Enright. It is early in the treatment, so the therapist chooses to hear but not comment on this revelation; at a later date, she might remark that Kate herself sometimes wishes to visit daddy when he is away from home, and begin to voice the inherent tension between Kate's emerging self-reliance ("I actually know how to get to daddy's office") and her regressive attitude toward toilet training.

THERAPEUTIC ACTION IN THE TWENTY-FIRST CENTURY

Contemporary psychodynamic notions about therapeutic action have shifted away from the primacy of the therapist's verbal insight-oriented work to include mutual aspects of the patient–clinician relationship (Blatt and Behrends 1987). Current theorizing recognizes multiple pathways toward patients' psychological growth; these include inter-related conscious and unconscious processes such as patient–therapist co-creation of meaning and narrative, their emotional reciprocity (including symbolically meaningful interactions such as **enactments**), and verbal interventions that seek to promote insight, integrate disavowed aspects of the self, and provide the patient with greater awareness of unconscious forces (Ablon 2005, 2014; Gabbard and Westen 2003; Michels 2007). A number of writers emphasize the potential of the unique patient–therapist relationship to unleash children's and adults' previously inhibited creativity, as well as to facilitate new interpersonal experiences, leading to moments of spontaneous discovery and surprise (Ablon 2000; Kieffer 2007; Mahon 2000).

In many ways, working with children necessitates a complex, multidimensional approach to therapeutic action that integrates traditional with more contemporary methods. Inevitably, the child therapist's interventions represent a blending of developmental knowledge, known information (some provided by parents and other caregivers) about the child's unique qualities and history, learned professional technique, and far more immediate, less conscious, interpersonal responsiveness to the child's rapidly shifting emotional signals, play, and behaviors. Clinician-led verbal techniques—labeling affects, connecting feeling states to behavior, and linking the child's defensive behaviors to warded-off emotions—are continuously adjusted to match with the child's evolving developmental capabilities for language, affect tolerance, insight, and self-control. Moreover, the child's status as a changing, developing individual powerfully shapes the therapeutic process, determining the potential benefits of verbal commentary; the forward pull of development often overrides the child's investment in the past, meaning that the therapist does not always seek to verbalize and make conscious to the child the impact of pivotal historical events (e.g., a sibling's birth, a divorce, a death) or the role of transference paradigms in the current therapeutic relationship (Abrams 1980; Abrams and Solnit 1998). In the vignette, Dr. Enright keeps private her many observations about the girl's hypothesized reaction to her brother's birth, her envy of the mother's pregnancy and of the parental bond, and the meanings of her stated belief that Dr. Enright has begun the session late and perhaps forgotten about her young patient.

Young children's normative levels of impulsivity create special challenges; indeed, the child's immature self-regulatory capacities and predilection for action frequently preclude optimal conditions for thinking and reflection, requiring that therapists rely on less cognitive means for knowing and understanding (Galatzer-Levy 2008; Molinari 2011). The nature of play itself, with its action-based orientation and its requirement for the therapist's full immersion and non-self-conscious participation, necessitates that the clinician embody an active, co-creative role and avoid a distanced, overly intellectualized stance in the playroom. Dr. Enright experiences internal discomfort and pressure as Kate reproaches her, turning the therapist into a potentially negligent adult figure ("I thought you forgot about me today. I had to wait for so long"). However, there is no time to grapple with Kate's perception and with her responding sense of unfairness and defensiveness; her verbal comment is lost in the ensuing action as Kate demands an immediate return to play.

In recent decades, the child psychoanalytic literature has reflected a shift toward broader appreciation for the role of relational processes in restoring children's developmental progression. Contemporary notions of therapeutic action include greater emphasis on the following: the mutative potential of joint therapist–child play, without additional verbal interpretation of the play; the benefit of fostering the child's capacity for **mentalization**, or mental state knowledge; growth-promoting aspects of the child–therapist here-and-now relationship, such as their implicit emotional communications, shared meaning-making, mutual affective regulation, and co-creation of play narratives; and the impact of the therapist's provision of developmental assistance, including limit setting and other ways of containing the child's affects (Harrison and Tronick 2011; Lyons-Ruth 2006; Mayes and Cohen 1993; Neubauer 1994; Slade 1994; Stern et al. 1998; Sugarman 2009).

Although we embrace an increasingly complex and inclusive view of therapeutic action, we continue to place special value on the therapist's verbal functions and on the evolving conversation between child and clinician. Play is the language we use, but the verbal components of play—inseparable as they are from action—nonetheless serve development in particular ways. The transformative power of words and narratives for sharing, modulating, and organizing the child's affective experience is well documented; we view the development of a mutual vocabulary for the child's inner states, the verbal expression of affects that are within and just outside of the child's consciousness, and the facilitation of therapist–child talk about feelings as fundamental to the therapeutic process (Blatt 2013). Within the developmental literature, shared adult–child emotional talk (naming feelings, narrating affect-laden events) is linked to acquisition of a mental state vocabulary and correlates with the development of emotional competence, including capacities for self-expression and self-regulation (Nelson 1996; Sales and Fivush 2005). Child psychoanalysts hypothesize that naming intense feelings and attaching them to storylines enables the child to reclaim disavowed, potentially overwhelming emotions and integrate them, in a more modulated form, with higher-order maturing ego processes (Bergman and Harpaz-Rotem 2004; Blum 2004; Knight 2003; Litowitz 2011; Loewald 1960; Rizzuto 2003; Vivona 2012).

Language-based interventions generally take place within the context of or at least closely connected to play: the therapist names and elaborates the characters' imagined inner states, child and therapist embody their play characters talking to each other, or both parties jointly plan and narrate the play scenarios. Conversation may also occur in moments outside of pretense, when the clinician directly addresses shifts in the child's mood or behavior; in the vignette, for example, Dr. Enright remarks on Kate's sudden change in facial expression ("You looked uncomfortable there for a bit"). Like many children, Kate ignores this initial comment; as their relationship develops, however, such comments can meaningfully underscore subtle changes in affect, abrupt play disruptions, or the use of action to handle intensifying feelings (e.g., near the end of a session, after a vacation), drawing the child's attention to emotional signals and the ways in which they represent inner states. Many children, as they gain comfort in the therapeutic situation and trust in the clinician, volunteer information about their activities, ask a question about the therapist, and begin to describe small but significant moments in their interactions with others, opening additional opportunities for shared talking and reflecting.

Of course, talking with children is vastly different from therapeutic conversation with adults: the child therapist is attuned to limits in language capacity (vocabulary and verbal abstraction) and to each child's unique style of emotional communication. In addition, the conventions of verbal exchange are distinctly less formalized than in adult treatment; the child's normative needs for self-protection and control lead to frequent incidents wherein the therapist's comments are initially sharply rebutted ("That's stupid!" or "Shut up right now!") or simply ignored, as in the case of Kate, who fails to respond to Dr. Enright's comment about her possible discomfort. Moreover, the content of therapists' conversations with children is distinguished by its increased focus on the here-and-now, including the play itself, with less emphasis on verbal reconstruction of past events and more judicious elucidation of nonconscious, repudiated mental contents (Sugarman 2003).

PLAY AND THE EXPANSION OF EMOTIONAL RESOURCEFULNESS

Imaginary play represents the predominant medium for therapeutic action in the treatment of young children. The multiple therapeutic functions of play include its provision of a unique window into the child's private world and a meaningful context for the therapist's verbal interpretations; indeed, therapeutic work within the displaced metaphors of play allows enhanced access to the child's inner processes without eliciting self-consciousness and fear of exposure (Cohen and Solnit 1993; Mayes and Cohen 1993; Neubauer 1994). The potentially growth-promoting and developmentally restorative value of play in the therapeutic situation was famously noted by Winnicott (1971), who hypothesized that both child and adult therapies embody special forms of mutual playing; when patients lack access to play, he proposed that the therapist's first task is to bring about a playing state.

Psychoanalysts postulate play as a mental process that is fundamental to social, emotional, and cognitive functioning. Emerging developmental achievements, such as reality testing, mentalization, and narrative competence, are practiced and consolidated as children develop storylines, experiment with trial thought and identifications, and negotiate play scenarios with a partner (Ablon 1994, 2014; Abrams and Solnit 1998; Bonovitz 2004; Mayes and Cohen 1993). Through play, the child acquires new perspectives, novel solutions, and a wider range of potential emotional responsiveness. Play with a trained practitioner, who is alert to the child's history and struggles and gradually shapes the pretense to reflect key inner states, illuminates through displacement the child's fears, wishes, and naïve interpretations; in addition, therapist and child together organize, integrate, and make meaning of inner states and affect-laden events (Lyons-Ruth 2006; Slade 1994). The metaphoric use of characters and plots helps render disowned aspects of the self more acceptable and knowable; these altered play representations can then be reclaimed and reassimilated by the child, contributing to an overall reduction in inhibitions and anxieties, and freeing the child to access evolving, age-appropriate affect tolerance and self-regulation (Birch 1997; Gilmore 2005; Mayes and Cohen 1993; Warshaw 2015). Indeed, a number of theorists propose that working inside the displaced metaphors of play, without more explicit interventions that directly address the child's conflicts, is often sufficient to achieve therapeutic benefit (Birch 1997; Cohen and Solnit 1993; Krimendahl 1998; Mayes and Cohen 1993; Rosegrant 2001).

The therapist's mobilization of the child's playing capacity and skill at sustaining and shaping pretense occupy a central role in the therapeutic process. Even when a child is capable of fluid play, as in the example of Kate, the quality of the clinician's playing stance—level of active engagement and absorption, non-self-conscious attitude, and spontaneous responsiveness to the child's signals—is a potent indicator, easily recognizable by youngsters, of the therapist's willingness to suspend reality and enter the child's private world (Gilmore 2011). Inhibition, hesitation, rigidity, or a censorious approach to the child's free-ranging fantasies may impede the child's freedom of self-expression. Not surprisingly, the therapist's integration of thinking (conceptualizing the unfolding treatment dynamics, keeping in mind the child's history, integrating the moment-to-moment play with previous sessions) with more intuitive and action-based modes of work represents a major challenge of play therapy (Rose 2002).

Once play begins to unfold, jointly created characters and storylines form a context for ongoing therapeutic action. The therapist is guided by the child's indicated play preferences, either by following explicitly stated preferences, mirroring the child's actions (such as when Dr. Enright mimics Kate's filling the house with babies or joins in the cacophony the babies create), or requesting direction when the child's wishes are ambiguous. At the same time, the clinician seeks opportunities to amplify certain affective moments (e.g., when Dr. Enright verbally reinforces how the babies are taking over the house), or to ask questions designed to elicit the child's naïve understanding of reality (as when Kate, in response to Dr. Enright's question about how babies are born, reveals her theory of human reproduction) so that individual distortions and fantasies can be verbalized and brought under joint reflection. In addition, the therapist shapes the unfolding narratives and animates assigned characters based on special knowledge of the child's circumstances and vulnerabilities. Dr. Enright's use of the older sister character is fluid and spontaneous, and does not appear overly intellectualized, but at the same time her personifications are clearly designed to represent Kate's suspected struggles over intense sibling feelings.

THE THERAPEUTIC RELATIONSHIP AS AN AGENT OF CHANGE

The child–therapist relationship is inseparable from therapeutic action. When working with young populations, the clinician fulfills roles that reflect the child's revived past relations, current experience of the therapist, and future potentialities; these separate but intertwined functions are embodied in the child's use of the therapist as a transference-based, real, and new object, respectively (Abrams and Solnit 1998) (see Chapter 5, "Basic Psychodynamic Concepts and Their Use in Play Therapy," for a fuller discussion of these components). In the vignette, Dr. Enright serves multiple purposes for Kate, including a recipient for perceptions based on the child's representations of early experience with parents (her interpretation that the therapist has forgotten her); a here-and-now playing partner and narrative co-creator; and an adult with whom she can identify, whose curiosity, composure, and reflective stance scaffold her own evolving ego capacities.

THE ROLE OF TRANSFERENCE

We view the clinician's gradual elucidation of the child's transference feelings and perceptions, through playing and talking, as central to such therapeutic goals as greater affect tolerance, increased awareness of mental states, reintegration of disavowed feelings and fantasies about the self in relation to others, and softening of rigid defenses that protect the self from painful relational experience. However, transference work with young children rarely occurs as a thoughtful mutual examination of the child's distant past; rather, it is often indivisible from the therapeutic dyad's here-and-now interactions. In play therapy, transference often appears wrapped into the quickly unfolding action of pretense, requiring that the therapist direct salient remarks to the play characters rather than to the child, discuss transference in terms of imaginary scenarios, and avoid prolonged verbal comments that might detract from their mutual immersion in play. More direct exploration of expectations and feelings that derive from early experience occupies a far less prominent role, particularly in the opening phases of therapy. Over time, however, the child's spontaneous remarks, expressed curiosity about the therapist's personal life, reactions to brief separations such as weekends and vacations, and other responses to the clinician's behaviors and attitudes open up additional opportunities for sensitive but more direct work on the child's transference-based experience.

In the vignette, Kate's spontaneous play represents a maternal object who is distracted and overwhelmed to the point of forgetfulness. Dr. Enright helps her elaborate this experience of self and other: the older children are forgotten and the babies are clearly to blame, the mother is simply overwrought, and the father is safely absent so protected from any responsibility for the chaotic scenario. Together, they name the older children's affects and reflect on their plight. Soon after, Kate's serendipitous early arrival and her naïve cognition (her 5-year-old sense of time) allow transference perceptions to center on Dr. Enright; as a result of their playing relationship, Kate is comfortable enough to express directly her fears that Dr. Enright is another adult who could forget about a small child. Over time, the expression of such perceptions coupled with the therapist's accepting response, and the integration of transference-based representations into play scenarios, will reduce the immediacy of Kate's affective experience and soften the more problematic ways in which she shields herself from interpersonal pain and loss (blaming greedy babies for her mother's distraction; identifying with babyish ways so as to maintain adult involvement).

THE NEW OBJECT RELATIONSHIP

The clinician's function as a new object facilitates emerging mental organizations by providing novel, growth-promoting interpersonal experiences and identifications for the child (Abrams 2003; Chused

1988). The therapist serves developmentally necessary roles that shift with the child's maturation; he or she is perceived at different times by the child as oedipal rival, desired object, or teacher and mentor. Moreover, the child's internalization of the clinician's attitudes and behavior (keen curiosity about mental states, reflectiveness, openness to imaginary play, affect tolerance) provides scaffolding for evolving capacities, such as mentalization and emotional self-regulation, which are essential for engaging developmental tasks. In this way, the therapeutic bond provides a necessary interpersonal framework, which may have been lacking in a child's original attachment relationships, with the potential to redress areas of cognitive-emotional deficit and resolve attachment-based inhibitions in thinking and reflecting (Fonagy and Moran 1991; Fonagy and Target 1996).

Indeed, the therapist's new object functions, including availability, willingness to enter into pretense, attunement to salient affects, and receptivity to projections, are often unique and unprecedented in the child's relational life. Such novelty creates opportunity for gradual modifications in the child's representations of self, other, and self-with-other experience; powerful mutative potential arises from the immediate, unfolding interactions between patient and therapist (Aron 2005; Birch 1997; Crenshaw and Kenney-Noziska 2014; Curtis 2011; Landreth 2012; Miller 2004). The intersubjective realms of therapist and child, as they share play, actions, and language, may be conceptualized as overlapping systems wherein unexpected shifts occur, allowing different self-organizations to arise (Benjamin 2004; Kieffer 2007). Moreover, the therapist's acceptance of roles created and assigned by the child opens a potential space for playing and thinking and provides a shared experience of meaning-making and dawning self-understanding (Bass 2012; Gomberoff 2013; Lyons-Ruth 2006; Slade 1994).

WORKING WITH DEFENSES AND INCREASING THE CHILD'S TOLERANCE FOR AFFECTS

Amelioration of rigid defensive patterns represents a major component of the therapeutic process. However, young children's limited tolerance for uncomfortable affects and their immature capacity for self-regulation shape the way in which therapists can effectively approach these self-protective mechanisms. Internal discomforts, such as guilt and its attendant conflicts, cause considerable anguish, especially in the context of the child's naïve cognition, categorical moral thinking, and fantasies of outsized punishments. The child's difficulty coping with inner tensions may be further exacerbated by the absence of a forgiving, tolerant, and restrained parental environment. Painful feelings often arise in connection with important attachment figures who evoke the child's deepest feelings, needs, and urges; in this way, issues of transference and defense are inextricably linked and arise together in the therapeutic situation. Conflicted feelings about parents and siblings, whom the child loves and depends on but who may also be the target of significant hostility or of unacceptable wishes (e.g., the oedipal child's romantic and possessive desires), can lead to extreme distress. Although the child's defense mechanisms serve the necessary function of maintaining unwanted feelings outside of the child's conscious awareness, such defenses may result in pervasive inhibition, loss of freedom and spontaneity, or widespread avoidance of potentially stimulating situations. In the case of Kate, her threateningly destructive sibling impulses, anger at her mother, desirous urges toward her father, wish to occupy the position of baby in the family, and concomitant fears of adult retaliation for all of the above contribute to a newfound passivity and complete avoidance of a normative developmental achievement—that is, toilet training; her naïve beliefs about procreation and an active fantasy life further reinforce the perceived need to reject the toilet at all costs.

In a therapeutic approach designed by Berta Bornstein (1949) for children in the early phase of latency, the clinician seeks to elaborate the child's defenses against painful affects without exposure of deep, underlying unconscious wishes and urges. The guiding principle of this analytic method—addressing the defensive process rather than focusing on contents of which the patient is completely unaware—is represented in adult psychodynamic treatments as well (e.g., Gray 2005) and aims at achieving an "experience-near" mode of mental exploration, one that collaborates with rather than overrides the individual's ego. The clinician's gradual, sensitive approach to a child's self-protective mechanisms and the emotions they seek to mask, often accomplished through the medium of play characters and scenarios, is well suited to young children's acute vulnerability to guilt, shame, and exposure. Rather than causing the child to feel that the therapist possesses magical abilities to see inside the mind or has invaded the child's privacy and stripped away autonomy and control, play-based defense work often strengthens the alliance by allowing the child to feel understood and by demonstrating via displacement that disturbing feelings can be safely talked about and shared. Making connections between distressing feelings and self-protective behaviors increases the child's tolerance for affective experience, supports mental state knowledge, makes meaning of seemingly incoherent and overwhelming experience, and ultimately improves behavioral self-control (Becker 1974; Bornstein 1951; Hoffman 2007, 2014; Sugarman 2003). Sugarman (2003) questions the value of traditionally defined insight-oriented work for child patients, suggesting that such therapeutic endeavors as making the unconscious conscious, via revealing repudiated contents and urges, impacts young children in an overstimulating, confusing, and distressing manner; he advocates for a process of "insightfulness" wherein the therapist aims to augment the child's natural curiosity about self and others and support the acquisition of mentalization capacities.

In the vignette at the start of this chapter, Dr. Enright carefully selects for emphasis the immediate feelings that cause Kate pain, while leaving aside the child's likely underlying rage, jealousy, and vengeful feelings toward her brother and mother; instead, the therapist focuses her comments on elaborating the frustration and loneliness of older children who must stand by while their mother is fully absorbed by babies' demands. Attempts to interpret murderous fantasies, incestuous desires, or other unconscious contents—even when these appear clearly in children's play scenarios—can threaten or humiliate the child, leading to disruptions in play and further entrenchment of defenses and inhibitions.

MULTIPLE MODES OF DEVELOPMENTAL ASSISTANCE

In work with young children, many of the therapist's behaviors and responses fall outside the realm of clearly defined interventions. Often, the clinician engages the child at whatever level is possible at a moment of affective arousal or avoidance, or employs a variety of means that hold promise for helping the child build and sustain a relationship and establish joint communication. These kinds of efforts are most prominent with children who require direct ego support as a preliminary step or as an ongoing adjunct to play therapy. Children who are easily overwhelmed and overstimulated by affective experience, who are extremely inhibited, who use primarily action-based outlets when they are emotionally aroused, or who lack access to developmentally expected levels of reality testing, language, symbolic play, or social reciprocity are not necessarily well served by more complex verbal interpretations of their defenses and emotional states (Fonagy and Moran 1991; Fonagy and Target 1996; Parks 2007). Ego-enhancing interventions, such as setting limits both verbally and physically, labeling affects that disrupt the therapy while containing the child's behavior, finding opportunities for pretense within sensorimotor activities, building on simplistic pretend schemas, and simply tolerating the child's avoidance and refusals, may be needed to help the child feel secure and discover motivation for sharing personal experience. The therapist's consistency, acceptance, nonthreatening stance, respect for the child's autonomy, and predictability are often key provisions that signal a safe and potentially nurturing environment.

We view the therapist's developmental assistance as an inevitable, ongoing component of the therapeutic process with all young children, including those whose developmental capacities meet or exceed expected ranges. Occasional eruptions of aggressive behavior are extremely common, and may represent a young child's efforts to halt the therapist's thinking and reflecting, or efforts to rid the self of unbearable, negative self-feelings (Fisher 1994; Fonagy and Target 1996). All children require the therapist's active ego support in the following ways (Fonagy and Target 1996; Knight 2003; Neubauer 2001):

- Identifying feelings and containing reactions when uncomfortable contents emerge in play, or when the inevitable frustrations of the therapeutic situation lead to disruption
- Facilitating fantasy, pretense, and narrative building
- Differentiating affective states
- Creating meaningful links between inner experience and outer behavior
- Occasionally setting limits when the child's anxiety, aggression, or exuberance leads to problematic actions

Even the therapist's acts of necessary physical restraint, which signal that nobody will be harmed in the playroom, may represent a form of nonverbal interpretation in which the child's underlying fears of omnipotence and destruction are acknowledged and assuaged (Sugarman 2009).

WORKING WITH PARENTS

Initial and ongoing work with parents represents a major component of therapy and is essential for restoring young children's developmental progress; in Chapter 10, "Working With Parents Over the Course of Treatment," we take up this topic and discuss ways to engage parents, maintain the child's confidentiality while providing parents with useful information, and talk with parents about the value of play and fantasy in their child's emotional life. In psychodynamic child treatments, major benefits of collaborating with parents are conceptualized to include the following: helping them envision the child as a separate, unique individual; assisting them in understanding the developmental needs and pressures of different phases; and facilitating their ability to recognize the impact of their own personal issues, including past relationships and unresolved conflicts, on their here-and-now parenting practices and attitudes.

THE STRUCTURE OF TREATMENT

Within psychoanalytic theory, the **therapeutic frame** represents a set of consistent, reality-based but also symbolically significant routines and practices such as the frequency and schedule of meetings, their duration, payment procedures, confidentiality, and the basic activities in which the patient and therapist engage. In child treatments, the regularity of meetings, including the clinician's predictable ending of sessions even when the child is unwilling to stop playing, any routines that mark the end of the hour (such as putting away toys, or safeguarding constructions in a special bin), and the consistency of the therapist's attitude and availability help to establish a feeling of safety and trust, and to promote the child's sense of affective regulation and containment.

Although psychodynamic psychotherapy may be practiced according to varying frequencies, we feel strongly that young children are best served by at least twice-weekly sessions to establish a sense of consistency, to allow the relationship and the play to deepen, and to offer the child adequate containment and support for the inevitable experiences of intense affect and stimulating contents during play. A number of outcome studies on psychoanalytic and psychodynamic psychotherapies point to the increased efficacy of more frequent and therefore intensive treatment; proposed benefits include the opportunity conferred by multiple weekly meetings to build up a trusting therapeutic relationship and to internalize aspects of the therapist's presence and work, including a tolerant attitude toward affects and a self-reflective posture (Fonagy and Target 1996, 2002; Frosch 2011; Tyson 2009).

SUMMARY

Contemporary ideas about therapeutic action encompass a wide range of verbal and nonverbal, conscious and unconscious processes. These include shared play, which expands the child's emotional resourcefulness; verbal interventions that help name and modulate painful, disavowed affects and mental states; the therapist's role as both a transference object and a new object, available not only to facilitate the revival of prior conflicts but also to provide novel relational experiences and growth-promoting identifications; work with the child's defenses against painful feelings; direct forms of developmental assistance to contain the child's affects; close collaboration with parents; and sufficient frequency of meetings to allow the relationship and the play to deepen.

KEY POINTS

- Contemporary psychodynamic theory posits multiple modes of therapeutic action, including verbal interventions as well as less conscious, implicit aspects of relational experience.

- Play represents the premier mode of therapeutic action in child therapy. Potentially mutative aspects of therapeutic play include the following: organization and modulation of affect-laden experience via language and narrative; use of trial identifications and perspective taking; devising of creative solutions for internal dilemmas; and the mutual experience of co-creating narratives and making meaning of interpersonal events.

- The child–clinician relationship, including the therapist's distinct but interconnected roles as transference, real, and new objects, is inseparable from the processes of therapeutic action. Transference-based work is often conducted through the development and expansion of play scenarios and characters. In their role as a new object, child therapists scaffold emergence of the child's mental organizations; the child internalizes the therapist's availability for play and emotional communication, containment, curiosity, and reflection. In addition, the novelty of the therapist's real attitudes and behaviors—affective openness and tolerance, and immersion in the co-creation of meaningful play scenarios—provides new ways for the child to experience the self and the self in relation to others.

- The therapist seeks to soften rigid defensive patterns that limit the child's flexibility and resourcefulness. Working with young children's defenses involves linking self-protective mechanisms to painful feelings, without undue exposure of unconscious wishes and impulses.

- The therapist serves multiple developmental functions that directly support ego capacities and help the child contain affective experience.

- Working with parents, particularly helping them to reflect on and empathize with the child's unique strengths, vulnerabilities, and developmental needs, is an important component of individual play therapy.

- The frequency of treatment is a significant factor in creating a sense of consistency and containment, deepening the treatment, and allowing the child sufficient opportunity to internalize the therapist's reflective and regulatory functions.

KEY TERMS

Enactment Symbolic patient–therapist interactions that reflect mutual unconscious processes.

Mentalization The capacity to understand mental states of self and others, usually demonstrable by about age 4 years. Within the empirical literature, theory of mind is a closely related concept.

New object relationship A component of the therapeutic relationship in which the child recruits the clinician as an object for identifications that are needed in order to complete developmental tasks.

Therapeutic action   Those therapeutic processes that are thought to contribute to improved psychological functioning.

Therapeutic frame   The regular, consistent structures of treatment including pragmatics, such as scheduling, duration of sessions, and payment, as well as the therapist's and patient's usual interactions, attitudes, and conduct.

●━━━━━━━━━━━━━━━━━●

REFERENCES

Ablon SL: "How can we know the dancer from the dance?" The analysis of a five-year-old girl. Psychoanal Study Child 49:315–327, 1994 7809292

Ablon SL: "Where work is play for mortal stakes": the good hour in child analysis. Psychoanal Study Child 55:113–123, 2000 11338984

Ablon SL: Reply to Blatt and Fonagy. J Am Psychoanal Assoc 53:591–594, 2005

Ablon SL: What child analysis can teach us about psychoanalytic technique. Psychoanal Study Child 68:211–224, 2014 26173335

Abrams S: Therapeutic action and ways of knowing. J Am Psychoanal Assoc 28(2):291–307, 1980 7381168

Abrams S: Looking forwards and backwards. Psychoanal Study Child 58:172–186, 2003 14982020

Abrams S: Transformation: identifying a specific mode of change: descriptive and conceptual considerations. Psychoanal Study Child 63:312–320, 2008 19449800

Abrams S, Solnit AJ: Coordinating developmental and psychoanalytic processes: conceptualizing technique. J Am Psychoanal Assoc 46(1):85–103, 1998 9565900

Aron L: Acceptance, compassion, and an affirmative analytic attitude in both intersubjectivity and compromise formation theory: commentary on a paper by Arnold Rothstein. Psychoanal Dialogues 15(3):433–446, 2005

Bass A: Negotiating otherness: the analyst's contribution to creating new ways of being and relating in the analytic process: commentary on paper by Frank Summers. Psychoanal Dialogues 22(2):162–170, 2012

Becker TE: On latency. Psychoanal Study Child 29:3–11, 1974 4475440

Benjamin J: Beyond doer and done to: an intersubjective view of thirdness. Psychoanal Q 73(1):5–46, 2004 14750464

Bergman A, Harpaz-Rotem I: Revisiting rapprochement in the light of contemporary developmental theories. J Am Psychoanal Assoc 52(2):555–570, 2004 15222461

Birch M: In the land of counterpane: travels in the realm of play. Psychoanal Study Child 52:57–75, 1997 9489461

Blatt S: The patient's contribution to the therapeutic process: a Rogerian and psychodynamic perspective. Psychoanal Psychol 30(2):139–166, 2013

Blatt SJ, Behrends RS: Internalization, separation-individuation, and the nature of therapeutic action. Int J Psychoanal 68(Pt 2):279–297, 1987 3583573

Blum HP: Separation-individuation theory and attachment theory. J Am Psychoanal Assoc 52(2):535–553, 2004 15222460

Bonovitz C: The co-creation of fantasy and the transformation of psychic structure. Psychoanal Dialogues 14(5):553–580, 2004

Bornstein B: The analysis of a phobic child: some problems of theory and technique in child analysis. Psychoanal Study Child 3:181–226, 1949

Bornstein B: On latency. Psychoanal Study Child 6:279–285, 1951

Chused JF: The transference neurosis in child analysis. Psychoanal Study Child 43:51–81, 1988 3227088

Cohen PM, Solnit AJ: Play and therapeutic action. Psychoanal Study Child 48:49–63, 1993 7694307

Crenshaw DA, Kenney-Noziska S: Therapeutic presence in play therapy. International Journal of Play Therapy 23(1):31–43, 2014

Curtis RC: New experiences and meanings: a model of change for psychoanalysis. Psychoanal Psychol 29(1):81–98, 2011

Fisher N: Therapeutic change: a clinical perspective. Psychoanal Inq 14(1):111–127, 1994

Fonagy P, Moran GS: Understanding psychic change in child psychoanalysis. Int J Psychoanal 72(Pt 1):15–22, 1991 2050481

Fonagy P, Target M: Predictors of outcome in child psychoanalysis: a retrospective study of 763 cases at the Anna Freud Centre. J Am Psychoanal Assoc 44(1):27–77, 1996 8717478

Fonagy P, Target M: The history and current status of outcome research at the Anna Freud Centre. Psychoanal Study Child 57:27–60, 2002 12723125

Friedman L: Who needs theory of therapeutic action? Psychoanal Q 76 (suppl):1635–1662, 2007 18286765

Frosch A: The effect of frequency and duration on psychoanalytic outcome: a moment in time. Psychoanal Rev 98(1):11–38, 2011 21466305

Gabbard GO, Westen D: Rethinking therapeutic action. Int J Psychoanal 84(Pt 4):823–841, 2003 13678491

Galatzer-Levy RM: The nuts and bolts of child psychoanalysis. Annual of Psychoanalysis 36:189–202, 2008

Gilmore K: Play in the psychoanalytic setting: ego capacity, ego state, and vehicle for intersubjective exchange. Psychoanal Study Child 60:213–238, 2005 16649681

Gilmore K: Pretend play and development in early childhood (with implications for the oedipal phase). J Am Psychoanal Assoc 59(6):1157–1182, 2011 22080503

Gomberoff E: Playing the game the child allots. Int J Psychoanal 94(1):67–81, 2013 23438985

Gray P: The Ego and Analysis of Defense, 2nd Edition. Northvale, NJ, Jason Aronson, 2005

Harrison AM, Tronick E: "The noise monitor": a developmental perspective on verbal and nonverbal meaning-making in psychoanalysis. J Am Psychoanal Assoc 59(5):961–982, 2011 21980139

Hoffman L: Do children get better when we interpret their defenses against painful feelings? Psychoanal Study Child 62:291–313, 2007 18524096

Hoffman L: Berta Bornstein's "Frankie": the contemporary relevance of a classic to the treatment of children with disruptive symptoms. Psychoanal Study Child 68:152–176, 2014 26173332

Kieffer CC: Emergence and the analytic third: working at the edge of chaos. Psychoanal Dialogues 17(5):683–703, 2007

Knight R: Margo and me, II: the role of narrative building in child analytic technique. Psychoanal Study Child 58:133–164, 2003 14982018

Krimendahl EK: Metaphor in child psychoanalysis: not simply a means to an end. Contemp Psychoanal 34(1):49–66, 1998

Landreth GL: Play Therapy: The Art of the Relationship, 3rd Edition. New York, Routledge, 2012

Litowitz BE: From dyad to dialogue: language and the early relationship in American psychoanalytic theory. J Am Psychoanal Assoc 59(3):483–507, 2011 21652513

Loewald HW: On the therapeutic action of psycho-analysis. Int J Psychoanal 41:16–33, 1960 14417912

Lyons-Ruth K: Play, precariousness and the negotiation of meaning. J Infant Child Adolesc Psychother 5(2):142–159, 2006

Mahon E: A "good hour" in child analysis and adult analysis. Psychoanal Study Child 55:124–142, 2000 11338985

Mayes LC, Cohen DJ: Playing and therapeutic action in child analysis. Int J Psychoanal 74(Pt 6):1235–1244, 1993 8138367

Michels R: The theory of therapeutic action. Psychoanal Q 76(suppl):1725–1733, 2007 18286769

Miller ML: Dynamic systems and the therapeutic action of the analyst, II: clinical application and illustrations. Psychoanal Psychol 21(1):54–69, 2004

Molinari E: From one room to the other: a story of contamination: the relationship between child and adult analysis. Int J Psychoanal 92(4):791–810, 2011 21843236

Nelson K: Emergence of the historical self, in Language in Cognitive Development: The Emergence of the Mediated Mind. New York, Cambridge University Press, 1996, pp 152–182

Neubauer PB: The role of displacement in psychoanalysis. Psychoanal Study Child 49:107–119, 1994 7809278

Neubauer PB: Some observations about changes in technique in child analysis. Psychoanal Study Child 56:16–26, 2001 12102011

Parks CE: Psychoanalytic approaches to work with children with severe developmental and biological disorders. Panel report. J Am Psychoanal Assoc 55(3):923–935, 2007 17915652

Rizzuto AM: Psychoanalysis: the transformation of the subject by the spoken word. Psychoanal Q 72(2):287–323, 2003 12718247

Rose C: Catching the ball: the role of play in psychoanalytic treatment. J Am Psychoanal Assoc 50(4):1299–1309, 2002 12580333

Rosegrant J: The psychoanalytic play state. J Clin Psychoanal 10:323–343, 2001

Sales JM, Fivush R: Social and emotional functions of mother-child reminiscing about stressful events. Soc Cogn 23(1):70–90, 2005

Slade A: Making meaning and making believe: their role in the clinical process, in Children at Play: Clinical and Developmental Approaches to Meaning and Representation. Edited by Slade A, Wolfe DP. New York, Oxford University Press, 1994, pp 81–107

Stern DN, Sander LW, Nahum JP, et al: Non-interpretive mechanisms in psychoanalytic therapy: the "something more" than interpretation. Int J Psychoanal 79(Pt 5):903–921, 1998 9871830

Sugarman A: A new model for conceptualizing insightfulness in the psychoanalysis of young children. Psychoanal Q 72(2):325–355, 2003 12718248

Sugarman A: The contribution of the analyst's actions to mutative action: a developmental perspective. Psychoanal Study Child 64:247–272, 2009 20578441

Tyson P: Child development and child psychoanalysis: research and education. J Am Psychoanal Assoc 57(4):871–879, 2009 19724068

Vivona JM: Is there a nonverbal period of development? J Am Psychoanal Assoc 60(2):231–265, discussion 305–310, 2012 22467444

Warshaw SC: Mutative factors in child psychoanalysis: a comparison of diverse relational factors. J Infant Child Adolesc Psychother 14(4):387–405, 2015

Winnicott DW: Playing and Reality. London, Tavistock, 1971

7

Play and Developmental Psychopathology, Deprivation, or Disability

OVERVIEW

Despite some controversy about play's developmental function, there is no doubt that play forms evolve with a child's emerging ego capacities. As each play form arises, it signals the acquisition of new cognitive, affective, socioemotional, and linguistic abilities, and arguably serves to exercise those abilities on a regular basis, facilitating their developmental evolution. Symbolic or pretend play, the premiere play form for play therapy, arises in tandem—and in dynamic concert—with important milestones in normal development: symbolic capacity, burgeoning language, expanded range of emotions (including ambivalence and guilt), evolving self-regulation, theory of mind, and a leap forward in the nature of object relations. To the extent that these milestones are affected by developmental delay, deprivation, environmental failure, or emerging psychopathology, the child's progressive development of the capacity to engage in symbolic play and other play forms is similarly impacted, derailed, slowed, or aborted. This is the basis for the use of play in a range of diagnostic measures, both clinically and in research protocols. Moreover, given that play is considered a facilitator of developmental progression, the characterization and treatment of play disturbance is an implicit goal in play therapy. In this chapter, we consider the interface between play and psychopathology, both in general and in regard to some specific diagnostic entities.

CORRELATIONS

As discussed in Chapters 2, "Play, Playfulness, and the Sequence of Play Forms in Development," and 3, "Pretend Play," whether or not play is considered a causal factor or is simply associated with developmental achievements, normal play follows a reliable progression as development proceeds through childhood and adolescence. Play forms that emerge later in adolescence and adulthood tend to be specialized according to the interests, capacities, and opportunities of the individual. Of course, play is always somewhat idiosyncratic in content, and even its unfolding forms show nuances that reflect the child's capacities and environmental provision. Regardless of the degree to which symbolic play provides practice, deepening, or evolution of emergent capacities such as self-regulation, mentalization, and differentiation of psychic and consensual reality (Tessier et al. 2016), symbolic play seems to arise and depend for expression on their intertwined developmental progression: a child's play is enriched by differentiation of emotions and tolerance of their intensity, stable and maturing defenses, adaptive strivings, nuances of relationships, sustained narratives, creative compromises, and so on. Similarly, all these emergent capacities are elaborated and consolidated by play.

Childhood disorders as depicted in DSM-5 (American Psychiatric Association 2013) are constructs derived from contemporary developmental psychopathology (Wicks-Nelson and Israel 2014), a model in ascendance since the 1970s. This is an interdisciplinary, multisystems approach (Cicchetti and Toth 2009) that considers psychopathology as disorders of developmental processes that are themselves complex systems with contributions from biology, genetics, psychology, family, epidemiology, culture, and society. From this perspective, developmental outcomes are manifestations of the nonlinear pathways and developmental cascades (Bornstein et al. 2010) produced by the interface of multiple influences and driven by maturation, whose adaptive success is measured according to the standards of a given culture and society. DSM-5, while still influenced by the polythetic dichotomous approach that was introduced with DSM-III (American Psychiatric Association 1980), is heavily informed by the notion of spectrum disorders rather than discrete entities (Regier et al. 2013; Shapiro 2009) and incorporates the dimensional-hierarchical scheme of behavioral adjustment initially proposed by Thomas Achenbach, the originator of the Child Behavior Checklist (Achenbach 1991), with the broadband categories of **externalizing and internalizing disorders** (Tackett 2010). The predictive power of these categories, their overlap or differentiation, and their consistency or patterned transformation over the course of development are all subject to ongoing scholarly debate (see Hink et al. 2013; Stone et al. 2015; Vachon and Krueger 2015).

Play capacity is mentioned as an aspect of DSM-5 diagnostic criteria for a number of childhood diagnoses in which its marked deviation from standard progression—whether by virtue of form, content, or timing—may be pathognomonic or at least strongly indicative of a particular disorder. The designated disorders can be divided into a few groups: the neurodevelopmental disorders, which deform development from the earliest months of life; the trauma-related disorders that interrupt a presumably typical premorbid developmental trajectory; and the particular entity of gender dysphoria, which cannot be readily placed in either category.

Even though highlighted in only two neurodevelopmental disorders—namely, attention-deficit/hyperactivity disorder (ADHD) and autism spectrum disorder (ASD)—almost all disorders in this diagnostic set show impairments in some form of play. These diagnoses are understood to have a more or less well characterized neurobiological substrate (Singletary 2015) that, from the earliest months of life, affect very young children's inborn responsiveness to environmental nutriment and readiness for playful engagement. Such interferences produce a cascade of impairments in the sequential emergence and consolidation of ego capacities that both support and are enriched by subsequent play, including language, cognitive development, capacity for theory of mind, and so on. The same capacities are, of course, the building blocks for object relations, interests and goals, emotional self-regulation, and educational progression.

In contrast, posttraumatic disorders occur in presumably normally developing children, although there are hypothesized premorbid characteristics that are more or less protective; resiliency is a factor, not yet fully characterized, that is postulated to modulate the impact of catastrophic events on personality development. Finally among the diagnoses highlighted in DSM-5 with play symptoms, gender dysphoria is unique because ego capacities are intact or advanced, play forms unfold as expected, but play content is heavily shaped by the child's gender feelings that contradict natal gender.

Even though an effect on play is not included in criteria for all types of childhood psychopathology, child clinicians regularly assess play as part of a comprehensive evaluation to characterize the child's level of development, the impact of the presenting problem on emerging capacities, the environmental impingements, plus mental representations, object relations, and core conflicts. Play is widely regarded as an indication of diagnostic severity, because its absence, curtailment, immaturity, or blocked progression leaves children without a vital righting mechanism and speaks to the degree to which their developmental movement is arrested, their resilience limited, and their capacity for pleasure diminished. Many psychodynamic clinicians believe that the level of play is a strong indicator of a child's current adaptation; similarly, play plasticity and progression over time are signs of the current and future potential benefits of treatment (Chazan et al. 2016; Tessier et al. 2016).

An early goal of treatment with the child who cannot play or whose play is constrained or fragmented by severe psychopathology is to foster play and help the child to find both meaning and enjoyment in playing (Gilmore 2005; Slade 1994); play is the way children make sense of experience and make thoughts thinkable (Bion 1962, discussed in Alvarez 1993). As children are more willing and able to show their inner world by entering a playing state with their therapists, they provide the medium where change happens; a child who develops the capacity to play with joy, narrative coherence, adaptive defenses, plot climax, and resolution in the course of play therapy (Main 1993) has been "restored to the path of normal development" (Anna Freud, quoted in Neubauer 1990, p. 112). The correlation between play and psychopathology, either as diagnostic criteria or as auxiliary evidence, has made play observation an intrinsic component of clinical and research assessments. Moreover, because play is understood by dynamic clinicians to be the language of childhood, far more revealing than a so-called grown-up interview (Birch 1997), play is valued as a window into the child's mind.

ASSESSMENT MEASURES

Many child specialists have proposed chronological taxonomies of play, because it is widely viewed as a reliable gauge of children's development and developmental deviation (Casby 2003). A number of instruments have been designed specifically to assess play as a developmental marker and/or as an indicator of therapeutic change. These include the Children's Play Therapy Instrument (CPTI; Kernberg PF, Chazan SE, Normandin L: "The Children's Play Therapy Instrument: Manual and Scale," unpublished paper, 1997; Kernberg et al. 1998), the Children's Developmental Play Instrument (CDPI; Chazan et al. 2016), and the Test of Pretend Play (ToPP; Lewis and Boucher 1997, 1998). The CPTI, developed by Kernberg and her colleagues, was designed to examine the impact of treatment on various play components, whereas its derivative, the CDPI (Chazan 2009, 2012; Chazan et al. 2016), was modified to assess the evolution of play in developmental progression. These instruments are based on the premise that pretend play serves as a representation of ego capacities, unconscious fantasy, core conflicts, interpersonal relationships, coping/defense mechanisms, and overall adaptation. Developmental and/or psychotherapeutic changes have been shown to be reliably reflected in performance on the measures when repeated over time (Chazan and Wolf 2002; Chazan et al. 2016). With both nonclinical and clinical populations, these instruments can signal progression, improvement, or deterioration. Unlike symptom checklists and other therapy assessment tools (e.g., the Child Psychotherapy Q-Set [Schneider et al. 2010]), the CPTI and CDPI focus exclusively on play, because, according to their developers, play provides the best picture of the child's mind and current state, as well as the meanings of his or her behavior in overall psychic organization.

The CPTI first documents the actual time spent playing compared with setting-up or other activities, and then uses a dimensional analysis, elucidating the structure of the play narrative—its affective, cognitive, dynamic, and development components—and its continuity over time (see outline in Appendix A at the end of this book). This dimensional format allows the observer to tease out and focus on a multiplicity of play elements that together indicate the degree of interference and conflict; the capacity to experience pleasure; the complex ability to construct coherent narratives; and the creative and collaborative use of toys, props, and other people to realize the play agenda. Children in therapy are categorized in clusters by virtue of their coping and defensive strategies as illuminated in the play segments; these clusters are adaptive, conflicted, polarized (rigid), and extreme anxiety. The CPTI underscores the value of the play analysis for diagnosis, assessment of current level of psychic functioning, and change over the course of treatment. It offers a useful frame for describing play in a standardized format so that it can be characterized in relation to psychopathology.

The CDPI, derived from the CPTI, yields a hierarchical typology of play styles that are considered state variables and not persistent differences between children. The categorization is intended to highlight the child's use of play as an expression of his or her experience of self and others at the moment of observation. Categories include the following play styles: adaptive, impulsive, conflicted/inhibited, and disorganized. Children may manifest more than one style within even a relatively brief sample. With trained observers, this measure has good reliability and can serve to document change in development and/or treatment. One other observational element is included, one that recurs throughout the literature as an important aspect of the capacity to play: that is, the child's own grasp of being in the pretend mode and its differentiation from consensual reality. In other words, scholars note the importance of children's awareness that they are playing (Chazan et al. 2016; Hobson et al. 2013).

The ToPP focuses on solitary play rather than play in interaction. This is an important distinction that is often not clearly isolated in literature examining play capacity in various populations. Most children play "better," by virtue of either imitation or enhancement, when playing with another person, especially an older peer or adult; this is captured in Vygotsky's (1978) famous phase: when playing, the child is a "head taller than himself" (p. 102). The ToPP measures three aspects of pretending: "the ability to substitute one object for another object or person, attribute an imagined property to an object or person, and make reference to an absent object, person or substance" (Hobson et al. 2013, p. 118). Thus, it closely examines the metarepresentational and symbolized process of pretending.

A few scales measuring **playfulness** have been developed in related disciplines, such as leisure studies and occupational therapies, originally in regard to children (Barnett and Fiscella 1985; Bundy et al. 2001) and subsequently applied to adults (Barnett 2007): these are

Barnett's (1990) Children's Playfulness Test (CPT) and Bundy et al.'s (2001) Test of Playfulness (ToP; see Appendix A at the end of this book). The constructs behind these instruments are slightly different from each other, as the ToP attempts to measure a "stable personality trait that expresses itself as a disposition to engage in play" (Muys et al. 2006, p. 160), whereas the Children's Playfulness Scale (CPS) uses descriptors, such as spontaneity, manifest joy, and sense of humor. There have been a number of conceptual problems with the scales (e.g., the failure to differentiate between environmental settings) and spotty correlations between them, but they continue to be refined and used to assess clinical populations. For example, the ToP has been a useful measure in understanding the play impact of autism (Muys et al. 2006) and attention-deficit/hyperactivity disorder (ADHD) (Leipold and Bundy 2000).

PLAY FORM AND CONTENT

Despite consistent developmental progression, a child's particular play themes and style always retain their unique and idiosyncratic elements, since play is a multiply determined activity that expresses a host of contributions from reality factors—family circumstances, culture, siblings, friends, school, and so on—and psychological factors—internal conflicts, oedipal constellation, defenses, object relations, drive endowment, superego development, and constitution. In previous chapters in this book, we illustrated the many layers of meaning that can be discerned in play and used in play therapy, such as the child's approach to treatment and the evolving relationship with the clinician, the child's capacity and motivation to play, the degree to which the play is spontaneous and expressive, the characteristic use of the therapist as playing partner, the central conflicts, the defenses employed, and self-regulation in the context of intense affects and impulses. Play is almost always a unique production wrought out of all these elements, but psychopathology similarly always finds an avenue for expression in play—by virtue of its impact on psychological, cognitive, and environmental elements. Because the child is in developmental process, it is often possible to observe and address the infiltration of psychopathology into emerging ego capacities and its effect on how the child meets new environmental demands from home and school, new requirements of relationships, and new expectations of self-regulation and control.

As noted earlier, gender dysphoria is a special case because ego capacities emerge as expected and these usually do not figure in parents'
reasons for seeking evaluation. Instead, the parents' focus is on the
child's gender-related behaviors, attitudes, and preferences that are dis-
cordant with natal gender. These are also the factors that impact play,
since it is one of very few arenas where the child's gender choices can be
freely expressed and exercised; opposite sex colors, clothing, leisure activities, and toys (as defined within a given culture) are readily observable in play roles and narratives, drawing attention to the child's state of
mind. Historically, many parents, family members, peers, and teachers
put pressure on such children to conform, compounding their feelings
of "difference" and even ostracism. Nonetheless, while gender dysphoric children may experience more or less external strife, internal
distress, and dissatisfaction about their bodies (Saketopoulou 2014), it
is usually their predilections and the **content** of their play, not their
emotional state, that are the immediate precipitants for consultation.

In this chapter, we discuss ASD and ADHD, and one traumatic syndrome, PTSD, in depth. It should be noted that, while not delineated
in DSM, intellectual disability, sensory impairments, and obsessive-compulsive disorder, among others, are syndromes also associated with
variants of symptomatic play showing both unique and common features—stereotypies, blunted play narratives, arrested progression, play
interruptions due to anxiety or other states, and so on. Depending on severity of the syndrome and the age at onset, affected children are often
blocked at the threshold of symbolic play: functional play is present but
does not evolve to the next step—that is, the child does not take the leap
of imagination and freedom of expression that "projects a supposed situation onto an actual one, in the spirit of fun" (Lillard 1993, p. 349).
For psychodynamic thinkers, this moment of arrest has broader significance still, since it is understood as an interruption in the development of *semiotic* capacity, which is vital for language, symbolic play,
autobiographical themes, trial identifications, theory of mind, and the
deepening understanding of emotion. Beginning around age 3 years,
the child is undergoing a quantum shift in mental organization as new
capacities emerge and a new agency, the superego, consolidates. Access
to pretending (or the *pretend mode*) helps children to master the powerful emotions of the oedipal phase; the child can "use signs for thinking and communicating thoughts and feelings" (Salomonsson 2011,

p. 91), begins to understand subjectivity of self and others, and gradually assumes the job of self-regulation. Symbolic play—with its narrative themes, complications, and resolution—provides the arena in which oedipal dynamics are expressed, signaling the capacity to grapple with triadic relationships, to bear ambivalence and guilt, to find ways to regulate the intense affects of this highly emotional phase of development, and to begin a long process of identifications and self-representation (Gilmore 2011). Children who stop short of this developmental step are handicapped further by the loss of the arena in which they can grapple with their conflicts and challenges on a smaller canvas, and within their control. To make matters worse, children with chronic and severe disorders cannot easily be drawn into the play of others because of their lack of *playfulness* or *playful disposition*, a capacity that allows them to protect their narcissism and feel a sense of agency. Some studies of children with these disorders suggest that lack of symbolic play is not necessarily a question of a globally failed developmental capacity, but rather a failure to spontaneously and playfully initiate and draw together the component capacities (Jarrold 2003; Rutherford and Rogers 2003), such as narrative development, creative compromise, and theory of mind, and a consequent failure to elicit environmental reinforcement and scaffolding that support the evolution of playing and its benefits.

AUTISM SPECTRUM DISORDERS

Emma was referred to Dr. Abraham just before her seventh birthday by a local special education school, because she seemed visibly depressed after her teacher took a maternity leave. She had been diagnosed at the high-functioning end of the autism spectrum (which, at the time of consultation in the mid-1990s, was referred to as Asperger's syndrome) at age 3, when her parents first sought an expert opinion to better understand Emma's poor eye contact, resistance to physical affection, and adamant dislike of doll or action figure play. In contrast to these deficits, she possessed an uncanny visuospatial ability, easily putting together 500-piece puzzles without noticing or using the picture of the completed puzzle. A neuropsychological evaluation at age 4, just before the birth of her brother, documented superior intellectual endowment, expressive language weakness, impaired executive capacities and motor planning, and extremely limited play. She received services including occupational therapy and social skills group therapy.

When Emma arrived for the first assessment session at age 6 years 8 months, she carefully and deliberately made eye contact with Dr. Abraham, who noted silently how hard it seemed for her. She came in the playroom readily, acknowledging her familiarity with therapy, and took in the room; then she announced without ceremony that she wanted to make something. She seemed preoccupied with creative ideas that she attributed to an older girl at school, and wanted to emulate her projects. It was clear that Emma was trying to make things that were too hard to construct out of the materials at hand, such as a bathtub and bathmat out of pipe cleaners; she did not avail herself of the toy objects available to create the bathroom scene and left feeling dissatisfied and self-critical without having ever played. Dr. Abraham told Emma's parents that although she had a feeling that Emma might benefit from play therapy, she would need an extended evaluation period to have more confidence in the recommendation. Dr. Abraham was encouraged by the following: Emma had shown her capacity to make use of other kinds of intervention, retaining her gains. She was verbal and openly manifesting depressive affect and thinking. Her recent decline coincided with the loss of a beloved teacher, suggesting her capacity to make attachments. Her parents reported that she was eager to play at home, raising the expectation that she would be able to bring play into her interaction with Dr. Abraham.

In the first several weeks of the assessment, Emma continued to construct things and played rarely. Occasionally, she brought in her Furby (a furry electronic pet that "learned" to talk through interaction with its owner) and put it out of sight even though it was calling for attention, wailing "Hungry, hungry!"

At about the 6-month mark, Emma began to explore the toys in the closet, and played rather monotonously with a collection of stuffed, bear-like figures from a toddler's television show, *Teletubbies*. She played out little scenes with the Teletubbies, with a slightly mocking and disparaging tone. Dr. Abraham had been told by Emma's parents that she had a history of "hating" stuffed animals and also Barbie dolls; she gave away all such figurative toys immediately if she received them as gifts. However, when she finally noticed a collection of Skipper dolls (Skipper is marketed as Barbie's little sister; she is clearly pubertal but slightly smaller and less developed than the classic Barbie) in the toy closet, she decided that she would assign each Teletubby its own Skipper, whom she designated a "dollple," meaning "something like people and something like a doll." This scenario, with an "owner" who owned and trained a lesser creature, a Skipper, to fight, bore a strong resemblance to her own favorite television show, *Pokémon*, in which Pokémon trainers prepare their Pokémon for sportlike contests. Unlike the Pokémon creatures, who battle by using their special powers, the competition in Emma's play centered on distinctly "girly" objectives: the dollples vied with each other about who was the best—the smartest, the prettiest, the best dresser. While playing out these contests with Emma, Dr. Abraham was invariably given the losing trainer-Skip-per pair to enact: she was instructed to express her Skipper's insatiable enviousness and despondency and to express the anger and disap-pointment of the manager, the foolish Teletubby Dipsy. Dr. Abraham observed to Emma what a relief it was to have a dollple who could al-ways be the loser and who had to take all the blame. She also wondered aloud about the idea of the dollple, something like a Furby, a kind of robot person but in Emma's game having all the bothersome and un-lovable feelings, while Dipsey was able to vent his relentless criticism and even overt aggression as if they were harmless. Very soon, the Tele-tubbies dropped away as if forgotten and the dollples became the main protagonists of the play, losing their humanoid designation. In the first story that emerged of their own, they not only competed about who was better but also had a rivalrous struggle for a boyfriend. In both dyadic and triadic configurations. Dr. Abraham became increas-ingly aware of the intense hostility and even cruelty of the rivals.

Emma is clearly on the high-functioning end of the autism spectrum; her play did have an element of pretending but was undeveloped and dis-avowed as babyish. Dr. Abraham was initially discouraged by the re-petitive and even boring interactions among the Teletubbies, but began to discern a glimmer of meaning in Emma's mockery of the babyish television show; this was a little girl who was contending with her jeal-ousy of a baby brother by demonstrating haughtiness and superiority. Emma was also showing how her characters used others, the robotic doll-ples, as objects or add-ons without recognition of their inner experi-ence (which a dollple is unlikely to have). Through Dr. Abraham's patient and tactful introduction of the Skippers' emotions, she implied that the dolls were not empty and that their thoughts and feelings differed from those of the Teletubbies (Rhode 2012). This process gradually served to advance the play into a more complex narrative line after a full year of play therapy. The harshness and sadism that emerged in Emma's play is a familiar feature in the play of verbal children on the autism spec-trum[1]; in our opinion, this play reflects a condensation of the highly

---

[1]Krass M: "Bullies and Bad Guys." Paper delivered at American Psychoana-lytic Association Scientific Meeting, January 2015; Gilmore K: Unpublished discussion of M. Krass's paper "Bullies and Bad Guys." Presented at Ameri-can Psychoanalytic Association Scientific Meeting, January 2015.

distorted parental objects (experienced as overstimulating, rejecting, demanding) and the child's own aggression.

With the publication of DSM-5 (American Psychiatric Association 2013), Asperger's disorder was subsumed into the broader autism spectrum concept, and diagnostic criteria for ASDs were expanded to encompass severe to mild (formerly Asperger's disorder) presentations while simultaneously streamlined from the DSM-IV "autistic triad" (deficits in social skills, deficits in communication, restricted and repetitive behaviors and interests; American Psychiatric Association 1994) to two behavior clusters (deficits in social communication and restricted behaviors) (Durand 2014). The latter category includes the famously distinctive disturbances in play alternately described in DSM-5 (p. 56) as "odd play patterns" or as "odd and repetitive behaviors" in the absence of play. These behaviors can incorporate "toys" but manifest as object fixations, repetitive actions without elaboration, and/or rigidly patterned and unchanging "play." Although not explicitly named in DSM-5, the failure to use toys symbolically figures prominently in other autism-focused diagnostic systems, such as the Autism Diagnostic Observation Schedule and Autism Diagnostic Interview (Lord et al. 2000). These features resonate with Kanner's remarkably prescient original publication in 1943 (Kanner 1943; Volkmar and McPartland 2014) in which he described 11 autistic children. In addition to noting motor stereotypies and repetitive actions, Kanner observed the children's devotion to objects over people and documented their monotonously "functional" play, without symbolic elaboration: turning light switches on and off, scribbling with a pencil, holding a telephone receiver to one's ear, and disconnecting and reconnecting the cars of a toy train. Even very high-functioning children with ASD, such as Emma, show some elements of these play disturbances.

Autism has generated a vast body of theory and multifaceted research into its origins, neuropsychiatric underpinnings, and psychology. Theories about the etiology of the disorder have come in and out of fashion since Kanner's (1943) paper, beginning with his description of the environmental impact of the refrigerator mother (which he recanted subsequently) to a delineation of neurocognitive defects affecting language and socialization and then back to disturbances in early attachments (Voran 2013). A majority of theorists in psychoanalysis and developmental science concur that it is "[t]ime to give up on a single explanation for autism," as recommended over a decade ago (Happé et al. 2006), and consider a multifactorial process that acknowledges the role of neuropsychiatric endowment *and* environment in the crucial interactions between parent and infant beginning in the first months of life.

Like other neurodevelopmental disorders, the autistic syndrome affects almost every aspect of the infant's interactions with other humans from birth, directly impeding the evolution of emerging ego capacities that both require and ensure ongoing environmental nutriment. These include mutual eye contact (Baron-Cohen et al. 1997), early attachment security, joint attention, social referencing, language, theory of mind, complex object relations, diversification of emotion, emotional self-regulation, and so on. The typical history of an unresponsive baby and of a mother who despairs of making contact sets off a cascade of self-perpetuating failed interactions that undermine attachment and communication from birth.

Contemporary psychodynamically inclined approaches to ASD are variations on this theme; they all emphasize the absence of playfulness and the importance of introducing a playing element in mother-infant and/or therapist–child exchanges. A prominent example comes from Stanley Greenspan (2007), who developed the Development, Individual-difference, Relationship-based (DIR) model and treatment approach based on the developmentally crucial cyclical interaction of infant and caretaker. His affect diathesis hypothesis suggests that pre-autistic infants are biologically challenged such that the parent–infant interaction fails to "co-regulate affective signaling" (Greenspan 2007, p. 200), referring to the connection of affects to sensory experience and motor discharge. The critical connection of sensory affect to motor experience that underpins intentionality and pleasurable activity does not evolve. For example, the perception of the mother's approach is usually associated with joy and the production of directed movements: turning the head, kicking the legs in synchrony, and excited vocalizations. Without the link of affect (joy) with sensory experience (auditory and visual perception of mother's approach), the infant's actions do not accrue intention (greeting mother). The mother, not receiving the expected enthusiastic, happy display, does not add on her own affective displays, such as using marked affect and motherese to show her reciprocal excitement, perhaps even including a plush toy puppy as a special guest in the exchange. The absence of this kind of developmental sequence impedes the evolution of meaningful sustained interactions and the development of symbolic function. Of note is that Greenspan's recommendation for treatment, the DIR model, uses *heightened pleasurable affect* to elicit meaningful behavior and engagement.[2] The method, as illustrated in his examples, involves the insertion and augmentation of affective associations, mostly through a playful addition or intensification of emotion, in order to interrupt stereotypies and engage the child; with younger children, the mother is continuously engaged in this process and extends it into daily life to draw the child forward. This is similar to the approach proposed by Sherkow (2011; Sherkow and Harrison 2013) which attempts to find meaning—to "make sense out of nonsense" (Bergman 2007, quoted in Sherkow 2011, p. 253)—in the disorganized or regimented actions of the autistic child, to translate for the mother, and to step up the activity into a playful interaction.

William Singletary (2015), another psychodynamic theorist, presents a slightly different understanding and approach to autism, although his synthesis is similarly based on the interface between infant neurobiological equipment and parental ministrations, and on the importance of reducing allostatic stress and stimulus deprivation by playfulness and expressive play. He incorporates and integrates two theories about autism: the **social motivation hypothesis** and the **excessive fear (intense world) hypothesis**. Both of these hypotheses arrive at a common recognition of the sense of environmental deprivation and aloneness that characterizes autistic children. The social motivation hypothesis suggests that a heritable neurobiological substrate creates vulnerability in the infant, impairing the capacity to engage with the caretaking environment; this, in turn, drives "maladaptive neuroplasticity," leading to the functional impairments that create the syndrome (Singletary

---

[2]He notes that heightened negative affective experience can also lead to the meaningful behavior of avoidance, but clearly this precludes further exchanges; moreover, negative intensity has a disorganizing effect on the infant's nascent capacity to develop a coherent mental representation of this experience. Recurrent reliance on avoidance, due to aversive exchanges with the environment early in life, precludes the use of the caretaker for self-regulatory support and consolidation (Greenspan 2007; Greenspan and Shanker 2004).

2015, p. 84). Such impairments further reproduce the experience of environmental deprivation; a vicious cycle ensues with disastrous effects on ongoing development. The excessive fear hypothesis suggests that problematic neurobiological endowment makes the experience of the environment equivalent to overwhelming sensory overload and stress, equivalent to a sensory assault. Such a response to the environment, even a benign one, leads to withdrawal and avoidance of social interactions, impeding or preventing the development of the social brain. Because the environment is felt to be so overwhelming, the child must retreat; paradoxically, the terrifying overstimulating world compels the child's withdrawal and ultimately produces the experience of environmental deprivation. These conditions give rise to a child who is imprisoned and isolated. Because the preautistic child is intolerant of joyful mother–infant exchanges, with their intense eye-to-eye contact and exaggerated affect, the infant loses precious moments of interpersonal and intrapsychic development that blossom in these same interactions: the evolution of playfulness, the experience of maternal attunement and state modulation, reciprocity, pleasure in relationships, and confidence in maternal ministrations.

A number of well-researched studies directly addressing play in the autistic child highlight the autistic impairment in imagination and pretend play (Jarrold 2003) and attempt to understand its dynamic relationship to the characteristic "behavioral manifestations of autism" (p. 379). In general, these studies aim to identify and characterize underlying cognitive defects that affect the play of autistic children, without attempting to postulate a primary etiological theory. A number of propositions have been generated by these investigations: that symbolic play in the child with autism is 1) delayed so that it appears much later than in a normally developing child; 2) deficient due to a disturbance of the "interpersonal intersubjective engagement" (Hobson et al. 2013, p. 115) that begins at birth and is the wellspring of empathy, joint attention, and play; 3) due to a problem of internalization such that the child cannot generalize or play alone, but is dependent on continuous scaffolding or prompting; 4) due to a cognitive limitation of **metarepresentation** (and implicitly language); and 5) due to a problem of generativity, motivation, or playful disposition (Charman and Baron-Cohen 1997; Hobson et al. 2013). Many researchers approaching autism through play observe the overall absence of playful pretense in autistic subjects (Hobson 2012), which in turn is understood as a lack of playful and gratifying interpersonal communication.

SYMBOLIC CAPACITY

Delay or impairment in symbolization has been studied as the major determinant of the late acquisition of language and emergence of pretense in autistic children. Many researchers have observed late-appearing language and some form of pretend play in high-functioning autistic children, although their pretending is clearly different from that of typically developing control subjects (Charman and Baron-Cohen 1997). However, studies attempting to isolate the missing feature of pretense have yielded some contradictory findings. Some results indicate that when matched with controls at the same intellectual level, autistic children do not actually produce fewer symbolic play acts; they can learn to symbolize at a comparable level and are able to go beyond functional play in structured settings (Sherratt 2002; Thiemann-Bourque et al. 2012). There is also evidence that autistic children can comprehend pretend acts (Jarrold et al. 1994). On the other hand, even when symbolic acts increase in autistic children "trained" in symbolic play, the real assimilation of an open-ended style, the generalization of "learned" symbolic playing, and especially the augmentation of the normal disposition to play (i.e., playfulness) have not been convincingly demonstrated to persist in daily life (Luckett et al. 2007; Sherratt 2002).

METAREPRESENTATION

Another conceptual approach to the lack of pretend play in children with autism grew from an idea proposed by Alan Leslie (1987) that both pretend play and theory of mind depend on a common underlying "cognitive metarepresentational capacity" (Rutherford et al. 2007, p. 1025). The ability to "represent another's representation"—that is, to simultaneously maintain two representations—is fundamental to understanding mental states and to symbolic play. This capacity originates well before it is testable in the classic **false-belief test**; it is understood to be present in nascent form in **joint attention** and can be discerned in the infant's early recognition that the mother is playing when, with marked affect, she launches into peek-a-boo or a pretend wail. It is also presumed to be present in the **visual cliff**, a test for **social referencing**, when the child reads the mother's facial expression as a signal of danger or safety. Despite their differences, the concepts of "mind blindness," deficits in the development of empathy (Baron-Cohen 1988, 2004), and failure to achieve mentalization (Fonagy and Target 1996a, 2000) all incorporate the idea of metarepresentation.

EMPATHY

Some experts suggest that impairments in empathy and joint attention reflect underlying deficits in imitation of, attention to, and identification with emotional displays of others in infants identified as at risk for autism (Charman et al. 1997). These children famously avoid eye contact (Klin et al. 2009) and do not seem to register other people's expressed distress or other emotional states. They cannot easily read facial expressions (Welchew et al. 2005) and tend to avoid looking at faces in general (Chawarska et al. 2010). All of these deficits bear a relationship—whether causal or correlated—to the impaired mother–infant connection and subsequent social difficulties. There is evidence that empathy has neural correlates in the "social brain"—that is, "a neuronal system whose design has evolved to…enable its possessor to interpret information about other individuals" (Brothers 1990/2002, p. 379); supporting studies show neurological impairments in this region in autistic individuals (Baron-Cohen 2004). Cognitively, empathy is understood to involve two major elements: "(1) the ability to attribute mental states to oneself and others, as a natural way to make sense of agents, and (2) having an emotional reaction that is appropriate to the other person's mental state (such as sympathy)" (Baron-Cohen 2004, p. 945). *Empathy* is the umbrella term that incorporates affect perception, theory of mind, and the "intentional stance." It is an important contribution to all the features of play—the understanding of perspectives and different subjective experiences, plus the self- and other-awareness of playing and meaning-making in concert—that are fundamental to playing with others. Its negative impact on the autistic child's capacity to attribute thoughts and feeling to dolls and actions figures is a consistent finding.

PLAYFULNESS AND SOCIAL PLAY

The origins of playfulness have been traced to the earliest exchanges between mother and infant; the mother intentionally uses playfulness to regulate her child's state, creating interest, engagement, and pleasure in the pursuit of sheer fun or to relieve distress. In these interactions, role-taking and exaggerated representations of emotions and mood can inform the child about the value of reading the other's state and engaging in communicative exchanges. These basic experiences are usually absent from the beginning of life for an autistic child, thereby reinforcing disengagement and avoidance of other potential playing partners. It is not surprising that autistic children show deficits in *social* pretend play, for which playfulness forms the backdrop. This play form, also known as *sociodramatic play*, emerges a year or two later than pretend play. As described in Chapter 2 ("Play, Playfulness, and the Sequence of Play Forms in Development"), such play is common in the typical kindergarten repertoire, involving two or more players who willingly exercise "collective intentionality" (Douglas and Stirling 2012, p. 35) by agreeing implicitly or explicitly to wrestle reality into a specific shape and arc, and to work together to achieve a shared (pretend) story or event, all while having fun (Hobson et al. 2013). Such "metacommunication" can be formally and explicitly achieved by the use of language, as in the phrases "let's pretend" or "this is *in* the game…" (i.e., statements made outside the frame that reinforce the frame), but has also been shown to occur nonverbally, intuitively, and within the frame, sustained by optimal adherence to "the illusion conservation rule" (Giffin 1984), a concept denoting children's ability to step outside the magic circle of the play briefly to renegotiate and then quickly resume the illusion despite the interruption. When play-related metacommunication is broken down to its component capacities, high-performing autistic children show an idiosyncratic array of competencies and deficits: strong conservation of illusion but little flexibility with their own play script (such that they resist incorporating elements introduced by the playmate) and resistance to moving in and out of the frame to clarify intentions. This lack of responsiveness to the other player may not be a problem of symbolization but rather a failure of disposition to play, metacommunication, and empathy.

Dynamic play therapy is a special form of social play, conducted between the child and a psychologically sophisticated adult player who seeks to follow the child's direction as much as possible. In order to take off, the playful exchange requires a degree of flexibility to tolerate compromise and the give-and-take of constructing a pretend scenario. An autistic child with severe intellectual and language limitations is unlikely to benefit from this format because the child's lack of language and comprehension preclude it. According to Shapiro (2009), there is little evidence that low-functioning autistic children are likely to derive benefit from standard play therapy technique; the therapist better serves these children by first helping their frustrated and despondent parents to mourn the idealized child of their dreams and come to terms with their disappointment in the child of reality. With this process under way, the therapist can help the parents to become more attuned and patient playing partners and to find opportunities to connect and engage even with a minimally responsive child. Parents usually require education and support to learn how to create moments of pleasurable exchange with their child through floor play that involves sitting on the floor at the child's level to make eye contact more likely; following the child's lead in simple exchanges that encourage reciprocity; and showing pleasure in minimal results. These sessions may restore parental engagement and optimize the possibility of connection.

Other psychodynamic contributors, including Stanley Greenspan, Susan Sherkow, and William Singletary, emphasize the potential benefit of very early intervention and believe that these measures can modulate adverse neuroplasticity and counter the isolation and deviance of the autistic child. These clinicians contend that psychodynamic play therapy can facilitate progress in autistic children, especially those with some language development, normal or high intellectual endowment, rudimentary play skills, and the capacity to learn both in school and in interpersonal exchanges. Of course, therapists must be cognizant of their own and the parents' therapeutic expectations, in order not to burden the treatment with excessive demands. These children require a careful and lengthy assessment for the therapist to be confident that the recommendations and projected benefits are reasonable and to determine which auxiliary therapies should be included. The play therapy itself can be oriented toward specific symptoms and areas of interpersonal and regulatory vulnerabilities. For example, in the vignette about Emma, the child responded well to a therapy informed by awareness of her deficits in playfulness, mentalization, and affective sensitivity, and her intolerance of intense affect. Interpretive comments are made primarily "within the play" and minimally abstracted from the play content; the introduction of more intense affects often produced a shift in her level of symbolization. The elucidation of multiple subjectivities, the explication of feelings and reasons for their presence, and the demonstration through the play of the many ways to contain affects and to manage and modulate their relationship to actions were important therapeutic interventions for Emma and for many other children on the autism spectrum.

Typically, the scripts of even high-functioning autistic children are rigid and static, limiting openings for clinicians, who must exercise tact and patience to find opportunities for therapeutic interventions "within the play" that allow them to introduce alternate subjectivities; address avoidances, rigidity, and defensiveness; and clarify their recruitment by conflict and anxiety. A recurrent observation in these children's play is the presence of a harshly punitive, critical, and powerful character (Krass 2015; see footnote 1); this firmly entrenched representation has been variously understood and addressed as an embodiment of the superego, the child's own "autistic brain" (Krass 2015; see footnote 1), a personification of the terrifying world, or a representation of the parent filtered through drastically elevated sensory defensiveness. Tactful interventions around these percepts might involve the slow introduction of a new, gently playful facet of the therapist's assigned character or the arrival of a different one to give voice to unarticulated feelings; this intervention allows for the gradual assimilation of repudiated emotions and the recognition that others may have different mental content. The therapist, when carrying out play interventions, needs to respect the autistic child's fear of intense affects and must titrate the level of interventions to the child's dawning capacity to tolerate them. In Emma's therapy, the connection of the savage attacks on weak characters to her rivalrous relationship to her brother or to deflected superego critiques of herself could not be broached for many months. Any therapeutic intervention, no matter how consistent with the child's narrative, can be disruptive for an autistic child, whose tolerance for both change and intense feelings is limited; a modulation of this low tolerance is another goal of treatment.

ATTENTION-DEFICIT/HYPERACTIVITY DISORDER

Four-year-old Aarush was known as an impulsive and inattentive child in his preschool class, but his skilled teacher found him manageable with a few techniques, such as seating him near her in circle time and using gentle touch and eventually a special hand signal to remind him to be quiet. However, his next teacher, for prekindergarten, was herself distractible, poorly organized, and easily overwhelmed by the many active boys in her classroom. Aarush began to resist going to school. At a special meeting with the teacher, the school psychologist, and the preschool director, his parents, the Desais, were distressed to learn that Aarush was a regular visitor to both the administrative and the psychologist's offices, sometimes on his own volition and sometimes at the request of his teacher. The Desais acknowledged that Aarush was very active, unable to sit at the dinner table, and disorganized in his play. They were encouraged to consult with a child psychologist, Dr. Washington. Dr. Washington first observed Aarush in the classroom and was immediately struck by the poor fit between Aarush and his teacher. In this overstimulating classroom, where the teacher strained to keep things under control, Aarush was distracting to other children, not able to keep his hands to himself at circle time, and visibly frustrated, sighing loudly and pulling his shirt over his face when he was repeatedly reprimanded for calling out. His clowning aggravated the teacher, who was not able to deflect it to better use. In what appeared to be an effort at self-regulation when clowning and joking failed, Aarush would disengage from the group, looking out the window or at a book when everyone else's attention was on the teacher.

In Dr. Washington's office, Aarush was restless and unable to settle on anything to play with, gravitating away from figurative toys toward the soft basketball and door hoop, despite his incoordination. He recognized Dr. Washington from his school visit and seemed ashamed. Dr. Washington offered the provisional diagnosis of ADHD to the parents, to be corroborated by neuropsychiatric testing. He recommended that testing be delayed for 8 months until Aarush's 6th birthday, when the results would be more reliable. Meanwhile, play therapy could begin at once, in order to address Aarush's distress and the school's concerns. Dr. Washington and Aarush began to meet twice per week.

In the opening months of play therapy, Aarush was a whirlwind of activity, restless and unable to fully engage in sustained play. When he selected a simple board game like Candyland, he managed to violate the rules: he collected all the cards that allow the player to advance rapidly and kept them to himself, for his use only. When he discovered the unfamiliar game Chutes and Ladders, he was very preoccupied with the moral lessons that explained why misbehaving children got chutes and super-good children got ladders. He began to talk about how his teacher was always sending him out of the room for "time-outs" but he had no idea why. Dr. Washington suggested that next time that happened, Aarush could ask the teacher. Aarush nixed that idea but said he wanted to make his own Chutes and Ladders, which doctor and patient set out to do. In his own version, it seemed clear to Dr. Washington that Aarush had some sense of his own transgressions: the precipitous chutes were the just deserts of children who mugged at the teacher or stood on their heads or tickled other children. There were no ladders.

Aarush's case is a typical referral from school, because ADHD symptoms bear directly on ego capacities necessary for school behavior and learning. Depending on their tolerance, parents sometimes are the first to seek help when their child is causing chaos, parent–child conflict, or extreme sibling friction at home. Depending on the degree of environmental structure, the child's poor self-regulation, intolerance of intense affects, impulsivity, and restlessness will be more or less evident and problematic. It is not unusual for the very young child with ADHD to have fluctuating behavior depending on even subtle changes in his or her environment, such as Aarush's different comportment with different teachers. For some children, the early years of preschool may provide a protective environment, because little concentrated attention and sustained focus are required and the frequent change of activities absorbs their restless scanning and limited perseverance. It is important for the clinician to remember that ADHD is a developmental disorder with presentations that fluctuate according to the child's age, the setting, the intrinsic and subjective interest of the activity, and the demands to perform; sometimes teachers or parents object to the diagnosis because the child is capable of sitting still and focusing in some circumstances (like playing a video game). The decline in opportunities to play and the uptick in actual academic demands in preschool may be among the factors that make first grade the signal year for the diagnosis of children with ADHD.

In the United States, an ADHD diagnosis is given to an astonishingly high proportion of clinic patients and of children in general: the American Psychiatric Association reports 5% of American children carry the diagnosis, and the Centers for Disease Control and Prevention estimates over twice that percentage (Holland and Riley 2014). Although the typical age at diagnosis is 7 years, symptoms may have manifested much earlier and are more or less problematic depending on the environment. DSM-5 has streamlined this diagnosis to two clusters: 1) inattention and 2) the condensation of hyperactivity and impulsivity, two formerly independent criteria. DSM-5 includes only one passing reference to play as a feature of the syndrome—"difficulty sustaining attention in tasks or play activities" (Criterion A1b)—and provides examples exclusively in the academic domain.

The diagnosis of ADHD encompasses a range of clinical pictures and a range of neuroanatomic findings on a continuum with the population at large (Baroni and Castellanos 2015). The neuroscientific research suggests multifactorial deficits and, on high-definition neuroimaging, documents anatomic correlates to some cardinal features of the disorder: deficits in inhibition and attention, reward-related processing, vigilant attention and reaction time variability, timing and synchronization, emotional regulation, and abnormalities of arousal—hyper and hypo—in addition to sleep abnormalities (Baroni and Castellanos 2015). Moreover, despite attempts to tighten up the criteria and rule out other neuropsychiatric insults, many cases in the literature have histories of foster care, poverty, traumatic loss, and possible or documented traumatic abuse (McCarthy and Conway 2011; Sugarman 2006; for examples, see Jones and Allison 2010). These factors can be understood as contributions to the symptom picture, which some believe is less a syndrome than a final common pathway of a range of insults in early development (Günter 2014). In particular, trauma has been implicated as a common element in the history of children with ADHD, explaining their vigilance, affective dysregulation, and poor concentration (Orford 1998).

PSYCHODYNAMIC CONTRIBUTIONS

There has been a small but steady and growing stream of psychoanalytic and psychodynamic contributions to the understanding of ADHD in the last decades. Despite many important differences, the conceptualizations of the disorder can be divided into two groups: 1) those that view ADHD as an umbrella construct (Castellanos et al. 2006), that is, a neuropsychiatric disorder with a range of etiological contributions (heredity, trauma, neuropsychiatry, etc.) and with widespread impact on developing ego capacities, affect processing, self-regulation, interpersonal relations, learning, and conflict and defenses (Gilmore 2000, 2002; Jones and Allison 2010; Sugarman 2006); and 2) those that suggest that ADHD has a primary psychogenic etiology (Günter 2014; Leuzinger-Bohleber 2010; Salomonsson 2011; Seitler 2011). For group 1, a treatment plan may include stimulants, but, as with group 2, the psychotherapeutic focus is on the disturbance in primary attachments, problematic self-regulation, and undeveloped mentalizing capacity (Conway 2015; Fonagy and Target 1997; Laezer 2015).

Psychodynamic theorists have been further divided into two camps, the ego psychological and object relational (Conway 2015). We believe that the distinction of these two camps is primarily one of emphasis; our developmental premise is that these two strands are entwined almost immediately in the newborn period: the early caretaking environment is essential for the emergence of ego capacities and optimal development, and the development of capacities such as the social smile, joint attention, and affective expression heightens the engagement of the interpersonal environment (Gilmore and Meersand 2014, 2015). Most of these different conceptualizations seem to converge on the deleterious transactional interface of infant and caretaking environment, in which two problematic vectors operate: 1) a depriving, traumatic, or otherwise deficient environment fails to help the baby manage motoric discharge and self-regulation, and 2) dysregulation or neurobiological disadvantage within the infant precludes attachment and attunement, perpetuating the parental failures and the disruption of emerging ego capacities. Thinkers from all schools note interference with self-regulation, impulsivity resulting from poorly contained and predominantly motoric discharge of intense affects and drives, and disturbances in interpersonal relationships with resulting lack of empathy (Conway 2015) and mentalization (Fonagy and Target 1994). A number of them assert that a history of trauma is the primary etiological factor in a majority of cases (Orford 1998; Sugarman 2010; Szymanski et al. 2011). Most children with ADHD benefit from play therapy that addresses the intrapsychic impact of the disorder on the evolution of ego capacities (Gilmore 2000, 2002), self-representations (Conway 2015), and subjective experience of the disorder as an inner state of agitation.

Where many of these writers diverge is in regard to the degree to which the neurobiological substrate is felt to represent a complex genetic predisposition or complex dynamic interaction of environmental insults and neurobiological vulnerability (Pozzi-Monzo 2012) rather than a reversible set of symptoms due to environmental insufficiency or overstimulation. This affects attitudes toward medication, which range from sharply critical to pragmatic. From our point of view, medication can be a useful adjunct that reduces chaos and fosters the breathing room for child and therapist to connect, to play, and to think.

PLAY AND PLAYFULNESS IN ADHD

ADHD symptoms inevitably reverberate in the evolution of the child's playing capacity. Disturbances in the development of mentalization, perspective taking, and empathy (Conway 2015; Fonagy and Target 1996b) directly affect play, especially social play, for which the capacity to read others and to collaborate in developing narratives is so essential. The developmental literature that specifically examines the play of children with ADHD is limited, but findings are consistent. Play, especially dyadic play, serves as a microcosm of the child's interpersonal difficulties elsewhere, reflecting interferences not only with the conduct of play but also with the normal pace of unfolding play forms (Alessandri 1992). Studies examining the play of children with ADHD, compared with typically developing control children, report the following features: less overall play, more shifting of activities, less sustained attention at play, disruptions of play, immature play (sensorimotor or functional vs. symbolic play of age-matched peers), lower levels of peer conversation (Alessandri 1992), and, in studies of play at school, more redirection and punitive interventions by teachers (Whalen et al. 1981). One study (Cordier et al. 2010) compared dyads in terms of the quality of the interaction: one type of dyad included a child diagnosed with ADHD playing with a typically developing control child; the other type consisted of two typically developing children. The findings showed the overriding influence of the child with ADHD on the course of the interaction: prosocial skills, including empathy, perspective taking, and discrimination of emotional states, in the typically developing children declined when playing with children with ADHD. This troubling finding was understood as a reflection of ADHD children's domineering, disruptive, and intrusive style, which usually elicits accommodation and/or a less mature play form from the typically developing playmate. This observation may explain the frequent finding of severe sibling friction in households with children with ADHD, because the sibling pair typically interacts at the level of the child with ADHD and readily regresses to immature and noncollaborative attempts to manage conflict. In contrast, in the dyadic play of typically developing children, the less mature child is typically drawn toward a higher level of play.

The notion of playfulness, which begins with parent–infant interactions and colors children's early object relations and lifelong pleasurable engagement with others, has been addressed specifically by the ToP (Leipold and Bundy 2000), which characterizes children's playfulness and its impact on play with peers. Children with ADHD had lower scores than typically developing control children, especially in regard to internal control, intrinsic motivation, and framing (referring to maintaining the mutual playing state and narrative). Not surprisingly, they scored higher on mischief, teasing/joking, and clowning (Leipold and Bundy 2000). Children with ADHD are frustrating to their playmates because they disrupt play, get distracted and derailed during brief play suspensions—that is, momentary interruptions when another child joins the game and had to be given a role, or when an adjustment in the physical boundaries of the game is necessary—and violate the mutual understanding of the play narrative or the declared "rules" of the play.

TRAUMA AND ASSOCIATED STRESS DISORDERS

Max, age 4 years, was referred for evaluation after he witnessed the fatal shooting of his mother by his father during a domestic quarrel. As far as could be determined, he had hidden from his parents during their fight and remained behind the living room sofa until the police entered the apartment. His father had fled the scene but immediately turned himself in at the local precinct. Max, who was silent and stunned when he was discovered in his hiding place, was immediately taken in by his maternal grandmother, who lived in the same building. She was initially overcome with grief and rage about the death of her daughter, screaming and crying uncontrollably, but quickly collected herself. The grandmother continued to visibly grieve but was very concerned about Max and brought him for an assessment a week after the murder.

Max was completely mute and dry-eyed when he and his grandmother arrived for evaluation by a male psychiatrist, Dr. Ali. Max showed minimal interest initially in the dollhouse and figures. However, during the initial conversation between Dr. Ali and his grandmother, which focused on Max's prior history and current state, Max quietly moved toward the toys, threw the children and mother violently behind the consulting room couch, retrieved them, and threw them again. He did not touch the father doll.

Over a series of meetings, some with the grandmother alone to discuss ways to help Max find words for his terrible experience and then with both Max and his grandmother, Dr. Ali slowly began a conversation with the grandmother in simple terms about what had happened to Max. For months, Max's "play" remained the same: ritualized, joyless, and unchanging. During one meeting, the grandmother appeared newly agitated, reporting that another shooting had occurred in the neighborhood; both she and Max panicked, and he began to scream "No! Not my baby!" She recognized her own anguished words that she had screamed repeatedly when entering the apartment immediately after the murder. In the room, Max became more agitated and frenetic in his throwing. Dr. Ali hoped to slow him down by joining him in throwing the figures, saying he knew how much Max had wanted to hide his mother and keep her safe too. His grandmother collected herself and said she was so glad and grateful that he hid himself. Dr. Ali then put the ignored father doll into the closet and said he would not come out until Max decided he could. Both therapist and grandmother knew that Max's relationship with his father would pose a huge challenge for Max, one that was not necessary to resolve at present. Over the subsequent months, Max's play became more disorganized and violent, opening an avenue to his identification with his aggressive father. During this phase, he was inadvertently exposed to some triggering footage of fundamentalist terrorists, and he correctly identified Dr. Ali as from the Middle East. He began to fight Dr. Ali, calling him a terrorist. As this play heightened in intensity, Max's real fear and panic reached intolerable levels. Dr. Ali felt compelled to intervene, saying Max was confusing him with some scary people; this was understandable because sometimes even people you trust confuse you by acting in scary ways. Max was able to deescalate his play and accept a warm high-five. This pattern recurred over the course of many months.

This tragic example of a boy who lost both parents in one moment of violence is unfortunately not rare in clinical reports of trauma (e.g., Kaplow et al. 2006), and certainly the death of a relative by shooting or acts of terrorism is common in today's world (see Chertoff 2009; Sossin and Cohen 2011). Traumatic experiences in children's lives take myriad forms and usually initiate a cascade of related deleterious events that transform the children's lives. At the very least, children's confidence in the reliability and continuity of daily life, the network of central attachment figures, and, in general, "the world as they knew it" for the years preceding the event is lost or ruptured. This can apply both when the trauma is a direct insult to the child and when it is transmitted through the parents or the caregivers' traumatization; severe grief and unresolved mourning in caregivers or parents can interfere with their "metacognitive monitoring" and their consistency in the parental caretaking role. With the caregiver absorbed in protracted bereavement, the child may become disoriented and attachment behaviors may become disorganized and insecure (Coates and Moore 1997). Moreover, both caregiver and child are subject to unexpected reactions to stimuli that resonate more or less clearly with the original event; in the child, these can occur even months to years after the trauma, often without the child's conscious recognition of any connection.

In Max's case, Dr. Ali was concerned that the child was in danger of recurrent retraumatization and compromise of a secure base in the grandmother because of the depth of her bereavement, however she struggled to hide it. Unsure of Max's prior level of language development, Dr. Ali also wondered if the timing of this profound loss might preclude representation in words. Furthermore, when Max was accidentally exposed to video clips of widely publicized terrorist attacks, Dr. Ali was immediately alert to the possibility that his own background would be drawn into Max's anxiety; like Max's father, Dr. Ali was a familiar man who could suddenly turn into a killer. This was used therapeutically with help from his grandmother, who, with explanation, understood the resonance in these events and the importance of her availability to Max.

CHILDHOOD TRAUMA

The topic of childhood trauma, specifically memories of childhood trauma by adults, has a complicated and controversial history in psychoanalysis and the mental health field at large, particularly in regard to its role in adult presentations of psychopathology, especially personality disorders. In childhood, when psychopathology emerges in the context of recent trauma, the impact on the biological stress systems and disruption of brain development are demonstrable and often permanent. Depending on the child's age, the type, severity, and duration of trauma, and the rapidity of the intervention intended to arrest deleterious processes, a range of cognitive functions—such as attention, memory, learning, inhibitory controls, executive capacity, and self-regulation—and their measurements—such as IQ or cerebral volume—are permanently derailed (De Bellis and Zisk 2014). Although the categorization of traumatic experience as cumulative trauma (Khan 1963), strain trauma (Kris 1956), or *shocklike trauma* is still in the literature, many traumatic experiences have extensive reverberations, self-creating a gradual and sustained series of insults, rather than a sudden singular event that depletes resources. The original concept of shocklike trauma refers to an experience that overwhelms the ego by an onslaught of stimuli, such that anxiety loses its function as a signal and usual defenses cannot be mobilized; severe anxiety about bodily and personality integrity can only be managed by extreme measures usually involving dissociative mechanisms (Brenner 1994; Chertoff 2009; Coates and Moore 1997; Varkas 1998), such as autohypnosis, altered consciousness, severe withdrawal, and fugue-like states. In every case of trauma, the sequelae are colored and shaped by the developmental timing; the source of the injury (personal, environmental, terrorism, and myriad others); the availability of caregivers to help, protect, or perpetrate; and the type of trauma. The age of the child at the moment of trauma is a crucial variable, because every developmental step brings with it a unique interface among developing systems, most importantly language and autobiographical memory. When the trauma predates a solidly established capacity for narrative autobiographical memories and/or exceeds the cognitive capacity for comprehension, the likelihood increases for a representation in bodily symptoms: "the body keeps the score" (van der Kolk 2015). Until roughly age 4 or even 5 years, children are less or not at all capable of verbal recall and typically have a "physiological memory" of an unmetabolized experience, which they can sometimes represent in drawings; most often there is somatic memory without conscious connection to the event. As children consolidate language and symbolic function, the traumatic experience finds its way directly into play, typically appearing as an organized repetitive reenactment of versions of the experience. These are not faithful reproductions, because the trauma immediately draws in all current developmental conflicts, neurotic anxieties, and so on; as time passes after the event, the likelihood of such elaboration increases. This is the case for Charlotte, discussed in Chapter 13 ("Play Therapy, Variations in Child Development, and Serious Psychopathology"), who was sexually abused when she was under 3 years old; she, like many other children, drew in order to "describe" trauma that had no verbal representation and was not available to consciousness (Coates and Moore 1997).

TRAUMA AND PSYCHOPATHOLOGY

A history of trauma is discoverable in many presentations of psychopathology, including conduct disorders, mood disorders, a host of anxiety disorders, ADHD, gender dysphoria, and personality disorders. In DSM-5, the criteria for PTSD are quite specific and include its manifestation in play—typically reenactments in play without conscious awareness of the referent. However, the vast variability of traumatogenic events and the unpredictable timeline to the outbreak of disturbance go beyond the guidelines of PTSD, because the recognizable set of symptoms does not always appear immediately and the contribution from trauma can only be suspected.

Lenore Terr (1979, 1981, 1983, 1988), an expert traumatologist and clinician who has seen hundreds of children after a wide range of traumatic events, uses a categorization that includes the idea of cumulative or strain trauma. She divides trauma into two types: Type I, "single blow," and Type II, "variable, multiple or long-standing" trauma (Terr 1991). These two variants can differ in terms of their overall impact on personality organization. Type I, the singular trauma, is associated with detailed memories, omens (also known as "reappraisals" [Terr 2009]), and misperceptions but lacks the global changes in personality seen in Type II. Type II inevitably begins with an unexpected event but is followed by long-standing disruption or recurrent exposures and is characterized by numbing and dissociation, rage, or "unremitting sadness" (Terr 1991, p. 16). There are many combined variations in which a singular horrific event transforms the child's life in ways that usher in subsequent trauma. Terr highlights four characteristics seen in variants of remembered childhood traumatization: strongly visualized memories, repetitive behaviors, trauma-specific fears, and changed attitudes about people, life, and one's own futures. Coates and Moore (1997, p. 287) present a different list of trauma effects, focusing on the intrapsychic transformations:

1. Intense unmetabolized affect
2. Distortions in self-structure and impairment in differentiation of self and other due to identification with the aggressor or an attempt to maintain a relationship with a lost object
3. Impairment in symbolic capacity and thus in the ability to play freely; reenactments rather than play are typical
4. Physiological memory of trauma
5. Hypervigilance

Terr's ideas highlight the impact of trauma in the immediate period and in future development: trauma can produce aberrant behaviors right after the event that appear directly linked to it, can set off a cascade of disturbance in many arenas of subsequent development, or can remain dormant until developmental transformation, an environmental trigger, or psychological factors reawaken the acute affect state. For example, if primitive defenses, such as somatization or frenetic action, are utilized to manage intolerable affects, these may persist as preferred defensive strategies and can interfere with the expression, and in many cases the awareness, of other emotions over the course of development. Affects transformed into bodily experience or impulsivity bypass representation in the mind. Children whose language development is in the early stages like Max are especially vulnerable: trauma derails their burgeoning ability to process and verbalize painful emotion. Moreover, phase-specific conflicts, physical development, drives, interpersonal relationships, and cognitive and motor capacities take on new idiosyncratic significance in the context of traumatic memory (Chertoff 2009). In Max's case, for example, his access to normal competitive aggression seemed to be contaminated by his observation of his father's violence, resulting in strong passive trends.

IMPACT ON PLAY

Specifically in regard to play, trauma directly interferes with the productive use of the pretend mode as a vital opportunity to express intense affects, evolving self-representation, and attachment needs in order to integrate them into a stable organization that ultimately emerges in latency, ready to grapple with consensual reality (Gilmore 2011). With trauma, pretending cannot serve such a function because it becomes a segue to dissociation and loses its playful quality (Fonagy and Target 2000). For example, in the aftermath of the 9/11 World Trade Center attack, distraught parents were less careful about television viewing and many children were "remotely" traumatized by the repeated imagery of the towers collapsing and the tense atmosphere at home and school. For children who lost a parent in the attack, the traumatic impact was massive. In one case, a 5-year-old boy was brought to a hospital clinic for treatment after his father presumably jumped to his death. Prior to the event, the boy was in the throes of oedipal rivalry, wanting his daddy to "go away" so he could be alone with his mother. The tragic loss of his father infused his competitive strivings with life-threatening aggression. This was represented repeatedly in therapy by the child wildly climbing the clinician's bookcase and then jumping off, creating enormous anxiety and fear that he would seriously injure himself right before her eyes. This can certainly be seen as a reenactment, but it is not "play"; it is real, dangerous, and disconsolate. It was impossible for this boy to think about minds—his own, his mother's, and his father's—because venturing into that domain courted terror and had to be denied. In this example, it was clear that trauma interrupted the use of fantasy and symbolization as coping mechanisms and thereby directly interfered with the productive use of play and thought, leaving the traumatic experience unmetabolized. In extreme cases and in preverbal children, trauma can hijack all play by a devastating interference in symbolic function; in the older child, it routinely deforms play in the service of repetitive reenactments that are compulsive and detached from conscious memory (Terr 1981). Psychodynamic play with traumatized children is a process of restoration of the spontaneity, joy, and meaning-making aspects of play. Some children's trauma may take years to appear in play (Kaplow et al. 2006). In contrast, both the little boy who lost his father on 9/11 and Max produced a reenactment of their version of the traumatic event almost immediately; in Max's case this was facilitated by the presence of his grief-stricken grandmother and his therapist's superficial resemblance to terrorists that Max saw "by accident" on the nightly news shows watched by his grandmother. For Max, the format of joint therapy allowed the grandmother to verbalize the loss they both experienced, and Dr. Ali's appearance, which became a trigger only after Max caught a glimpse of TV news footage about a terrorist attack elsewhere, gradually allowed him to "contextualize" the story and "play it differently." For the other boy, the relentless exposure to television footage of the 9/11 attacks forced this imagery into his mind. His therapist also used a parent (caretaker)–child format during the treatment when she felt that his mother was stable enough to help him.

Repetitive reenactments by traumatized children can be numbing to the therapist, re-creating the child's own feelings in the countertransference. Clinicians must stay alert to the states that the child's play induces. If examined closely, these enactments can become valuable windows into the distortions, misperceptions, and misunderstandings in the child's mind in the wake of the traumatization and can be useful entry points to help the child develop more flexible and self-determined narratives.

Finally, it is worth noting that the degree to which a given event is traumatic for its victims is highly individualized, because their role during the event (e.g., helpless victim, resourceful caretaker, passive bystander) and their preexisting personalities differ (Terr 1979). Early in the history of developmental psychopathology, the observation that certain children were able to overcome illness, adversity, and trauma led to the study of *resilience* (Garmezy 1993; Masten and Obradovic 2006), also conceptualized (slightly differently) as "invulnerability" (Anthony and Cohler 1987). Resilience was initially felt to be an inborn trait that protected the individual from the impact of stressed environments (Garmezy 1985). Contemporary thinkers conceptualize resilience as the outcome of multiple systems, including internal regulatory and motivational systems, attachment categorization, available caregivers, and cultural supports, such as religious institutions, school, and peer group. Moreover, the possibility that resilience is not a fixed attribute within the child but is potentially "reprogrammable" increases the therapeutic potential of early intervention following traumatization (Fritz 2015).

SUMMARY

Many of the neurodevelopmental disturbances of childhood, as put forth in DSM-5, are similar in regard to their impact on play. Excluding severely affected children on the autism spectrum whose language and intellectual development are profoundly limited and whose play is absent, children with ASD, trauma histories, and ADHD commonly demonstrate the following characteristics of play:

1. Poorly developed symbolic function, such that the pretend mode is not consistently available
2. Predominance of functional play
3. Avoidance, dysregulation, and disruptions in play with affect-laden scenarios
4. Impairments in mentalization, affecting the capacity to role-play
5. Deficient intuitive understanding of the illusion of pretending
6. Limited narrative development

7. Rote, repetitive, and joyless play
8. Problematic self-representations

These common features lead some investigators to think that there may be overlapping etiologies or at least common disordered developmental processes, even with a range of disparate neurobiological underpinnings. On the other hand, all of these disorders interfere with basic aspects of development that originate in early childhood, and inevitably their expression impacts the same fundamental arenas: the experience of the nurturing caregiver; the evolution of reciprocity, attunement, regulation, and ultimately self-regulation of states; the emotions of love, joy, and safety in the experience of the other; the pleasure in exploration of the body and things in the world and in mastery and competence; and so on. It is not surprising that there are similarities in their impact on play.

KEY POINTS

- Play originates in the earliest mother–infant relationship; neurobiological disorders, environmental insults, deprivation, or trauma typically disturb that interaction from birth. In addition, these noxious events or processes directly affect the array of evolving ego capacities that emerge in universal sequence in the first months of life that are required to ensure the ongoing loving ministrations of the caretaker.

- In affected children, the unremediated misattunement between the child's neurobiological equipment and the environment perpetuates deleterious impact on mental development in regard to object representations, affect regulation, intentionality, mentalization, and other ego capacities.

- Despite specific pathognomonic play features that are associated with autism spectrum disorder, posttraumatic stress disorder, and attention-deficit/hyperactivity disorder, the play impairments of these disorders share a number of key elements. This is because they act on the same emerging capacities that are required to elicit environmental nutriment. The optimal interaction between baby and the human environment determines play and sets the paths and potentials of future development.

- The full flowering of pretend play is rarely seen in children with these disorders but can be scaffolded and supported in play therapy. The degree to which play in therapy generalizes to play with others and evolves into a real "disposition to play" (Luckett et al. 2007) continues to be debated.

- Quality of play and progression of play are frequently used as measures of severity of psychopathology and of benefits from treatment.

KEY TERMS

Excessive fear (intense world) hypothesis   A theory about the etiology and evolution of autism, which postulates that the core neurophysiological pathology is excessive neuronal information processing and storage in local circuits of the brain. Affected infants shut down and become unresponsive because their experience of caretaker and environment is overwhelming, painful, and aversive, in contrast to normally developing infants, who find such encounters playful or comforting (Markram et al. 2007).

Externalizing and internalizing disorders   Broadband dimensions of behavior used clinically and in research. *Internalizing disorders* are those in which the primary symptoms involve inner emotions and the self, such as anxiety, depression, and somatic complaints. These fall on a continuum, tend to be covert, and are difficult to detect. *Externalizing disorders* involve external behavioral symptoms characterized by acting out, aggression, impulsivity, and disruptiveness. Despite their differences, the two types can coexist (Nezhad et al. 2011).

False-belief test   Test used to assess the child's achievement of theory of mind by examining whether the child can understand that another individual will not "know" something has been displaced unless he or she witnesses the move. Children under age 4 do not typically possess the capacity to recognize that others can maintain false beliefs (i.e., can have a different subjectivity).

Functional play   A play form appearing in the sensorimotor period that precedes symbolic play but continues onward in development. It involves "practicing" play, in which objects are used as they are intended in a repetitive fashion; there is no imaginative use of objects to represent something else.

Joint attention   The capacity to use pointing to direct attention to the same object; this is demonstrable in the 9-month-old infant who can follow the caretaker's pointing finger to join in the attention to the object of interest (Stern 1985).

Metarepresentation   The capacity to represent a representation that develops in the third year of life. For example, when a toddler observes that his mother is pretending to be hiding behind a pillow even though she is completely visible to him, he understands her relationship to that pretense—that is, that she is pretending to be hidden—and then they can both pretend surprise and delight when she reveals her face and "appears."

Playfulness   Defined differently by different scholars and different assessment measures, but generally considered to reflect a disposition to lightheartedness; used instinctively by parents to ease their child's adaptation to reality.

Social motivation hypothesis   A hypothesis which asserts that children with ASD do not "overimitate" adult behaviors, although a universal tendency of typically developing children is to copy every action of an adult, even those actions extraneous to the objective. This remarkably consistent finding in typically developing children has been understood to reflect *social motivation* to "be like" the adult; it is presumed to be the vehicle for identification and the proliferation of cultural characteristics and skills. Children with ASD, seemingly lacking social motivation, are posited to imitate only the task-oriented actions, although recent research has not supported this differentiation (Nielsen et al. 2013).

Social referencing   The infant's reliance on the caretaker's facial expression in situations of uncertainty to "know" if it is safe to proceed, such as in the visual cliff situation. The intersubjective aspect of this development allows for nonverbal shared understanding and meaning-making.

Visual cliff   A test that examines the infant's capacity to use social referencing in a danger situation. The test exposes a crawling infant

(6–14 months) to a situation of uncertainty: a crawling surface is made to look as if it drops off suddenly (the illusory "cliff"); the typically developing infant uses the caretaker's face for information as to how to proceed. If the caretaker is smiling and encouraging, the baby continues to move forward; if the caretaker looks worried or scared, the baby stops (Emde 1990).

REFERENCES

Achenbach TM: Manual for the Child Behavior Checklist/4-18 and 1991 Profile. Burlington, University of Vermont, Department of Psychiatry, 1991

Alessandri SM: Attention, play, and social behavior in ADHD preschoolers. J Abnorm Child Psychol 20(3):289–302, 1992 1619135

Alvarez A: Making the thought thinkable: on introjection and projection. Psychoanal Inq 13(1):103–122, 1993

American Psychiatric Association: Diagnostic and Statistical Manual of Mental Disorders, 3rd Edition. Washington, DC, American Psychiatric Association, 1980

American Psychiatric Association: Diagnostic and Statistical Manual of Mental Disorders, 4th Edition. Washington, DC, American Psychiatric Association, 1994

American Psychiatric Association: Diagnostic and Statistical Manual of Mental Disorders, 5th Edition. Arlington, VA, American Psychiatric Association, 2013

Anthony EJ, Cohler BJ (eds): The Invulnerable Child. New York, Guilford, 1987

Barnett L: "Winners" and "losers": the effects of being allowed or denied entry into competitive extracurricular activities. J Leis Res 39(2):316–344, 2007

Barnett L, Fiscella J: A child by any other name…A comparison of the playfulness of gifted and nongifted children. Gift Child Q 29(2):61–66, 1985

Barnett L: Playfulness: definition, design, and measurement. Play & Culture 3:319–336, 1990

Baron-Cohen S: Social and pragmatic deficits in autism: cognitive or affective? J Autism Dev Disord 18(3):379–402, 1988 3049519

Baron-Cohen S: Essential Difference: Male and Female Brains and the Truth About Autism. New York, Basic Books, 2004

Baron-Cohen S, Wheelwright S, Jolliffe T: Is there a "language of the eyes"? Evidence from normal adults, and adults with autism or Asperger syndrome. Vis Cogn 4:311–331, 1997

Baroni A, Castellanos FX: Neuroanatomic and cognitive abnormalities in attention-deficit/hyperactivity disorder in the era of "high definition" neuroimaging. Curr Opin Neurobiol 30:1–8, 2015 25212469

Birch M: In the land of counterpane: travels in the realm of play. Psychoanal Study Child 52:57–75, 1997 9489461

Bornstein MH, Hahn CS, Haynes OM: Social competence, externalizing, and internalizing behavioral adjustment from early childhood through early adolescence: developmental cascades. Dev Psychopathol 22(4):717–735, 2010 20883577

Brenner I: The dissociative character: a reconsideration of "multiple personality." J Am Psychoanal Assoc 42(3):819–846, 1994 7963232

Brothers L: The social brain: a project for integrating primate behavior and neurophysiology in a new domain (1990), in Foundations in Social Neuroscience. Edited by Cacioppo JT, Berntson GG, Adolphs R, et al. Cambridge, MA, MIT Press, 2002, pp 367–384

Bundy AC, Nelson L, Metzger M, Bingaman K: Validity and reliability of a test of playfulness. Occup Ther J Res 21(4):276–292, 2001

Casby M: Developmental assessment of play: a model for early intervention. Communication Disorders Quarterly 24(4):175–183, 2003

Castellanos FX, Sonuga-Barke EJ, Milham MP, et al: Characterizing cognition in ADHD: beyond executive dysfunction. Trends Cogn Sci 10(3):117–123, 2006 16460990

Charman T, Baron-Cohen S: Brief report: prompted pretend play in autism. J Autism Dev Disord 27(3):325–332, 1997 9229262

Charman T, Swettenham J, Baron-Cohen S, et al: Infants with autism: an investigation of empathy, pretend play, joint attention, and imitation. Dev Psychol 33(5):781–789, 1997 9300211

Chawarska K, Volkmar F, Klin A: Limited attentional bias for faces in toddlers with autism spectrum disorders. Arch Gen Psychiatry 67(2):178–185, 2010 20124117

Chazan SE: Observing play activity: the Children's Developmental Play Instrument (CDPI) with reliability studies. Child Indic Res 2(4):417–436, 2009

Chazan SE: The Children's Developmental Play Instrument (CDPI): a validity study. International Journal of Play 1(3):297–310, 2012

Chazan SE, Wolf J: Using the Children's Play Therapy Instrument to measure change in psychotherapy: the conflicted player. J Infant Child Adolesc Psychother 2(3):73–102, 2002

Chazan SE, Kuchirki Y, Beebe MA, et al: A longitudinal study of traumatic play activity using Children's Developmental Play Instrument (CDPI). J Infant Child Adolesc Psychother 15(1):1–25, 2016

Chertoff JM: The complex nature of exposure to early childhood trauma in the psychoanalysis of a child. J Am Psychoanal Assoc 57(6):1425–1457, 2009 20068246

Cicchetti D, Toth SL: The past achievements and future promises of developmental psychopathology: the coming of age of a discipline. J Child Psychol Psychiatry 50(1–2):16–25, 2009 19175810

Coates S, Moore MS: The complexity of early trauma: representation and transformation. Psychoanal Inq 17(3):286–311, 1997

Conway F: Current research and future directions in psychodynamic treatment of ADHD: is empathy the missing link? J Infant Child Adolesc Psychother 14(3):280–287, 2015

Cordier R, Bundy A, Hocking C, et al: Empathy in the play of children with attention deficit hyperactivity disorder. OTJR 30(3):122–132, 2010

De Bellis MD, Zisk A: The biological effects of childhood trauma. Child Adolesc Psychiatr Clin N Am 23(2):185–222, vii, 2014 24656576

Douglas S, Stirling L: Metacommunication, social pretend play and children with autism. Australasian Journal of Early Childhood 37(4):34–43, 2012

Durand VM: Autism Spectrum Disorder: A Clinical Guide for General Practitioners. Washington, DC, American Psychological Association, 2014

Emde RN: Mobilizing fundamental modes of development: empathic availability and therapeutic action. J Am Psychoanal Assoc 38(4):881–913, 1990 2286743

Fonagy P, Target M: Who is helped by child psychoanalysis? A sample study of disruptive children, from the Anna Freud Centre Retrospective Investigation. Bulletin of the Anna Freud Centre 17(4):291–315, 1994

Fonagy P, Target M: Playing with reality, I: theory of mind and the normal development of psychic reality. Int J Psychoanal 77(Pt 2):217–233, 1996a 8771375

Fonagy P, Target M: Predictors of outcome in child psychoanalysis: a retrospective study of 763 cases at the Anna Freud Centre. J Am Psychoanal Assoc 44(1):27–77, 1996b 8717478

Fonagy P, Target M: The problem of outcome in child psychoanalysis: contributions from the Anna Freud Centre. Psychoanal Inq 17(suppl 1):58–73, 1997

Fonagy P, Target M: Playing with reality, III: the persistence of dual psychic reality in borderline patients. Int J Psychoanal 81(Pt 5):853–873, 2000 11109573

Fritz GK: Psychological resilience in children. Brown University Child and Adolescent Behavior Letter 31(2):8, 2015

Garmezy N: Stress-resistant children: the search for protective factors, in Recent Research in Developmental Psychopathology. Edited by Stevenson JS. Oxford, UK, Pergamon Press, 1985, pp 126–146

Garmezy N: Children in poverty: resilience despite risk. Psychiatry 56(1):127–136, 1993 8488208

Giffin H: The coordination of meaning in the creation of a shared make-believe reality, in Symbolic Play: Development of Social Understanding. Edited by Bretherton I. Orlando, FL, Academic Press, 1984, pp 73–100

Gilmore K: A psychoanalytic perspective on attention-deficit/hyperactivity disorder. J Am Psychoanal Assoc 48(4):1259–1293, 2000 11212190

Gilmore K: Diagnosis, dynamics, and development: considerations in the psychoanalytic assessment of children with AD/HD. Psychoanal Inq 22(3):372–390, 2002

Gilmore K: Play in the psychoanalytic setting: ego capacity, ego state, and vehicle for intersubjective exchange. Psychoanal Study Child 60:213–238, 2005 16649681

Gilmore K: Pretend play and development in early childhood (with implications for the oedipal phase). J Am Psychoanal Assoc 59(6):1157–1182, 2011 22080503

Gilmore K, Meersand P: Normal Child and Adolescent Development: A Psychodynamic Primer. Arlington, VA, American Psychiatric Publishing, 2014

Gilmore K, Meersand P: The Little Book of Child and Adolescent Development. New York, Oxford University Press, 2015

Greenspan SI: Levels of infant-caregiver interactions and the DIR model: implications for the development of signal affects, the regulation of mood and behavior, the formation of a sense of self, the creation of internal representation, and the construction of defenses and character structure. J Infant Child Adolesc Psychother 6(3):174–210, 2007

Greenspan S, Shanker S: The First Idea: How Symbols, Language, and Intelligence Evolved From Our Primate Ancestors to Modern Humans. Reading, MA, Perseus Books, 2004

Günter M: Attention deficit hyperactivity disorder (ADHD): an affect-processing and thought disorder? Int J Psychoanal 95(1):43–66, 2014 24628222

Happé F, Ronald A, Plomin R: Time to give up on a single explanation for autism. Nat Neurosci 9(10):1218–1220, 2006 17001340

Hink LK, Rhee SH, Corley RP, et al: Personality dimensions as common and broadband-specific features for internalizing and externalizing disorders. J Abnorm Child Psychol 41(6):939–957, 2013 23474797

Hobson JA, Hobson RP, Malik S, et al: The relation between social engagement and pretend play in autism. Br J Dev Psychol 31(Pt 1):114–127, 2013 23331110

Hobson RP: On the nature and standing of psychoanalytic psychotherapy. Psychoanal Psychother 26(3):179–198, 2012

Holland K, Riley E: ADHD by the Numbers: Facts, Statistics, and You. Healthline Media, September 4, 2014. Accessed August 7, 2016.

Jarrold C: A review of research into pretend play in autism. Autism 7(4):379–390, 2003 14678677

Jarrold C, Carruthers P, Smith PK, et al: Pretend play: is it metarepresentational? Mind Lang 9(4):445–468, 1994

Jones B, Allison E: An integrated theory for attention-deficit hyperactivity disorder (ADHD). Psychoanal Psychother 24(3):279–295, 2010

Kanner L: Autistic disturbances of affective content. Nerv Child 2:217–250, 1943

Kaplow JB, Saxe GN, Putnam FW, et al: The long-term consequences of early childhood trauma: a case study and discussion. Psychiatry 69(4):362–375, 2006 17326730

Kernberg PF, Chazan SE, Normandin L: The Children's Play Therapy Instrument (CPTI): description, development, and reliability studies. J Psychother Pract Res 7(3):196–207, 1998 9631341

Khan MM: The concept of cumulative trauma. Psychoanal Study Child 18:286–306, 1963 14147282

Klin A, Lin DJ, Gorrindo P, et al: Two-year-olds with autism orient to non-social contingencies rather than biological motion. Nature 459(7244):257–261, 2009 19329996

Kris E: The recovery of childhood memories in psychoanalysis. Psychoanal Study Child 11:54–88, 1956

Laezer K: Effectiveness of psychoanalytic psychotherapy and behavioral therapy treatment in children with attention deficit hyperactivity disorder and oppositional defiant disorder. J Infant Child Adolesc Psychother 14(2):111–128, 2015

Leipold EE, Bundy AC: Playfulness in children with attention deficit hyperactivity disorder. OTJR 20(1):61–82, 2000

Leslie A: Pretense and representation: the origins of "theory of mind." Psychol Rev 94(4):412–426, 1987

Leuzinger-Bohleber M: Psychoanalytic preventions/interventions and playing "rough-and-tumble" games: alternatives to medical treatments of children suffering from ADHD. International Journal of Applied Psychoanalytic Studies 7(4):332–338, 2010

Lewis V, Boucher J: Manual of the Test of Pretend Play. London, Psychological Corporation, 1997

Lewis V, Boucher J: The Test of Pretend Play. London, Psychological Corporation, 1998

Lillard AS: Pretend play skills and the child's theory of mind. Child Dev 64(2):348–371, 1993 8477622

Lord C, Risi S, Lambrecht L, et al: The autism diagnostic observation schedule-generic: a standard measure of social and communication deficits associated with the spectrum of autism. J Autism Dev Disord 30(3):205–223, 2000 11055457

Luckett T, Bundy A, Roberts J: Do behavioural approaches teach children with autism to play or are they pretending? Autism 11(4):365–388, 2007 17656400

Main M: Discourse, prediction, and recent studies in attachment: implications for psychoanalysis. J Am Psychoanal Assoc 41(suppl):209–244, 1993

Markram H, Rinaldi T, Markram K: The intense world syndrome—an alternative hypothesis for autism. Front Neurosci 1(1):77–96, 2007 18982120

Masten AS, Obradovic J: Competence and resilience in development. Ann NY Acad Sci 1094:13–27, 2006 17347338

McCarthy J, Conway F: Introduction: attention deficit hyperactivity disorder in children and the psychoanalytic process. J Infant Child Adolesc Psychother 10(1):1–4, 2011

Muys V, Rodger S, Bundy AC: Assessment of playfulness in children with autistic disorder: a comparison of the Children's Playfulness Scale and the Test of Playfulness. OTJR 26(4):160, 2006

Neubauer P: First day. Bulletin of the Anna Freud Centre 13:79–122, 1990

Nezhad MAS, Khodapanahi MK, Yekta M: Defense styles in internalizing and externalizing disorders. Procedia Soc Behav Sci 30:236–241, 2011

Nielsen M, Slaughter V, Dissanayake C: Object-directed imitation in children with high-functioning autism: testing the social motivation hypothesis. Autism Res 6(1):23–32, 2013 23166017

Orford E: Wrestling with the whirlwind: an approach to understanding ADD/ADHD. Journal of Child Psychotherapy 24(2):253–266, 1998

Pozzi-Monzo M: Ritalin for whom? Revisited: further thinking on ADHD. Journal of Child Psychotherapy 38(1):49–60, 2012

Regier DA, Kuhl EA, Kupfer DJ: The DSM-5: classification and criteria changes. World Psychiatry 12(2):92–98, 2013 23737408

Rhode M: Whose memories are they and where do they go? Problems surrounding internalization in children on the autistic spectrum. Int J Psychoanal 93(2):355–376, 2012 22471636

Rutherford MD, Rogers SJ: Cognitive underpinnings of pretend play in autism. J Autism Dev Disord 33(3):289–302, 2003 12908832

Rutherford MD, Young GS, Hepburn S, Rogers SJ: A longitudinal study of pretend play in autism. J Autism Dev Disord 37(6):1024–1039, 2007 17146707

Saketopoulou A: When the body propositions gender: reply to commentaries. J Am Psychoanal Assoc 62(5):823-833, 2014 25352346

Salomonsson B: Psychoanalytic conceptualizations of the internal object in an ADHD child. J Infant Child Adolesc Psychother 10(1):87–102, 2011

Schneider C, Midgley N, Duncan A: A "motion portrait" of a psychodynamic treatment of an 11-year-old girl: exploring interrelations of psychotherapy process and outcome using the Child Psychotherapy Q-Set. J Infant Child Adolesc Psychother 9(2–3):94–107, 2010

Seitler BN: Is ADHD a real neurological disorder or collection of psychosocial symptomatic behaviors? Implications for treatment in the case of Randall E. J Infant Child Adolesc Psychother 10(1):116–129, 2011

Shapiro T: Psychotherapy for autism. J Infant Child Adolesc Psychother 8(1):22–31, 2009

Sherkow S: The dyadic psychoanalytic treatment of a toddler with autism spectrum disorder. Psychoanal Inq 31(3):252–275, 2011

Sherkow SP, Harrison MM: Autism Spectrum Disorder: Perspectives From Psychoanalysis and Neuroscience. Lanham, MD, Rowman & Littlefield, 2013

Sherratt D: Developing pretend play in children with autism: a case study. Autism 6(2):169–179, 2002 12083283

Singletary WM: An integrative model of autism spectrum disorder: ASD as a neurobiological disorder of experienced environmental deprivation, early life stress and allosteric overload. Neuropsychoanalysis 17(2):81–119, 2015

Slade A: Making meaning and making believe, in Children at Play: Cognitive and Developmental Approaches to Meaning and Representation. New York, Oxford University Press, 1994, pp 81–107

Sossin KM, Cohen P: Children's play in the wake of loss and trauma. J Infant Child Adolesc Psychother 10(2–3):255–272, 2011

Stern D: The Interpersonal World of the Infant: A View from Psychoanalysis and Developmental Psychology. New York, Basic Books, 1985

Stone LL, Otten R, Engels R, et al: Relations between internalizing and externalizing problems in early childhood. Child Youth Care Forum 44(5):635–653, 2015

Sugarman A: Attention deficit hyperactivity disorder and trauma. Int J Psychoanal 87(Pt 1):238–241, 2006 16635870

Sugarman A: Convergences and divergences in treatments of so-called ADHD children. Int J Psychoanal 91(2):395–398, 2010 20536866

Szymanski K, Sapanski L, Conway F: Trauma and ADHD—association or diagnostic confusion? A clinical perspective. J Infant Child Adolesc Psychother 10(1):51–59, 2011

Tackett J: Toward an externalizing spectrum in DSM-5: incorporating developmental concerns. Child Dev Perspect 4(3):161–167, 2010

Terr LC: Children of Chowchilla: a study of psychic trauma. Psychoanal Study Child 34:547–623, 1979 504534

Terr LC: Psychic trauma in children: observations following the Chowchilla school-bus kidnapping. Am J Psychiatry 138(1):14–19, 1981 7446775

Terr LC: Chowchilla revisited: the effects of psychic trauma four years after a school-bus kidnapping. Am J Psychiatry 140(12):1543–1550, 1983 6650683

Terr L: What happens to early memories of trauma? A study of twenty children under age five at the time of documented traumatic events. J Am Acad Child Adolesc Psychiatry 27(1):96–104, 1988 3343214

Terr LC: Childhood traumas: an outline and overview. Am J Psychiatry 148(1):10–20, 1991 1824611

Terr LC: Using context to treat traumatized children. Psychoanal Study Child 64:275–298, 2009 20578442

Tessier VP, Normandin L, Ensink K, Fonagy P: Fact or fiction? A longitudinal study of play and the development of reflective functioning. Bull Menninger Clin 80(1):60–79, 2016 27028339

Thiemann-Bourque KS, Brady NC, Fleming KK: Symbolic play of preschoolers with severe communication impairments with autism and other developmental delays: more similarities than differences. J Autism Dev Disord 42(5):863–873, 2012 21720725

Vachon DD, Krueger R: Emotion and the joint structure of personality and psychopathology. Emot Rev 7(3):265–271, 2015

van der Kolk BA: The Body Keeps the Score: Brain, Mind, and Body in the Healing of Trauma. New York, Penguin Books, 2015

Varkas T: Childhood trauma and posttraumatic play: a literature review and case study. Journal of Analytic Social Work 5(3):29–50, 1998

Volkmar FR, McPartland JC: From Kanner to DSM-5: autism as an evolving diagnostic concept. Annu Rev Clin Psychol 10:193–212, 2014 24329180

Voran M: The protest of a 6-month-old girl: is this a prodrome of autism? J Infant Child Adolesc Psychother 12(3):139–155, 2013

Vygotsky LS: Mind in Society: The Development of Higher Psychological Processes. Cambridge, MA, Harvard University Press, 1978

Welchew DE, Ashwin C, Berkouk K, et al: Functional disconnectivity of the medial temporal lobe in Asperger's syndrome. Biol Psychiatry 57(9):991–998, 2005 15860339

Whalen CK, Henker B, Dotemoto S: Teacher response to the methylphenidate (Ritalin) versus placebo status of hyperactive boys in the classroom. Child Dev 52(3):1005–1014, 1981 7026186

Wicks-Nelson R, Israel AC: Abnormal Child and Adolescent Psychology: Pearson New International Edition. London, Pearson Education, 2014

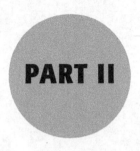

PART II

Technique of Play Therapy

8

The Logistics

Planning a Practice and Arranging for Office Space

Immediately following her child psychiatry fellowship, Dr. Green worked full time as an inpatient attending physician on an adolescent unit. After 3 years, she decided to cut back to part-time work in order to develop a private practice, with an eye toward eventually leaving her hospital position and having more control of her hours. She was approached about joining a suite with three colleagues; two were good friends from her psychiatry residency class who worked with adults, and the third, Dr. Lee, was a child psychologist who did her internship at the same time that Dr. Green was doing her child training. Dr. Lee was eager to have Dr. Green join the group for a number of reasons: she wanted the child psychopharmacology backup; she was interested in developing a psychoeducational testing practice that would attract referrals from other child therapists; and she felt that another child clinician who was already acquainted with her suitemates would tilt the balance toward a more child-friendly atmosphere. Dr. Green had reservations about the arrangement, however, because she knew that the two adult psychiatrists were rather formal and, in fact, might not welcome another child therapist with unruly patients.

Child therapists setting out to begin a practice contend with a number of considerations unique to their specialty. Although every clinician hopes for a convenient and comfortable office arrangement, the issues

217

multiply where children are involved. Children cannot be expected to seamlessly comply with the usual expectations of psychotherapy offices. Children are potentially disruptive, messy, and excessively curious. The caregiver in attendance, whether a parent, nanny, or other person, may take the view that the therapist's office is a place where his or her close supervision and the enforced maintenance of social constraints are unnecessary. The waiting room, the bathroom, and the office itself are all subject to the child's level of socialization, disinhibition, and current state, as well as the extent to which these are monitored and contained by their adult escort. A well-functioning practice that is visited by children and adults, even if the latter are only the caregivers of child patients, must weather these disruptions and transitions without requiring that clinicians expend energy and time on continuous monitoring. If a therapist is joining a suite with adult-focused clinicians, these issues begin in the waiting room and extend from there to the bathroom and the individual office itself.

MODIFYING THE WAITING ROOM AND BATHROOM

Dr. Green visited the suite and was immediately struck by the "grown-up" waiting room; the only child-oriented diversion was a box of crayons and some printer paper discreetly stashed on a bookshelf. The layout of the suite put her potential office at some distance from the bathroom, requiring a long trek past everyone else's consulting rooms. Worse yet, the bathtub was piled with office and bathroom supplies hidden by the shower curtain. The soundproofing of the space was unimpressive, and there was no carpet in the hall. She shared these observations with Dr. Lee, who agreed, acknowledging that she, as the only child person, had been reluctant to insist on changes. Now that there might be two of them, she felt emboldened to join Dr. Green in a discussion with the two adult therapists. Because Dr. Green had trained with the other doctors in the suite and knew them quite well, she was able to lead a frank discussion about concerns on both sides and to discuss what she perceived as essential steps to modify the waiting area. Minimal adjustments would be a child's table and chair in the waiting room, a stepstool in the tiny bathroom for children's hand washing, a storage cabinet to get the office supplies out of the bathtub, and more advanced noise reduction. After some thought, the adult psychiatrists expressed uneasiness about the changes, which they realized were important for a child practice. In the end, all parties agreed that despite personal collegiality, having Dr. Green join the practice was unlikely to work. The two child clinicians decided to look for their own suite; they were confident that they could tolerate what they knew would be some level of chaos in the shared space.

A collection of child-friendly books and materials for drawing are not major impositions on the decor of the waiting room but can be viewed as a departure from a preferred atmosphere, even if satisfying the goal to keep the child patient (or sibling) occupied and quiet. Adult therapists often feel that these objects are infantilizing to their patients and/or inconsistent with the office ambience. Although child and adult clinicians can coexist, it can be a huge relief to child clinicians to know that suitemates will likely understand if a patient is having tantrums or has not flushed the toilet. Many child clinicians also see adults, but the latter are presumed tolerant unless they say otherwise; comments about the child-oriented books, objects, misbehavior in the waiting room, and so on, continue but not in a consequential way.

No matter what the composition of therapists and patients is, the shared territory of the waiting room requires collaboration; for example, staggered session times may help to keep the number of waiting children to a minimum. If a patient or sibling is noisy, disruptive, and not easily settled by a book, the therapist may need to ask the accompanying adult to bring something entertaining and/or avoid lengthy waits. The ultimate luxury is to have a play area in the waiting room that can weather spills and scratches and can muffle sound. Unfortunately, dedicated play space within the waiting or consulting room is hard to arrange, and child therapists must consider how to configure their offices in ways that allow children freedom of expression and provide access to play materials.

One solution is to mark off an area in the consultation room designated as the play space, even if only demarcated by its proximity to the toy chest and a colorful mat. Putting such an area adjacent to a closet where a rollout table and toy boxes can be stored can solve the toy storage problem and create a sense of privacy. With limited space to preserve constructed scenes and the specific toys that a given child is using for the current play theme, a private box for each young patient to store important figures or objects may be helpful to reestablish the ongoing action at the next visit. Not surprisingly, such a box can become a place where children hoard toys and deprive rivals; this then becomes a therapy issue.

Drs. Green and Lee had the good fortune to join up with another child psychiatrist, Dr. Vargas, who had just completed an infancy fellowship. Dr. Vargas was a real asset, with special training in infancy and mother-infant work, and also provided the opportunity to refer within the group to a Spanish speaker and to a man, as occasionally requested by pubertal boys. The three clinicians found a suite with an L-shaped waiting room and four decent-sized offices, each with a large closet with sliding doors and some shelving. The fourth office accelerated the group's interest in seeking another compatible clinician; all three of the original group felt convinced that the addition of a therapist specializing in cognitive-behavioral therapy (CBT) and dialectical behavior therapy (DBT) would prove useful and add to the diversity of services they offered. Dr. Lee had in mind a colleague, Dr. Reed, who was finishing a postdoctoral fellowship. Dr. Reed had just taken her licensing exam and hoped to begin a practice once she was sure she had passed and had completed her requisite supervised clinical hours. She was a skilled individual CBT and DBT therapist, who had expertise in treating eating disorders.

EQUIPPING THE OFFICE WITH THE RIGHT TOYS

As Dr. Green observed, the individual offices, while not spacious, were light-years better than office space at the hospital. Happy to discard her old hand-me-down toys from the clinic, she now was faced with the challenge of equipping her office within her budget. She was eager to see young children but she knew that she would likely have more latency-age and adolescent referrals. She decided that directing her child patients away from her desk was a priority because the computer was too alluring, and she was uncertain about how she would handle the anticipated demand for video gaming. She found a small table and fold-up chairs that could be stowed in the closet, boxes so each patient could have one, drawing supplies, basic paper craft items such as scissors and transparent tape, a few very simple board games, a pack of cards, a couple of baby dolls, and some figurative toys. She loved dollhouses but they seemed very expensive and bulky. She decided to go for the type of figurative toys with associated scenes, such as rooms, markets, and outdoor settings, that could easily be set up and put away. She also chose a few popular action figures and a removable basketball hoop.

When a single office is being equipped for a practice that may include kids of all ages and adults, stow-away space is a huge asset. If a closet is not available, a toy chest and an opaque box assigned to each patient diminish clutter. Some adolescents may be more bothered than adults if the office appears too childish, but they do appreciate objects to play with, like the so-called "executive toys"; these desktop playthings, such as worry beads, pendulums, or magnets, absorb fidgetiness and diminish the pressure for continuous eye contact when a teenager is discussing charged topics. Basic supplies for younger kids should include toys that lend themselves to narrative development such as figures and play sets. Although gender neutrality would seem to cover everyone's requirements, children, especially in **latency (or latency phase)**, tend to prefer gender specificity. Other essentials include drawing and basic craft supplies, building sets, and a few simple games (e.g., cards, checkers, Connect 4). Many board games are now available that call on the child to verbalize conflicts or dominant affects, but these games should be used with caution; some are very adaptable to a child's agenda, but others are not. In dynamic play therapy, defenses are considered a primary focus because of their role in symptom formation and should not (cannot) be swept aside. Although part of the work of play therapy is to help the child understand his or her inner life and attach words to experience and emotions, opportunities to do so are most productive when affects emerge spontaneously in the relationship or play.

Reserving some of the toy budget for current popular toys ensures that the items selected are relatively familiar and well liked. It is impossible for the practitioner to keep pace with every new toy craze, but an occasional purchase to make the collection contemporary is helpful to engage children. As time passes, very old and broken toys should be removed.

PRINCIPLE 1

To the extent possible, the clinician should create a setting, including waiting room, colleagues, and office, that is conducive to the groups' primary focus on their patients. Sound-proofing, suitemates with compatible practices, simple but interesting toy supplies, and easy storage are key components.

SEEKING REFERRALS AND SCHEDULING CONSULTATIONS

All the clinicians in the newly created suite were trained in the city where they opened the practice, so they assumed that their mentors and colleagues in the area would refer patients to them. Dr. Vargas had done an infancy fellowship and wanted to do some mother–infant work; he hoped that Dr. Reed might be a source of young child referrals following or even during CBT. Both psychiatrists, especially Dr. Green, made use of psychoeducational testing and especially liked Dr. Lee's cogent, dynamically sophisticated assessments of learning profiles. The three decided to include Dr. Reed in the preliminary meetings as they weighed the options of various group practice models versus a working collaboration among clinicians who functioned independently. They settled on the latter model, agreeing to revisit this decision periodically. For now, they wanted to maintain separate practices and calendars and different phone numbers. After reviewing electronic medical records, they realized they would save money by investing together in a program they could all use that allowed them to operate their calendars, notes, and billing separately. They decided that when Dr. Reed joined them in a few months, the group would be able to support an assistant for a few hours per week, to do insurance submissions, handle calls for refills, and do some essential paperwork.

This meeting also led to a decision to send out an announcement as a group, since together they offered an array of services that might appeal to referring doctors and potential patients. All the clinicians except Dr. Reed had accrued a few ongoing cases, but they still wanted to expand their referral sources. Their announcement designated the group as the Fox Meadow Practice, named after their street address. They also brainstormed about further expanding their referral circle. Dr. Lee reached out to two local nursery schools, whose directors she had met in the course of her early childhood training. Based on her experience with the directors, she decided an introduction to the faculty and parent body through two short lecture series would be welcome. In the first series, she and Dr. Vargas spoke on toddler issues and separation anxiety during the first school experience, and in the second series, they spoke on the management of **gender dysphoria** in nursery school. These lectures were eagerly accepted and became a yearly tradition in one of the two schools. Dr. Lee also contacted a classmate from her doctoral program who was now the school psychologist at a nearby K–12 school. Dr. Green accompanied her to a meeting because the school psychologist said she was looking for a psychiatrist to take on a difficult case that potentially included medication. Dr. Reed also anticipated that she would be able to tap the adolescent partial hospitalization program and hospital-based eating disorder program as referral sources when she finished her postdoctoral fellowship.

With this foundation, the child clinicians felt less anxious about their practices. They decided to coordinate their open hours so that they could meet for 90 minutes every 2 weeks and discuss cases. They agreed that on the alternate weeks, the 90-minute opening slot would be a good time to meet with new parents for intake or to schedule other appointments that needed more than 45 minutes; for Dr. Green, it was an excellent block to schedule a follow-up with parents about testing. The four also decided to collaborate on the development of an annotated database of helpful resources, such as parent guidance books, educational programs for parents, special-education schools and programs, and referral sources and recommended professionals, such as tutors, occupational therapists, specialized remediators, and parent-training experts.

Clinicians who begin private or faculty group practice often worry about filling their hours. Introductions to local schools and colleges are helpful for developing a referral network. Outreach programs, such as the lecture series Dr. Lee created, are rarely remunerated but can consolidate relationships with neighboring schools, school psychologists, and other professionals. The varied opportunities to cross-refer within this suite—for medications, work with preschoolers, CBT, DBT, and psychoeducational testing—made the group into its own referral source. Moreover, the opportunity to discuss cases, often abruptly curtailed when a clinician transitions from training to practice, was built into their schedules and proved mutually enriching even when their practices expanded. Peer supervision creates bonds, generates ideas, and improves patient care.

A database like the one the group developed is immensely helpful to child clinicians, because patients often require a range of services. If the parents are directed to providers of services such as occupational therapy or parent counseling by other friends or a school, the clinician should have contact information to coordinate care and should consider adding these other professionals to the roster if they are collaborative and skillful. Time spent developing relationships is usually more than compensated by invaluable and collegial services down the road.

PRINCIPLE 2

Child clinicians beginning practice need referrals from child clinicians, educators, pediatricians, and others, and also need these other professionals as resources to provide various services to their patients. This interactive network evolves over a period of years and is synergistic; for example, relationships with school psychologists can lead to referrals as well as names of well-regarded testers, remediators, and tutors. Then all of the latter lead to referrals and shared cases. Child clinicians are almost always part of a team and need to nurture relationships with other child professionals.

CONDUCTING THE CONSULTATION AND FORMULATING RECOMMENDATIONS

Dr. Green's visit to the nearby school did indeed result in a referral from the school psychologist. Mr. and Mrs. Park, both busy and successful professionals, called almost immediately and requested a consultation about their 5-year-old daughter Ellie; they were jolted into action when the regularly scheduled parent–teacher conference turned into a meeting with teachers, school psychologist, and head of the preschool. They had been aware of the school's recent concerns about Ellie; over the previous few months, the teacher had been e-mailing to let them know about recurring episodes of impulsive aggression directed at her peers. At the conference, the teacher and psychologist had described a change in Ellie's state; her former enthusiasm for play and learning seemed to have disappeared over winter break, and she seemed irritable and disagreeable. The Parks felt that Ellie had never posed a behavioral problem at home; her development was, if anything, advanced; her mood was steady and upbeat, albeit sometimes bossy. They were unpleasantly surprised by this meeting.

OVERVIEW OF THE PROCESS OF CONSULTATION

Consultation in regard to a child is very different from a consultation with an adult patient. Evaluating a child is a multistep process, typically requiring contact with a number of adults beyond the parents for observations and supplemental assessments.

Whatever the source of referral, the first step in the evaluation of any child under age 15 or 16 is almost without exception consultation with parents, ideally with both parents and without the child in attendance.[1] There are several commonsense reasons why the clinician and parents meet before an introduction to the child; most of these are self-evident. For instance, parents must screen the professional to whom they are entrusting their child. A good rapport from the outset is helpful because there will likely be hard times ahead if the treatment proceeds. Parents want to feel that their perspective is honored. They have always been the "experts" on their child, but now their confidence may be shaken and they may be anxious and defensive. If the referral comes from the school, the parents often feel not only that they have been mistaken in their understanding of their child but also that they have failed. Clinicians usually have several agendas in the first meeting, but the most important may be to address the parents' sense of failure and establish an alliance with them, if at all possible. While gathering a developmental history, the clinician can also learn more about the parents' views of their child, past and present; assess their agreements and disagreements; and get a sense of the family dynamics as represented in the room and from the parents' report. The rationale for requesting that the parents come to the first meeting without the child is to protect the therapist's future rapport with the young patient. If children are left in the waiting room while the "grown-ups meet," there is already potential for them to feel they are in trouble and have been excluded. Parents hopefully understand this even if it causes inconvenience and seems to them unlikely that the child will be troubled by waiting. If the child's presence is unavoidable due to distance from the clinician's office, babysitting coverage, or some other reason, it is usually helpful if the therapist greets the patient, explains what is going to happen, and spends a little time with the child.

Spelling out the assessment process to parents from the outset, at the first meeting or even during the phone contact to set up the first appointment, establishes reasonable expectations about the length

---

[1]With adolescents, the first meeting may be with the teenager himself or herself; sensitive parents recognize that they need to stand back initially to allow their older child to make the connection to the doctor, before they participate in the process.

and depth of a comprehensive assessment. The clinician can indicate the likely need to include other sources of useful information (e.g., nannies, tutors, teachers) and the possibility of referrals for ancillary evaluations, such as by occupational therapists, psychoeducational testers, speech and language therapists, and so on. The clinician can assure the parents that this process of information gathering will yield a more complete and multifaceted picture of the child. Obviously, urgent consultations inevitably arise and may demand immediate intervention, in which case some steps in the assessment will need to be postponed; even in these circumstances, however, it is helpful for parents to know beforehand what assessments might be needed after the crisis is over.

USING THE INITIAL CONSULTATION TO ASSESS THE CHILD AND ESTABLISH RAPPORT WITH PARENTS

The group decided to create a development form for general use in the practice; based on common sense and their familiarity with routine assessment questionnaires in training, they crafted a comprehensive form that each clinician could modify as desired. Dr. Green asked Mr. and Mrs. Park to complete the form and return it before the first meeting, giving her the opportunity to look it over in advance. With the basic developmental background information and no red flags, Dr. Green was able to focus on the presenting problem. She began by asking the parents about their understanding of the school's concern and their own experience of Ellie's current state. They said they were feeling somewhat harassed by the school, with frequent calls from the head teacher and school psychologist since Ellie's return to school following winter break. This was in stark contrast to the smooth transition to school and the relatively happy adjustment she seemed to make initially. As far as they knew, there was no change in Ellie; the family had been away together during the holidays visiting the paternal grandparents, as was their custom. The grandparents are very traditional and primarily speak Korean despite having adequate English skills; Ellie understands almost everything and usually enjoys these visits. However, this was the first such visit with Ellie's new little sister, who was now 11 months. Her parents didn't notice any change in the grandparents' attention to Ellie; they had all been sensitized to Ellie's need to be recognized in spite of the draw of the cute baby. The end of vacation and return to the usual routine meant a sharp reduction in Ellie's time with both parents, but this was inevitable and usually well tolerated.

The Parks acknowledged that managing two children, given their busy professional lives, was more challenging than they had expected. Mrs. Park had gone back to work after 3 months of maternity leave. Mr. Park's job had always required a lot of travel but was even more demanding in recent months. Coverage was available: either Mrs. Park or Ellie's lifelong nanny, Susie, was always at home in the evenings. Nonetheless, Dr. Green sensed the parents' defensiveness and wondered whether something was going on that they weren't telling her. She offered a general comment about the many factors that help support children's self-regulation and mood: parents, siblings, nannies, school, and friends—even for a child at such a young age, they are all vital to maintain and nurture the child. She suggested a second meeting to consolidate her connection to the parents before proceeding with the assessment of Ellie.

Although the initial consultation period is focused on collecting information about the presenting complaint and obtaining a developmental history, it is also an opportunity to understand the parents' state of mind and, if indicated, to address their sense of failure. Dr. Green's experience of the Parks' defensiveness led her to slow down to offer some psychoeducation and support.

In the course of a child evaluation, the therapist can help parents immeasurably by tolerating and defusing their anxiety, their urgency, and their anger at their child, thereby setting a measured pace for the assessment. Parents are fearful about blame, about their causal role in their child's difficulties, and, by the time they seek consultation, about their demonstrated helplessness to fix the problem. Of course, parents approach a referral for their child with their idiosyncratic preconceived ideas about psychotherapy, and it is helpful for the clinician to explore, acknowledge, and address these ideas. Some parents turn to the therapist with relief and gratitude, hoping for a "cure" for their child; some seek help for their own conflicts and needs. Others feel offended and resentful, blame the school or teacher, and approach a consultation with their minds made up. Whether the parents are hopeful or bitter, the referral marks a nadir in parenting confidence. Parents' defensiveness around perceived failure may be expressed in anger and aggression, toward each other, the child, and the clinician.

Parents, the parental relationship, and the parents' independent relationships with their child all have complex meanings and dynamics, but they are also an intrinsic part of the growing child's mind. The child's

object representations are in construction and undergoing modification throughout childhood; they are foundational to mental structure, and thus primary objects such as parents continue to play a central role in their child's development, shaping the child's identifications, relational templates, value system, and myriad other aspects of personality. This reality, in addition to parents' crucial role in sustaining the pragmatic aspects of treatment, makes parents vital collaborators who can make treatment work or interfere with its progress. The therapist's first goal should be to establish a cooperative relationship with the parents of the prospective patient, providing them a place to vent their frustration and disappointment while augmenting their understanding of their child's inner life.

In situations of separation or divorce, meeting both parents at once is important for determining their ongoing ability to work together for the sake of their child. Parents who say they cannot meet together, whether due to acrimony or inconvenience, are inadvertently obscuring the details of an important dynamic in the child's life; poor communication and rapport between feuding parents creates a huge challenge for the child who has to bridge the divide; it also exposes the therapist to considerable pressure to take sides, thereby diminishing the value of the consultation. Maintaining neutrality and being open to each parent's suffering is never easy but is crucial to the clinician's ability to work with the child. Such neutrality does not mean that clinicians are oblivious to the specific experiences of each parent, which are often vital for understanding the child's experience. In addition, meeting together with parents, including divorced parents, at least once gives the therapist a vivid picture of the child's day-to-day challenges.

Sometimes the very fact of the referral creates such a negative atmosphere, due to narcissistic injury, shame, and a sense of failure, that the parents' externalization is unrelenting. They can spend many preliminary meetings defensively railing against the school, the teacher, one another, or the child. A tactful and sympathetic approach is often hard to sustain for the clinician; however, giving the parents credit for their efforts not only builds the collaboration but also eventually makes it safer for them to explore their contribution to the child's difficulties. Parents are often depicted as the hardest part of child work, and working to establish rapport from the outset may pay off in the long term, because there are likely to be ups and downs in the course of working together. A willingness to understand each parent's point of view is crucial for the success of any treatment.

When faced with any appearance of childhood pathology, parents often try a range of solutions, such as instituting consequences, reward systems, and behavioral plans that may have been suggested by other parents, family members, the child's teacher, or the popular parenting literature of the day. Despite the reasonable nature of many of these approaches and the parents' commitment to them, parents often find them hard to maintain and/or resort to ultimatums or threats. Nonetheless, the therapist's respectful inquiry into the history of both the symptoms and the parents' attempted solutions reduces the parents' sense of loss of status as the experts on their child. The therapist must keep in mind that referral to a child psychotherapist is often understood by parents as the ultimate negative referendum on their parenting. The visit to a mental health professional's office is usually the last resort, arrived at with anger, impatience, and/or despair. If the backdrop to the child's symptoms is marital conflict, unemployment, parental illness, or any other situation that potentially feels shameful, the threat is not only to the parents' success as parents but also to their privacy. Occasionally, parents take the position that their issues are not part of the conversation about their child. Even if ultimately willing to talk openly with the consultant, parents may consider disclosure to the school unnecessary, rationalized by their high-profile positions, their conviction that the school will mishandle the information and prejudice teachers against their child, or their denial of relevance.

PRINCIPLE 3

The child clinician should approach parents with respect and empathy. The operating assumption, until proven otherwise, is that they want the best for their child, whether or not the clinician agrees with their notion of what the "best" is. Listen to their version of what led them to seek consultation and address their concerns.

UNDERSTANDING MOMENTS OF REFERRAL

For young children, peak referral times can occur at normative critical junctures in childhood—birth of a sibling, extensive parental absence, parental discord, and entry into kindergarten or grade school—or in times of crisis—parental illness or death, divorce, sibling illness, and other traumatic experience. The referral itself is usually initiated by one of a handful of sources: the school (e.g., toddler programs, nurseries, early grade school) via the psychologist, administrator, or teacher; the pediatrician; the parents themselves; or a concerned relative. Schools make a significant proportion of referrals, and it is therefore essential for the clinician to develop a working relationship with schools and school personnel. The clinician can aid the relationship with a school by attending school meetings about the patient and by forming relationships with the administration and school psychologist. However, it is not always possible for the clinician to make the time, so establishing appropriate expectations is also crucial, especially in regard to recurring meetings.

If the request for consultation originates from school, because of a child's unrelenting separation anxiety, aggression, academic struggles, or distractibility, parents are typically already under siege as they field frequent phone calls from teachers and are summoned for special school conferences. Unfortunately for the parent–child relationship, the child begins to embody parental shame and helplessness as he or she is singled out due to behavioral dysregulation, cognitive disability, socialization, or evident mood disturbance. If the precipitant appears to be the birth of a sibling, marital troubles, or extensive parental absences (e.g., travel, primary caretaker's return to work), the parents may be reluctant to discuss these issues; sometimes the parents claim they cannot "see" the connection even though they are clearly uneasy about the situation. It may require several meetings for the clinician to achieve a relationship with the parents that is comfortable enough to address such sensitive topics.

Unless there is a true emergency, the therapist's first task is to try to reduce the atmosphere of desperation and sketch the course of the consultation, emphasizing the value of a thorough evaluation that may include testing, school reports, and contacts with other concerned adults. Following the assessment, the clinician should provide parents with a diagnostic impression and recommendations.

Dr. Green met with both of Ellie's parents for a second time. She gathered more history about each parent's own experience growing up, their families, and their birth order. She knew that as second- and third-generation Korean Americans, they might be reluctant about seeking psychiatric help, which might explain their guardedness. She told them that she would need their tolerance and guidance in terms of cultural differences, especially because she had had little experience with people of their heritage. In this context, Mrs. Park observed that her return to work had elicited some disapproval from Mr. Park's parents; he concurred with this assessment and admitted that it worried him too, now that Ellie was symptomatic. This would be a recurrent topic between Mrs. Park and Dr. Green; Mrs. Park felt safe to discuss the issue with another professional woman, especially now that her husband was aware it was in the conversation.

During this second meeting, Dr. Green also underscored that she wanted to understand the Parks's impressions of the school and especially Ellie's teachers. She felt it was important to emphasize that her primary commitment was to Ellie and to them. She explained that having consulted to a school while she was a fellow, she knew well how varied and unpredictable the student–teacher match could be and how differences in teaching style could be transformative for a given student. The parents seemed much more relaxed in the second consultation. They reported that they had loved the school up to this point, but now had concerns that Ellie's current classroom seemed less structured and that morning drop-off took longer than last year; Ellie seemed a little lost and aimless. They liked her teachers but wondered if Ellie needed more active engagement. By the end of the appointment, the Parks enthusiastically agreed to Dr. Green's suggestion that she make a school visit before meeting Ellie in the office because it would be easier to get a true picture as a neutral observer.

Ellie's parents revealed a number of possible precipitants and/or contributions for Ellie's referral, such as the birth of her little sister, her mother's return to work, or some school-related difficulty. Such common events are all suspect in a child consultation because they constitute a significant disruption of the child's prior adaptation.

THE BIRTH OF A SIBLING

Many young children feel and express their grief at the arrival of the intruder immediately after their sibling's birth. Others may show no initial response, but with the increasing mobility and emerging personality of the baby, the older sibling may manifest a disturbance in functioning such as regressive behavior or overt aggression. In either situation, there is typically a mixture of emotions, including possessiveness, affection, resentment, jealousy, and pleasure in or dislike of the new role of "big brother" or "big sister." When negative feelings predominate, parents complain of feeling unprepared for "double trouble" and can experience a sharp reversal of their formerly tender relationship to the older child. Care for the newborn can dominate the focus of the primary caregiver—be it mother, father, relative, and/or nanny, compounding the older child's sense of powerlessness and loss of status. If the child cannot modulate the mixed emotions and defends against them with maladaptive defensive strategies, symptoms may appear at home and/or school.

Sibling conflict is a normal and expected part of childhood, but even before the younger sibling is born or has a personality to speak of, the older brother or sister senses that the new baby is a harbinger of change. Regression such as revivals of sleep problems, demands to be babied, preoccupation, and possessiveness of the pregnant mother are typical reactions and reflect the child's efforts to manage strong emotions. It is only when the child's state unravels—for example, when the previously established mood or self-regulation seems to have disappeared—that the response is deemed problematic.

CONSULTATION IN DIVORCE

Another frequent precipitant for referrals occurs in the context of escalating marital problems and divorce. This is a particularly complex challenge for the clinician, depending on where in the process the family is when arriving for consultation. In very acrimonious circumstances, it can be difficult to establish rapport with both parents. Because children in such situations are trying to protect themselves and manage their feelings as their world crumbles, they may not be available to truly engage with the therapist. As Anna Freud famously observed, treatment "performed on a battlefield" may be impossible (quoted in Downey 1988, p. 279). Divorced parents who have settled into new lives with new partners may still not be collaborating smoothly, but in most circumstances they have worked on compromising enough to be able to cooperate around treatment. In the throes of imminent marital collapse, the situation is often so tumultuous that the battlefield becomes a minefield. Even in these cases, however, there are parents who manage to cordon off their discord to work together; in such situations, treatment can proceed.

> Becky Singer's recently divorced parents contacted Dr. Lee about the 6-year-old's increased bedtime anxiety and distractibility at school. They agreed to meet together for an initial appointment, although the couple's prolonged negotiations over the date resulted in delays of several weeks; each parent privately expressed, through separate phone calls to Dr. Lee, that the other was "impossible to deal with." At their first meeting, Dr. Lee began the session by thanking them for the joint meeting and asking for a description of their concerns about Becky. A grudging civility prevailed as each parent detailed a mostly consistent report of their daughter's sudden refusal to sleep alone and her teachers' comments about lack of focus in the classroom. Mr. Singer studied his phone as his wife spoke, and vice versa, but both paid attention when Dr. Lee asked questions or made preliminary observations. A momentary breakthrough of anger on both sides occurred when Dr. Lee asked how Becky was handling the transitions between the two households: Mrs. Singer immediately referenced Mr. Singer's new girlfriend, insisting that she not be introduced to Becky; Mr. Singer retorted that the overall lack of routine and structure in his wife's home was the main source of the child's problems. Dr. Lee intervened quickly to bring the discussion back on track, focusing on an area of shared concern where coordination between households could be mutually supportive—in this case, resistance to sleep. She reminded the two that Becky was manifesting similar sleep problems in both of their homes. The couple relaxed slightly and allowed themselves to be reengaged in a more child-focused conversation.

In consulting with a family where marital breakup is imminent, the therapist may have to clarify the boundaries of his or her jurisdiction, knowledge, and experience. Because the child's well-being and custodial arrangements are entwined and at stake in divorce proceedings, and because experts are often asked to weigh in on the court's decisions, parents may expect that the consultation will lead to a report or a court appearance. Therapists who have no forensic training and no interest in developing a court-based practice should make the limits of their expertise known. Even with the best of intentions and confidence in the assessment, an inexperienced and untrained clinician is at a huge disadvantage handling an appearance on the stand; this may, in turn, have deleterious impact on the outcome. Moreover, if there is an indication for play therapy with the consulting clinician, an active role in decision making is problematic. The potential therapist to the child is already subject to pressures from both parents and cannot remain receptive to all parties if compelled to participate in major decisions that affect the day-to-day life of the potential patient. If the clinician is strongly polarized from the outset, he or she may not be able to engage both parents in the course of the work with the child. Establishing a clear boundary around the child's visits to the therapist, by underscoring that the child's visit is protected and private, may reduce some complications.

Many children in the throes of parental separation yearn for an adult to talk to who is not involved. The parents may have lost both their idealized position in the child's mind, because of mutual hostilities, and their authority as they quarrel and question each other's decisions. Depending on children's understanding of the drama unfolding, they may feel protective of the parent perceived as more vulnerable. When one parent shows extreme distress, the child can be cast in a parentified and caretaking role. The child's own struggle may not be evident. As in regard to many crises created by environmental stressors, the impulse to automatically put a child into treatment, however well-meaning, may be counter-productive, because the child may be managing adequately and may feel even more unfairly relegated to the care of others by being packed off to an unknown psychotherapist. However, many children do become symptomatic during this period, either at home or at school, which leads to a referral.

PRINCIPLE 4

Acrimonious and/or divorcing parents who come for a consultation about their child can be very challenging. From the outset, the clinician may be compelled to set firm boundaries around the consultation and establish the extent of his or her involvement in future deliberations. Not taking sides is not always easy, but if it is possible, better communications can result.

CONSULTATION AROUND GENDER DYSPHORIA

After Dr. Vargas gave his lectures on gender dysphoria, he received a call from the Greenhills, parents of Beno, age 4 years 7 months, who had been complaining about being a boy for over a year. The Greenhills reported that he was always a "sensitive" baby, highly reactive to loud noises and harsh light. Sometime after his second birthday, he seemed to veer toward playing with his older sister Sara and was much less interested in his older brother Jake, her twin, than he had been just weeks earlier. He eagerly sought the part of the baby when Sara played house with her friends and begged to be dressed up as a baby girl, in a pink bonnet, holding his favorite prop, a pink blankie. His mother, a wedding planner, initially enjoyed Beno's interest in her activities; she was delighted he wanted to tag along when she went to scout out new bridal boutiques and scour wedding tradeshows for new ideas. He was the favorite of the two assistants at her studio, where he would dive into racks of bridal and bridesmaids' gowns, blissfully surrounding himself in clouds of pale, delicate lace and gauzy chiffon. Mr. Greenhill was very upset when he arrived at the studio one afternoon and found Beno playing wedding dress-up with the assistants while his wife was meeting with clients. In the consultation he told Dr. Vargas, "It's fine with me if he's gay, but dressing him up as a girl is not okay." The parents had soon after put an end to the baby play with Sara, and Mr. Greenhill made an effort to spend more time alone with Beno, teaching him to ride a Micro Mini Scooter. However, Beno continued to tag along with Sara and her friends and was discovered trying on her ballet tutus several times. Mrs. Greenhill became increasingly worried because she noticed that Beno hid his penis between his legs in the bathtub and frequently complained that he didn't like it.

Dr. Vargas met with the Greenhills, took a history, and went to observe Beno in school before seeing him at his own office. In the classroom, Beno was happy to play in the dress-up corner with two girls he liked, and he seemed relatively comfortable and attentive at circle time. On the rooftop playground, he avoided the boys who were playing out a Clone Wars scenario, and hung out with the girls who were engaged in what appeared from a distance to be sociodramatic play combining freeze tag and magic spells.

Dr. Vargas met with the Greenhills several more times, separately and together. He wanted to understand their feelings about Beno's apparent dislike of his maleness. He tried to reframe the issue of whether he was "gay." He explained that, in his opinion, sexual orientation was not Beno's main concern at the moment. He was struggling with his feelings about his body and how that jibed with what he felt about himself. Dr. Vargas told them that what Beno was feeling, called *gender dysphoria*, was something that psychotherapists and scholars were still trying to figure out, not to mention parents and people who grew up with this feeling. He told them that how it would develop over time for Beno was also uncertain, but that he would recommend that they not pressure him into acting "more like a boy." He also said that he couldn't tell from their description whether it was them or Beno who was in conflict with what was going on at the moment. If Beno was really suffering because he hated his body or was picked on at school or anything like that, Dr. Vargas would be happy to work with him; if the parents were having a lot of trouble with the situation, he would meet with them. He volunteered to go to school for a faculty meeting to discuss how the school was communicating with Beno and with his classmates.

After a few meetings, the Greenhills felt certain that Beno was struggling; even after the parents had quit pressuring Beno, they felt he was unhappy with his preference for girls' things "since everyone else didn't like it," and he frequently cried about not being able to choose what he was. So he began working with Dr. Vargas, at first once weekly and then twice per week. The parents were seen weekly and then every other week.

Beno arrived in the office for his first visit wearing his favorite yellow corduroy overalls and carrying the "play" pink blankie. He recognized Dr. Vargas and was shy but friendly. He wanted to play with Dr. Vargas's collection of baby dolls and a stroller; this became a recurrent scenario in his play, in which he was the mom, Dr. Vargas was the dad, and the baby was a little girl who happened to be in yellow corduroy overalls, an amazing coincidence that Beno found very funny. Beno named her Betty. He told Dr. Vargas that they needed to play this from the beginning of every session and that Dr. Vargas should call him Bea and talk about him like he was really the mommy "so Betty would understand who was who." After several months of supermarket shopping, they began to shop for clothing. It was at this point that Bea told Dr. Vargas that his own dad didn't like it when kids acted like babies. He talked at length about how much he used to love playing the baby, just like Betty. Dr. Vargas wondered if maybe his dad was worried about the Betty part, even more than the baby. Then Beno/Bea disclosed that his dad really wanted him to be a boy, but he just couldn't do it. It didn't feel right. Dr. Vargas said, "It must be very hard to feel like your dad is disappointed. What do you say to him?"

Treatment of children with gender dysphoria has become highly politicized and controversial; sticking close to the clinical material is not a guarantee of a therapist's neutrality. Whatever their ultimate developmental trajectory, in terms of sexual orientation and gender acceptance, there is no doubt that children with gender dysphoria suffer, and not just by virtue of conflicts with the environment. The material reality of the body exacts a tremendous toll on the mental life of the child, who cannot come to terms with the concrete equation gender=genital (Saketopoulou 2014) and who often cannot figure out a comfortable way to live with it.

> Dr. Vargas made clear to the Greenhills that he wanted to help Beno come to terms with whom he himself felt he was, and then help him figure out how to deal with his body which may be asserting, by its fixed anatomy, something different. Dr. Vargas wanted to advise them in advance that the process of discovery was different for every child and every family; he anticipated that they would need to meet regularly to talk through their own feelings and reactions. He made it clear that he would not approach Beno with a preconceived agenda, and wanted them to be "on board" with that stance.

The growing visibility and activism of the transgender community in the twenty-first century has raised awareness of the complexities of childhood gender dysphoria; play therapists who treat such children need to be cognizant of the current dialogue, available services, and alternative schooling (such as schools specifically dedicated to LGBT children). Maintaining an alliance with the parents around the therapeutic stance of exploration rather than what often amounts to pressure or coercion from relatives, school, or peers may protect the child from repeated traumatic experience—for example, from public shaming, forced gender compliance, and other harsh measures—and fosters a collaboration open to new information. Learning about the child's mental life through play and enactments within the treatment may expose experiences that have been implicated historically in gender dysphoria in the psychiatric and psychoanalytic literature: an occult trauma, an **attachment disturbance** (Coates and Moore 1997), or compliance with the preferences of a depressed mother—all or none of which may be contributions to the conflict. Despite its intensity and typically early onset, this disorder is like many others in that a singular etiology is unlikely. A therapist who is open to learning from parents and child, in addition to colleagues and the transgender community, is best also to negotiate these complexities.

PRINCIPLE 5

Child clinicians should not expect to tell patients or parents "why" the child has this or that difficulty (Gilmore 2008). It is important, especially when working in an arena that has stirred controversy and disagreement, to approach parents as collaborators. Of course, parents' minds may already be made up, so the initial work should involve getting them to see and hear their child.

REFERRAL FROM THE SCHOOL

Entry into school, even into a play-oriented school setting for very young children with minimal academic demands, may trigger an onset of symptoms. Because very young children typically show separation anxiety when first beginning school, most nursery schools expect parents to participate in a gradual phase-in for all very young children, regardless of history or apparent difficulty. Parents of the children who proceed without distress are usually able to shorten the phase-in period. Because school adjustment is usually viewed as a normative crisis, referrals among this age group are relatively rare. If the child cannot adjust, the parents or school may decide the time is not right for the child to begin school, and they delay for another year to allow for the child's natural developmental progression in self-regulation and object constancy. Separation anxiety may forecast subsequent school refusal, but the latter syndrome is less prevalent in primary school than in secondary school (Heyne and Sauter 2013).

Children from prekindergarten and elementary school grades are referred for a range of issues: socialization, defiance, frequent meltdowns, attention deficit disorder (hyperactive type), sensory integration disorders, developmental delays, and failure to meet academic expectations. Because academic demands are now beginning even in prekindergarten, the young child may manifest behavioral distress to avoid struggling to meet expectations that tap ego capacities that have not yet emerged, such as reading readiness, socialization, and group cooperation. In early childhood, uneven development is commonplace, and relative weaknesses, which are typically self-correcting over time, can become a source of trouble at school. For example, a simple two-step direction ("Wash your hands and then come to the snack table") can be challenging for children with neurodevelopmental unevenness that affects sequencing. Similarly, circle time in preschool demands awareness of personal space and focus on the teacher in a sea of stimulation, and thereby poses challenges to children with attentional problems or incipient sensory integration disorders. Boys' development is especially uneven in early childhood, and boys may experience frequent reprimands, confusion, or failure even though they are likely to "catch up" by age 6.

A school referral for a preschool-age or older child should always raise a question about a developmental or cognitive contribution to the child's problem. Many cognitive, motoric, attentional, and executive function disabilities are unmasked by academic, organizational, and self-regulatory challenges associated with each phase of schooling. On the other hand, overzealous diagnosis may pathologize a child with a slower developmental pace. The clinician is faced with determining whether neuropsychiatric or psychoeducational testing is indicated and likely to be helpful; testing is costly and time-consuming, good testers often have long waitlists, and parents can manifest strong opinions, pro or con, about testing. Moreover, some testers are reluctant to take on a child under age 6 (the lowest age for which the Wechsler Intelligence Scale for Children is standardized), so it may be beneficial for the clinician to cultivate relationships with testers who have expertise in early childhood. If the clinician strongly believes that the child's learning profile is contributory, testing must be presented as part of the recommendations. However, other parts of the comprehensive evaluation can proceed without a precise picture of the child's cognitive profile; it is often helpful for preliminary supports to be in place before a report is available in cases where testing is delayed. When the index of suspicion for learning disabilities is high, it helps to remind everyone involved that the possibility of specific findings on testing may require modification of the treatment recommendations.

Other developmental lags can be assessed more rapidly. These may be observed in play, vividly described by other adults, or documented in evaluations by other specialists. Fine and gross motor delays (e.g., poor pencil grip, balance problems, incoordination), visuospatial weakness (e.g., poor block building skills), language delays or speech pathology, and apraxias are the domain of affiliated professionals whose findings may be available sooner than the full battery of neuropsychiatric testing can be performed; ultimately, all of these results should be in place to provide the fullest picture of the child's strengths and weaknesses.

We may be stating the obvious, but child therapy, unlike work with adults, includes contact with parents, caregivers, and a wider circle of other professionals (e.g., occupational, physical, and speech-language therapists; teachers; testers; tutors), each of whom is likely to have useful observations and information to share with the clinician both at the time of initial consultation and during treatment. Therapists should be prepared to attend a school meeting if their participation is requested. Often a child is referred after the school has sounded the alarm multiple times. The school personnel may be reassured simply by knowing there is a concerned clinician on the team.

If the clinician's picture of the child is too jumbled or contradictory by virtue of the multiplicity of opinions, it is helpful to observe the child at school. When the child is already acquainted with the treating clinician, it is almost impossible for that person to sit in the classroom as a neutral observer. Sometimes the school psychologist can perform this function, but parents may be concerned about the biases of school personnel. A descriptive narrative report of the child at school (see Appendix C at end of book), conducted by someone who is not on the school staff, can be valuable. Training a student or supervisee to perform such observations is minimally time-consuming and has a big payoff, because therapist and parents can look afresh at a factual and relatively neutral description of the child during the school day. This kind of narrative is often revelatory to all parties involved. It may even shed light on the kind of academic tasks that disorganize the child, thereby supporting the need for further testing; alternatively, it may identify a classroom organization that is particularly ill-suited to the child being observed.

PRINCIPLE 6

The child clinician should seek information from all adults involved with a child and, if necessary, arrange a school observation to augment or resolve contradictory reports. If the clinician's presence in the classroom might disrupt his or her burgeoning relationship with a child, it is helpful to induct a trainee into the art of narrative reporting "without prejudice" in order to obtain a description of the child as seen by a naïve observer (see Appendix C). Reasons for school referrals can vary, but it is important for the clinician to at least consider a cognitive or developmental component to the problem.

Following her meetings with Mr. and Mrs. Park about their daughter Ellie, Dr. Green arranged a morning visit at Ellie's school and observed Ellie's arrival with her nanny, Susie. The child seemed tired and irritable; at best, she appeared uninterested in the other children and clearly annoyed by some of them. She separated without reaction from Susie, who gave her a quick squeeze nonetheless, and got in line to go to her classroom. She showed very little animation and, in Dr. Green's opinion, seemed more like a depressed adult than a 5-year-old. Dr. Green greeted the teacher, Kim, with whom she had arranged the visit. Because visitors were common in the classroom, Kim introduced Dr. Green and explained simply that she was a child specialist interested in their classroom. The room was large and, to Dr. Green, a bit chaotic, with lots of separate stations for different activities. Although this arrangement had the benefit of allowing Dr. Green to stay in the background, it was not optimal for children like Ellie who had little enthusiasm and seemed aimless. Dr. Green spent the next 2 hours observing and writing a narrative report, which described the events of the morning and how Ellie responded to tasks, other children, and the teacher. Here is an excerpt from her report:

> At Circle Time (8:30–9:00) the children assumed preassigned spots in a circle on the carpet surrounding Kim, who was going to discuss the letter of the day. The letter was P, and Kim told the children that it could be found all over the classroom, always in pink. One child called out, "Pink starts with P!" and Kim nodded in agreement. She engaged the children in naming things starting with P. During this time, Ellie sat a little outside the circle, not facing Kim, and did not participate. She was twirling her hair and seemed preoccupied. Children began to scan the room, clearly excited, but Ellie continued to sit and twirl. She became clearly angry and pushed away another girl who pointed to her (Ellie's) head and said, "Ponytail!" The teacher observed this exchange and went over to Ellie, who cried briefly; the teacher attempted to comfort her by complimenting her shiny ponytail and reminding her that even her last name began with P.

Dr. Green had already spoken to Kim but had a moment before leaving to clarify the extent to which this was a uniform picture for Ellie. Kim explained that Ellie was able to show more life at recess and was not irritable with the adults; however, she had definitely declined in terms of energy and joyfulness, according to the teachers who had known her the previous year.

The first appointment for Ellie was planned for the following week. When Dr. Green came out to the waiting room, Ellie was sitting close to her mom and seemed mad about being there. She immediately said she had already met Dr. Green, and Dr. Green said yes, they had met on the "P is pink" day. She told Ellie that she was a feelings doctor (a description decided with the parents) and suggested that Ellie come in the office to play with her, saying that her parents had asked for this meeting because she seemed sad. Ellie didn't smile, hid her head behind her mother, and announced in a muffled voice that her mom had to come in with her. Her mom agreed but said she would have to do some e-mail work while there. They entered the room together. Ellie scanned the "play area" for toys of interest and approached the Playmobil house with a glimmer of enthusiasm; she sought out the house furniture and family figures. At each discovery, she wanted to show her mother. Dr. Green commented, "It's nice to have all your mom's attention and be able to share everything with her." The session was spent with Ellie positioning furniture in the Playmobil house. She established two sleeping areas and had a baby in the mom and dad's bed while the big sister slept alone. Dr. Green made some further light commentary: "That baby is lucky to get both parents! What about the big sister? Is she okay sleeping by herself?" Despite some forays into narrative by Dr. Green, Ellie couldn't seem to generate a story, but the premise seemed clear to the adults in the room. When it was time to stop, she did not protest but she did agree to another visit.

Before the first meeting with a child, the clinician should coordinate with the parents. They can discuss how the therapist will be introduced and what the child will be told is the reason for the visit. Depending on the family's subcultural milieu, the child and/or the parents may prefer to use the therapist's first name; in our opinion, accepting the version of the name that the child or family selects yields interesting content and almost always gives the child a sense of control in a worrisome situation. Although children are accustomed to adults talking about them in their presence and out of it, they seem alert to the special circumstances of visiting a child clinician. Occasionally, children will protest and say that they do not want a feelings or playing doctor and that their parents can help them just fine. Therapists can reassure the children that parents are part of the team trying to figure out what is wrong; they will all be talking together. Toys and other materials are ideally in sight so that the play area is appealing; an invitation to play is often unnecessary but certainly should be made if the child hesitates. The first meeting is burdened by a few tasks extraneous to actual play therapy. Clearly, further diagnostic considerations are on the agenda. Data to gather in this unstructured setting include observations of the child's approach to the therapist, and the child's play itself may hold diagnostic significance. The child's management of time, separation, and interruption (if playing) are all of interest dynamically. Acclimating the child to the therapist and the setting are important. But children, especially those who are slow to warm up, will sometimes require several meetings and reassurance that playing together is the best way to "get to know you."

PRINCIPLE 7

The primary goal of the first meeting with the child is an introduction to the setting and the clinician. The child may want to be accompanied by a parent into the office; if treatment proceeds, there is plenty of time to understand what purpose the parent's presence serves. The child may be unable to do too much in the first meeting; some children feel that this visit is happening because their parents and/or the school are displeased with them and they are constrained by a wish not to incur any further punishment. Playing with children by following their lead and respecting their defenses is a solid beginning.

In the case of Ellie, the picture at home and the view at school were consistent. Although Dr. Green knew there was more to the story, she felt she could offer something to the parents. The initial assessment was complete, and a follow-up with the parents was scheduled.

DISCUSSING THE FINDINGS AND MAKING THE RECOMMENDATION OF PLAY THERAPY

The evaluation phase concludes with a conversation with parents about findings and recommendations. Initial impressions are usually presented as open to further clarification and information, in part because developmental momentum is an unknown variable that can be, in and of itself, a righting process. It is often extremely reassuring to parents for a clinician to show sincere confidence in the developmental process, not to override the need for treatment but as an important ally to dynamic therapy.

The conversation at the conclusion of the evaluation is necessarily influenced by the source of the referral and the parents' reasonable need to hear a plan that includes an approach to the identified problem in addition to other problems. Parents may be under fire from the school and may, in turn, demand solutions from the evaluation process, for example by insisting that certain behaviors be eliminated at once. The assessment should document the child's strengths and weaknesses and include recommendations for whatever array of therapeutic interventions and accommodations (at school and at home) may be helpful. Play therapy is often only one of a number of such recommendations and will make more sense to parents if other areas of vulnerability and psychopathology are addressed by a multifaceted approach. Indeed, play therapy is not really directed at the extinction of symptoms, although this is a natural outcome of therapeutic work. Psychodynamic play therapy has much more to do with the synthetic function of the ego and, regardless of a specific diagnosis, promotes such basic capacities as self-regulation, object relations, the management of anxieties, self-representation, and so on. The parents' capacity to understand the need for play therapy depends in part on the clinician's ability to be clear about its goals.

The recommendation of dynamic play therapy may be surprising to parents, especially if they are generally unfamiliar with treatment modalities or are more familiar with behavioral interventions. The therapist should be prepared to discuss other forms of treatment, their pros and cons, and the reason for advising play therapy (which may be the single recommended treatment or only a part of the treatment package). If other referrals, such as parent training or parent guidance by a different clinician, tutoring, occupational therapy, or physical therapy, are likely to be made, mentioning these at the beginning prepares the parents for a referral down the line. Regardless, it is crucial to emphasize that the parents are an important piece of the therapy; meeting regularly with them both deepens the child work in most cases and improves the parents' capacity to understand their child. Ideally, the work with parents is presented and understood as an intrinsic part of the child's treatment. Inevitably, the therapist will be faced with questions about "what to do" in both the consultation and going forward. Most therapists prefer not to be an active agent in the patient's real life for two reasons: 1) although therapists may help parents consider important decisions, the parents' preferences and ultimately their choices have to be honored; and 2) the therapist's role is to help the child understand and come to terms with the decisions made by the adults around him or her. Too much active participation by the therapist in the decision-making process, whether in concert with or in opposition to parents, may make it difficult for the clinician to remain attuned to the child's feelings.

EXPLAINING PLAY THERAPY TO PARENTS

Play therapy is only one of many therapies currently available, and parents may need to be educated about its indications and benefits relative to other modalities. The fact that play therapy can be helpful in a wide range of circumstances regardless of diagnosis only heightens the need for explanation, because diagnosis typically dictates therapeutic modality, such as CBT, physical therapy, occupational therapy, tutoring, medication, or special educational accommodations, and conforms to expectations based on a medical model.

One compelling explanation clinicians can give parents is that play therapy addresses the child as a whole, rather than an isolated symptom or behavior. Because development is so rapid in childhood and so many building blocks of personality are being put in place, children's sense of self, identifications, affect tolerance, impulse management, and object relations can become caught up in the current turmoil, taking them off track developmentally. Approaching children's difficulties through playing, especially in early childhood, supports a vital developmental capacity that promotes self-regulation, adaptive defenses, anxiety containment, and tolerance of painful feelings. Even while acknowledging that some behaviors need modification, the therapist should emphasize that the child's inner life (e.g., self-representation, interpersonal templates, curiosity and energy for learning, defenses) has generated the problematic adaptation and therefore is the rightful domain of therapeutic concentration.

Because most adults have lost access to their playing selves and have trouble connecting to the passions and preoccupations of childhood, parents are often skeptical about play as a medium for therapeutic change. They doubt its therapeutic benefit, in part because playing has not seemed to provide solutions for their child so far and sometimes is even part of the problem; to them, play therapy seems like a flimsy and even whimsical approach to a child in serious trouble. It is helpful for the therapist to point out to parents that play is the language of childhood and that it contains more information in its themes, its formal elements, and its interpersonal expressions than the young child is capable of putting into words; playing with a psychodynamically trained clinician is entirely different from solitary play or social play, however salutary that may be. Playing makes a child "a head taller than himself" (Vygotsky 1978, p. 102), and the clinician who scaffolds that stretch helps the child progress toward optimal adaptation. During latency, when symbolic play may be relatively limited compared with game playing, children are still action oriented; even when playing is consigned to drawing, throwing a basketball, video games, board games, or cards, glimpses of children's inner struggles are usually discernible in how the activity is organized and conducted, how winning and losing are tolerated, how the therapist is used, how feelings are expressed, and what the specific idiosyncratic content is. The school-age child has plenty of language, but self-reflection is still fragile and defenses in latency are a powerful impediment to the verbal expression of conflict. For these reasons, treating the latency-age child in a setting that has access to toys and games is conducive to the emergence of the inner tensions and emotions that shape the current problems. Working in **displacement**—that is, using toys or games as an indirect vehicle for the expression of mental content—is a safe context in which the child typically exposes far more inner conflict than in conversation (Neubauer 1994).

SUMMARY

Child practices are not easy to integrate into adult psychotherapy offices, because waiting room and office requirements are often incompatible with the usual adult setting. Waiting rooms must be child friendly, individual offices must have space for a play area, the bathroom must be easily accessible, and suitemates must have high tolerance for chaos and noise. An important goal in setting up a new practice is for child clinicians to feel comfortable allowing their child patients freedom for self-expression without censure from others in the suite and from adult patients within their consulting rooms.

Developing a network in the local communities that serve children is important for a referral base. Offering a lecture or seminar (or a series of them) to local schools, developing a socialization group, attending school meetings about patients, and taking a highly regarded psycho-educational evaluator out for a coffee are excellent outreach activities. Child mental health is usually a team effort and requires the collaboration of parents and school personnel (e.g., teachers, administrators, school psychologists), plus nannies, pediatricians, camp counselors, occupational therapists, physical therapists, neuropsychiatry testers, tutors and remediators, grandparents, and neighbors.

KEY POINTS

- Thinking through the particularities of a child practice—the inevitable noisy and toy-strewn waiting room, messy bathroom, and limited time to put away all the toys before seeing adult patients—can and should dictate the choice of office space and suitemates.

- When like-minded clinicians establish an office practice, it is advantageous to think ahead and to establish an infrastructure consisting of flexible systems for collaboration, cooperation, and backup (e.g., electronic medical record system, hiring of bookkeepers or assistants, a contact file of recommended ancillary services). This coordination creates an efficient and mutually supportive atmosphere.

- Outreach to other individuals, institutions, and organizations that provide services to children is time well spent in terms of a developing network of colleagues and referral sources.

- A diverse practice with a variety of clinicians creates in-house resources and opportunities to share cases and learn from each other. This does not mean that everyone in the suite refers only to each other; parents can become apprehensive about limiting their options and want to feel that recommendations are based on what is the best possible fit for their child.

- A practice should first invest in basic toys, games, and supplies and then add others as indicated by patients' needs. Providing current toys that children actually play with is advisable. Toys and supplies to start with include crayons and markers, scissors, colored and plain paper, transparent tape; building toys, such as basic sets of blocks or interconnecting sets (e.g., magnetic tiles or Legos), that allow children to create their own playthings and scenarios, and figurative toys, such as dolls, stuffed animals, puppets, action figures, or play sets that include little figures (e.g., Playmobil, superheroes, or collections of jungle animals, dinosaurs); a few games, such as checkers, playing cards, Connect 4, and Sorry; and some low-key indoor sports items, such as an indoor door-mounted basketball hoop and a Nerf or Koosh ball. If very young children are seen in the practice, then baby dolls with accessories, such as bottles, pacifiers, and strollers, are popular.

- A comprehensive evaluation is a complex, multipart process that involves data collected from a range of sources (e.g., parents, teachers and school administrators, nannies, neuropsychiatric testers, other therapists). A narrative school observation can be a helpful document that allows parents and clinician to share a "fly-on-the-wall" description of the child in school.

- Common instigators for referrals of young children include birth of a sibling, parental discord and divorce, gender dysphoria, separation following a parent's return to work or entry into school, and difficulties at school.

- First meetings with parents should establish child clinicians as interested and committed professionals who want to understand the parents' viewpoint and their concerns. Most important is therapists' communication that they are there to discover and protect the best interests of the children involved.

- The use of play therapy is not dependent on diagnosis, even though diagnosis or explanation of the symptoms should be part of the consultation. Play therapy is a more global intervention that seeks to set in motion the child's capacities to move forward developmentally, resolving conflicts and areas of maladaptive solutions by integrating positive potentials into a more mature personality organization.

KEY TERMS

Attachment disturbance   A term used here to refer to the attachment categories developed by Mary Ainsworth and Mary Main, based on John Bowlby's theoretical contributions. In research examining infant reactions to the strange situation paradigm, babies are categorized as 1) secure, 2) insecure (avoidant or resistant/ambivalent), or 3) disorganized (see Main 2000); Nos. 2 and 3 reflect attachment disturbances. None of these imply the presence of a reactive attachment disorder, a highly, typically persistent pathological syndrome seen among deprived or traumatized children and included in DSM-5 (American Psychiatric Association 2013).

Displacement   The mechanism whereby conflicts are transferred to another context in order to find solutions for them. It is an aspect of normal development, a defense proper, and a component of other defenses. Unlike many other defenses, the conflict is not repressed but rather relocated to allow more productive solution seeking. Children's play is the quintessential manifestation of displacement as an adaptive process (Neubauer 1994).

Gender dysphoria   The DSM-5 term for a state formerly given the diagnosis of "gender identity disorder." Because its etiology and possible biological basis are as yet unclear, the term attempts to avoid the category of "disorder." It refers to children who as early as 24 months show a preference for colors, clothing, toys, and activities that are "typical" of the other sex. These children often suffer as they move into grade school because gender sorting becomes more widespread; children's anxieties about their own gender identity and their attempts to differentiate themselves tend to produce rigidly binary views, isolating the gender dysphoric children.

Latency (or latency phase)   The period of development that corresponds roughly with the grade-school years (i.e., ages 6 through 10 or 11), wherein most children manifest a significant increase in cognitive, social, and emotional maturation as demonstrated by greater autonomous self-regulation, awareness of reality, a capacity for logical thinking, and a decisive turn toward the peer group.

Object representation   A complex, multilayered psychic representation of a significant other, such as a parent, that is available in evocative memory. Object representations evolve over the first decades of life; they are vital to attachments in infancy, a source of identifications, and the subsequent re-creations of relationships that appear in transference, in friendships, and in romantic relationships throughout life. Mental representation is a precondition for object constancy.

REFERENCES

American Psychiatric Association: Diagnostic and Statistical Manual of Mental Disorders, 5th Edition. Arlington, VA, American Psychiatric Association, 2013

Coates SW, Moore MS: The complexity of early trauma: representation and transformation. Psychoanal Inq 17(3):288–311, 1997

Downey TW: The disavowal of authority in a child of divorce. Psychoanal Study Child 43:279–289, 1988 3227077

Gilmore K: Psychoanalytic developmental theory: a contemporary reconsideration. J Am Psychoanal Assoc 56(3):885–907, 2008 18802135

Heyne D, Sauter F: School refusal, in The Wiley-Blackwell Handbook of the Treatment of Childhood and Adolescent Anxiety. Edited by Essau CA, Ollendick TH. Chichester, West Sussex, UK, Wiley, 2013, pp 471–517

Main M: The organized categories of infant, child, and adult attachment: flexible vs. inflexible attention under attachment-related stress. J Am Psychoanal Assoc 48(4):1055–1096, discussion 1175–1187, 2000 11212183

Neubauer PB: The role of displacement in psychoanalysis. Psychoanal Study Child 49:107–119, 1994 7809278

Saketopoulou A: Mourning the body as bedrock: developmental considerations in treating transsexual patients analytically. J Am Psychoanal Assoc 62(5):773–806, 2014 25277869

Vygotsky LS: Mind in Society: The Development of Higher Psychological Processes. Cambridge, MA, Harvard University Press, 1978

9

Getting Started, Creating an Alliance, and Facilitating Play

Eight-year-old Jeremy McAlvin's vehement opposition to therapy assumed multiple forms in the first weeks of treatment. His parents anxiously warned Dr. Vargas that their son "doesn't think he needs therapy" despite a recent increase in his anxiety and defiant behaviors, as well as an expansion in his morning and nighttime rituals. In addition, on the day of the boy's first appointment, Mr. McAlvin e-mailed Dr. Vargas that although he and his wife had intended to prepare Jeremy for the visit, the couple had argued over when to tell him; the result was that they hastily informed him that very morning, as he was getting ready for school, that he had an appointment that afternoon.

Initially, Jeremy simply refused to leave his mother's side in the waiting room and wanted her to accompany him into the playroom. Once they were in the playroom, he glared at his mother angrily and maintained a stony silence except for mumbling, "This is so stupid," under his breath. After a few sessions, he grudgingly agreed to enter alone, but his nearly mute presentation precluded much interaction. His few communications were scathing critiques of Dr. Vargas's room: "Are these nineteenth-century toys?" or "This is the most boring place I've ever been." He also insisted on frequent bathroom or water breaks, taking his time about reentering the room. Dr. Vargas, rather than responding to Jeremy's innumerable complaints and criticisms, quietly empathized with the difficulties of having to share personal material with a stranger, the experience of feeling that his parents had betrayed him by divulging his secrets (especially his rituals), and how being brought to treatment against his will felt like a punishment rather than an offer of help. He noticed that Jeremy attended to these comments, although they did little to stop the flow of protests.

251

During the first few weeks, worried phone and e-mail communications from Jeremy's parents intensified: "Is he doing anything at all in there? He says he just sits and stares at the floor and that we are wasting our money! Do you think we should consult with someone else?"

Initiating play therapy requires patience, resourcefulness, and knowledge about children's unique perceptions of the therapeutic situation. There are many reasons why a child might feel reluctant to engage in treatment. Although these may derive from the child's individual personality and experience (shyness, rigidity, fear of "the doctor," recent parental divorce), they often represent developmentally normative trends. A preschooler's separation anxiety, a 7-year-old's fear of losing recently acquired capacities for self-control, and a 10-year-old's dread of dependency are familiar age-appropriate concerns that require the therapist's tact and sensitivity (Freud 1966). Fears over loss of autonomy, the prospect of an unfamiliar adult's intrusive scrutiny, and the risk of potentially mortifying self-exposure are powerful impediments to the child's comfortable entry into the unknowns of a therapeutic relationship. Parents' behaviors, including their explanation for the initial visit, can contribute to the child's reluctance and protests. In Jeremy's case, his parents, who often shrank from confrontations and their son's ensuing angry reactions, failed to inform him about the initial meeting until the morning of the appointment; their previous extended consultation with the therapist, in which they had discussed ways to help prepare Jeremy for treatment, seemed to have been forgotten under the immediate pressure of having to deal with a resistant child. Not surprisingly, Jeremy responded with outrage, leading to a late arrival at school that morning; these outbursts were reprised when his mother picked him up at dismissal, ready to escort him to the therapist's office for his first visit. His shock, sense of betrayal, loss of autonomy, and extreme anger at his parents further impeded a beginning alliance with Dr. Vargas.

Negative reactions to therapy are certainly not universal, and there is some empirical evidence to suggest that children attach positive expectations to beginning treatment (Carlberg et al. 2009). However, although some children request to be taken to a "feelings doctor," most often it is parents who decide that there is a problem requiring intervention. Frequently, the child feels little conscious discomfort because internal conflicts are generally relieved through the very manifestations (disruptive or controlling behaviors, withdrawal from environmental challenges) that disturb parents and teachers; indeed, the child is often highly motivated to maintain the status quo and avoid any examination of feelings below the surface (Salzberger 1963). To make sense of the therapeutic relationship and its unfamiliar elements, children sometimes equate the therapist with a teacher who will scrutinize and evaluate their responses; moreover, a young child may view the therapy as punishment for bad behavior. These various perceptions and concerns lead to **early resistances**, forms of avoidance or protest that are designed to ameliorate the child's initial fears of the clinician and the therapeutic situation by maintaining a feeling of control and autonomy. They are differentiated from **later resistances** that arise in response to a deepening of the therapy and the emergence of painful issues; working with later resistances will be discussed more fully in Chapter 11, "Deepening Play Therapy: Verbalizing Inner States, Expanding Narratives, and Working With Transference and Defense."

Historically, child analysts dealt with early resistances via an introductory period in which the child's positive feelings were actively encouraged; special toys, snacks, and the therapist's engaging behaviors were all marshaled in an effort to bypass potential negative responses (Chused 1988; Harley 1986). Clinicians were trained to present themselves as "benevolent providers" (Chused 1988, p. 53) and to avoid eliciting the child's sense of frustration or deprivation. Thoughts about how best to initiate treatment have shifted, and child therapists now employ a range of interventions to build an initial **working alliance** and deal with early resistances; these include such varied but interrelated processes as the following (Chused 1999; Keable 2011):

- Creating an alliance
- Facilitating a mutual state of play
- Containing the child's overwhelming affects
- Verbalizing the potential meanings of the child's behavior
- Setting limits when necessary
- Commencing gentle, sensitive work with the child's defenses against painful feelings

The child's initial resistance is sometimes verbalized (as when Jeremy said, "This is the most boring place I've ever been" and "This is so stupid") but more frequently manifests via action. Common early demonstrations of resistance include refusals to separate from the parent or caregiver, excessive activity in the playroom, aggressive behavior toward the therapist, a mute stance, avoidance of eye contact, or frequent excuses to dash out of the room. Older children might communicate their negative feelings about treatment by using the session to do homework, or bringing cell phones and other technology into the room and then proceeding to busy themselves with their screens. Adolescents who attend therapy alone might choose not to show up, demonstrating the ultimate resistance while simultaneously communicating their normative need for action-based responses and autonomy. Although direct acts of aggression might require the therapist's immediate intervention, most manifestations of a child's underlying distress are best viewed as meaningful communications that potentially inform the clinician and move the treatment forward. Accepting and tolerating the child's verbal protests and actions, using them to reflect on the child's expectations of the treatment and the therapeutic relationship, and finding ways to articulate the underlying anxieties—for example, loss of control, fear of exposure, perception that the therapy is a form of punishment for badness—are far more conducive to the initial working alliance and to the larger goals of therapy than seeking to shut them down.

Outside of the sessions, children often recruit parents in the service of avoiding treatment, as Jeremy does, by complaining incessantly about the uselessness of therapy or the ineptitude of the clinician. In such instances, the therapist's work with the parents is essential, both to prepare them for the child's potential resistances and to help them find ways of maintaining and supporting the treatment without exacerbating family conflict. As therapy progressed with Jeremy, Dr. Vargas realized that the parents needed more help anticipating and managing their son's vociferous reactions. Indeed, now that he was a target of Jeremy's substantial anger, Dr. Vargas achieved greater empathy with the parents' feelings of helplessness in the face of the boy's rage. Moreover, he realized the importance of verbally expressing, containing, and deescalating Jeremy's intense anxiety rather than taking on his angry accusations and complaints. Dr. Vargas communicated to the parents how frightened and out of control their son felt, and explained that Jeremy's worries were increased when adults appeared passive, allowed him to argue them into submission, or responded with anger and futility. They discussed ways to soften Jeremy's morning and evening rituals, which included his demands that one of his parents stay with him in the bathroom while he brushed his teeth and washed his face, and his insistence that a parent sit in his bedroom until he fell asleep at night. At times, parents' management of their child's various reactions and resistances reveals the need for additional clinicians who can deal more directly with individual or couples issues. Ultimately, Jeremy's parents, who were extremely distressed over their ineffectiveness in the face of the boy's struggles, accepted a referral to a marital counselor with the goal of diminishing their conflicts and achieving a unified response to their son's difficult behaviors.

Not all early resistances present as obvious opposition to the aims of therapy. Some children approach therapy with a pseudo-adult, intellectualized, and overly compliant stance.

> Highly verbal and precocious 7-year-old Yael was referred to Dr. Green for the emergence of sudden nighttime anxieties; she insisted that one of her parents stay in her room until she fell asleep and often called them in the middle of the night, complaining of bad dreams. Her parents suspected that the recent hospitalization of Yael's grandmother, who had fallen ill while visiting the family, was a main source of the girl's fears. On the first day of treatment, Yael introduced herself and entered the playroom independently, politely asking what she should call the therapist. She took a seat at the arts and crafts table, and announced that she knew she was there "because of my bedtime issues." With composure, she assured Dr. Green that the sleep problems were getting much better, that she knew her fears were "not real, because Grandma is old and I'm not," and that her parents did not need to worry about her so much. She eagerly provided descriptions of some of her classmates' less rational orientations, shaking her head in a parental way over their persistent beliefs in such entities as ghosts, Santa Claus, and tooth fairies. Yael displayed no interest in play but asked what Dr. Green thought they should talk about next.

Like Yael, some children may eschew play, insist from the outset on adult-like levels of conversation, or engage in other seemingly cooperative but controlling behaviors in order to ward off deeper engagement in the emotional aspects of treatment (Kabcenell 1993). Although such exhibitions are inherently less disruptive and may be reassuring to parents (their child "is talking" and appears to be engaged), these defensive maneuvers are equivalent with action-based resistances in their potential to keep the child's deeper emotions and conflicts outside of the playroom. Indeed, because of their seemingly pleasant and cooperative qualities, quieter self-protective stances may initially escape the clinician's notice. Dr. Green at first experienced Yael's precocious demeanor as charming and assumed her high intelligence would function as an asset in treatment; only after some sessions had passed did Dr. Green become aware that the relationship felt superficial and that her understanding of the child was not deepening at all. With this realization in mind, she was better able to attend to Yael's efforts to control the course of sessions and deflect focus on her own internal tensions via animated, somewhat dismissive descriptions of others. Dr. Green began to observe aloud that Yael seemed to talk about other people when she herself experienced a moment of discomfort. In addition, after a few weeks of pointedly ignoring the toys, Yael manifested clear interest in a set of attractively decorated nesting dolls; agreeing that they were quite unique, Dr. Green tactfully moved them closer in a way that suggested she herself, rather than Yael, desired to touch them. Yael soon suggested that they could pretend the dolls came to life and were amazed to encounter a world of humans.

Often, the initial period of adjustment to therapy elicits the entire family's individual and shared anxieties. The child patient, siblings, and parents are all vulnerable to intense wishes for quick solutions and the fear of disappointing outcomes; the emotional challenges of integrating a new individual into a familiar, preexisting family constellation; feelings about divulging private family matters; and competitive reactions to the special bond between the therapist and one member of the family. Orienting parents to the role of play, managing their treatment expectations, and preparing them for the child's inevitable resistances is discussed more fully in Chapter 10, "Working With Parents Over the Course of Treatment."

THE INTRODUCTORY PERIOD: CREATING A WORKING ALLIANCE

Initial treatment goals center on facilitating the child's sense of trust in the therapist, feeling of security in the play environment, freedom of self-expression (through words, actions, and play), and gradual understanding of the unique therapeutic relationship. Unlike adults, who have already engaged in a series of self-aware, efficacious, and collaborative actions (realizing the need for treatment, pursuing an initial evaluation, agreeing to a proposed plan of therapy), children often arrive at a first appointment without much sense of why they are there or what to expect. Before adolescence, children simply lack the developmental capability to reflect on their internal problems and assume responsibility for resolving emotional or social challenges (Chused 1999; Sandler et al. 1980). Creation of a working alliance, which involves the child's basic sense of trust, willing participation in treatment, and beginning capacity to identify with the therapist's reflective stance, represents a major objective during the early phase of therapy. A clinician's actively involved but nonintrusive attitude, willingness to engage at the child's level of available communication, and tolerance for various manifestations of discomfort—such as the child's reluctance to enter the playroom without a caregiver—indicate a setting in which the child can build a mutual relationship while retaining a sense of autonomy. Indeed, for many young children, the dread of helplessness constitutes a real threat; their knowledge that the clinician will avoid controlling, overwhelming, and invasive actions and comments is key for developing the early therapeutic bond (Chused 1999).

In the treatment of young children, *the process of playing is the best way to build an alliance*; the therapist's capacity for mutual pretending signals interest, willingness to enter the child's world and share meanings, and responsiveness at the level of the child's needs and capacities. In the early phase of treatment, play fulfills a number of essential functions: it allows for the safe displacement of private worries and wishes without directly addressing the child, thereby assuaging the child's fears of scrutiny and exposure; it indicates that the therapist is willing to be guided by the child's imagination, without attempts to impose or direct, suggesting that the child may retain individuality and control; and it fosters, through the mutual state of pretending, a sense of shared meaning and subjectivities. No less importantly, play helps foster the child–therapist relationship as it demonstrates to the child, via a normative and nonthreatening venue, the potential of the treatment to bring relief from powerful internal pressures. Using the child's play characters and scenarios, the clinician begins to label and elaborate affective experience, attach chaotic feelings to narratives, and make links between emotions and behaviors; such gentle, initial work on the child's defenses—conducted through pretense, without expecting the child to assume ownership of displaced feelings and self-protective reactions—helps reduce the intensity of inner demands and strengthen the child's tolerance for uncomfortable affects (Chused 1999; Hoffman 2007).

The therapist's opening explanations, during the first play therapy session, need not be extensive but represent an opportunity to set the tone of treatment. A tactful, sensitive approach, based on the child's developmental capacities, avoids unduly raising anxieties; addressing a young child's symptoms or problems directly runs the risk of eliciting unnecessary discomfort and embarrassment before a sense of trust is established. Potentially challenging questions, such as "Do you know why you are here?" "Do you know who I am?" or even "Can you tell me about your nighttime worries?" may arouse feelings of shame and exposure, heighten defenses, or give the impression that there is a correct answer (i.e., one that will please the therapist). It is often sufficient to make a few straightforward remarks about having met with the parents, referencing their concerns about how the child is managing strong feelings, and to introduce oneself as a person who helps children cope with worries and emotions. To ease the child's concerns about what to expect, a simple statement suggesting that the therapist and child will get to know each other by playing and talking together can suffice. At this point, school-age children may want to add their own comments, including protests about the inaccuracy of parental reports or elaborations of their worries and fears. Therapists should be transparent about their intentions to meet with the parents or to speak with others involved in the child's care and education; in addition, they will want to clarify the role of confidentiality (i.e., that the child's direct statements or specific games will not be revealed, but that any concerns about safety will be shared with parents).

None of these preliminaries need to be delivered in the manner of a prepared speech or in the first few minutes of the initial meeting. Indeed, prelatency children often immediately gravitate toward toys and immerse themselves in play, requiring little in the way of formal introductory statements. In such cases, it is not necessary to impede the child's natural inclinations; there may be an opportunity to say a few words later in the session, or even in subsequent meetings. Older children, who are more threatened by regressive play, may benefit from the presence of a few more structured options, such as art materials or rule-bound games; the therapist may wish to suggest an ice-breaking activity, such as drawing a picture of the family, if the child appears stuck or very uncomfortable. Following the child's lead, avoiding comments that evoke a sense of scrutiny and invasion, and helping to assuage initial inhibitions are principles that should take precedence over other specific goals for the first few sessions. The most useful data for the therapist rarely take the form of the child's initial answers to structured questions or come from direct talk about personal problems and symptoms; rather, the child's emotional tone, potential for reciprocity, and quality of play represent more valuable sources of information.

Reluctance to leave caregivers is best addressed by allowing the child some degree of control over the separation process. The therapist's suggestion of showing the parent or babysitter the playroom may be sufficient; after a few minutes, the child is often able to say good-bye and remain alone with the clinician. If children insist on having an attachment figure remain in the playroom, however, there is little to be gained from enforcing that individual's departure. Many treatments with young children commence in unique ways: in the waiting area, with the child concealed behind the parent's chair; in the hallway between waiting room and playroom; or in the playroom, while the child clings to the caregiver and refuses to look at the therapist. Often, even after the initial separation occurs, children continue to check in with the adults, traveling back and forth between playroom and waiting area at moments of increased anxiety. There is value in allowing young children to set the pace of separation during the introductory phase of treatment. Such behaviors represent important information about the children and the nature of their attachments; beginning to discern the meanings of a child's actions, and the precipitants of anxious responses, is far more important for the treatment than controlling their expression.

> Lisa, age 3½ years, was having trouble adjusting to preschool, often creating intense alliances with one other girl and excluding all others from their play; she reacted to circle time, or any form of group activity, with tears and refusals to participate. Although the initial referral was made to Dr. Lee, she suggested her suitemate, Dr. Vargas, because of his specialty in infancy and early childhood development. On the first day of treatment, Lisa firmly grasped her father's hand and insisted that he accompany her into Dr. Vargas's playroom. Once inside, she eagerly

commenced pretend play with her parent, contentedly arranging cups and plates and preparing dinner. Her father somewhat tentatively suggested that he might leave in a few minutes, "to take a phone call," but Lisa shook her head vigorously. Dr. Vargas, who had seated himself on the floor at a slight distance from the cooking activity, signaled to the father that the current arrangement was fine, adding aloud that Lisa did not know him well enough yet to feel comfortable alone with him. Initially, Lisa completely ignored Dr. Vargas, excluding him from the cooking game; however, when he admired the supper she relented slightly and answered one or two questions, allowing the psychiatrist to peer inside a pot and view the contents of what she was preparing. "Do you want to give Dr. Vargas one of the plates so he can eat with us?" asked her father. Lisa ignored this question, but a few minutes later she asserted that Dr. Vargas could help her prepare dessert. Lisa insisted on beginning the next few sessions similarly, exclusively focused on her father and their game of cooking. Dr. Vargas began to engage more actively, playfully complaining about his hunger and his feelings of being left out; Lisa responded enthusiastically, encouraging him toward more lively representations of these deprived states. Over the course of a couple of months, the cooking game shifted to include Dr. Vargas in a more active way; soon, Lisa began to enter the room alone.

In this example, Lisa's initial anxiety is expressed by her insistence on her father's presence. Both he and the psychiatrist follow her lead when she rejects the suggestion that her parent leave after a few minutes, allowing her to control the timing of separation. Dr. Vargas hangs back, showing interest and availability without intruding on or interrupting the play in progress. Once Lisa has had a chance to scrutinize this new adult from the safe base of the father–daughter dyad, she is ready to accept the clinician's gradual participation.

PRINCIPLE 1

The major goals of the introductory period are facilitating the child's sense of comfort and trust, and building an early therapeutic alliance. These goals are best met by allowing each child's unique needs and relational style to determine the pace of engagement and the specific manner in which the early sessions unfold. The clinician should try to avoid controlling events or hurrying the process. For example, a therapist should not insist that a parent or caregiver leave the playroom, require the child to answer specific questions, or attempt to insert himself or herself into the child's play too quickly if not invited.

ESTABLISHING A MUTUAL PLAYING STATE

For many young children, the presence of toys conducive to pretense and the therapist's unique availability are sufficient for play to begin. Often, a directly vocalized or implied invitation of "Let's pretend" gets the treatment started, and the clinician's responsiveness fosters a gradual co-creation of play themes and scenarios. Initially, the main tasks for the therapist include following the child's lead, noting affective expressions and shifts, accepting preliminary assigned play roles, and enlivening characters according to the child's overtly stated or more subtly conveyed wishes; fulfilling these assignments rests on the therapist's personal capacity for wholehearted pretense as well as tolerance for the child's disavowed affects and rejected self-representations which are often allocated in play to the clinician (Birch 1997; Gilmore 2005). Moreover, the therapist's patience and restraint are particularly valuable as the early child–clinician relationship begins to unfold. The clinician's eagerness to begin meaningful work, in the form of discovering and elaborating the child's psychological dynamics, must yield to therapeutic tact. Indeed, if the child has already begun to play freely, the clinician's main objective is to avoid play disruptions in the form of unnecessary comments, premature verbal links between the child and the play characters or scenarios, and direct remarks about the child's difficulties.

The introductory phase of play treatment is best characterized as receptivity to the child's imaginary ideas; the therapist's initial remarks are largely confined to the play itself and designed to facilitate an ongoing state of mutually engrossed, non-self-conscious pretense. In the case of Lisa, introduced in the previous section, Dr. Vargas is careful to avoid stating that the child herself desires to play the role of insider; he never overtly comments on Lisa's longing to form an intimate, exclusionary couple with her father, and to disown the mortifying role of omitted other. The therapist stays within the boundaries of the play but finds ways to comment on the difficulties of triadic relationships and the inevitable feelings of jealousy and deprivation they evoke. In this displaced form, which nonetheless reflects Lisa's innermost wishes and angry feelings, the child is able to tolerate Dr. Vargas's preliminary remarks, and the play continues without interruption. The subsequent phase of treatment, in which the therapist gradually expands pretend narratives, explores roles and characters, and develops a mutual language for the child's affective states and self-protective behaviors, is explored more fully in Chapter 11.

How does the therapist proceed when children are too anxious, inhibited, distracted, or overstimulated to initiate pretense or independently sustain coherent play narratives, or when developmental limitations lead to play that is solitary, chaotic, or severely restricted, with little apparently meaningful content? Often, children who arrive at therapists' offices suffer a level of distress and developmental disruption that manifests in hindered, disordered, or nonmutual play. In such cases, the therapist finds alternative ways to engage with the child and build a relationship, while simultaneously laying the groundwork for the emergence of a shared playing state. Facilitating the child's sense of security, containing affects, and establishing forms of mutual communication take precedence when pretense is not yet available as a tool for self-expression. The therapist may approach preliminary work in the following ways: participating in rote or sensorimotor play (e.g., a child simply stacks blocks and knocks them over, or pounds playdough without creating recognizable forms) and gradually introducing narrative opportunities; accepting an extended period of exclusion from the child's solitary stance, while seeking moments for brief nonintrusive connection; setting limits on behavior when necessary; or attempting to label the child's affective states and connect them to seemingly chaotic, confusing behaviors.

Older latency-age children, between ages 8 and 10, often present a specific developmental dilemma. Many in this age group avoid pretend play due to conscious fears of babyishness and less-conscious anxieties about regressive potentials; for the school-age child, imaginary play represents a potentially threatening situation in which recently mastered infantile wishes and impulses may find self-expression. Because of these fears of latency-age children, along with their cognitive maturation and greater interest in reality, these children begin to veer toward rule-bound games and goal-focused activities. When they enter treatment, they often display a preference for board games, rote tasks, or projects; indeed, the child may need engagement in such activities to retain a sense of security, self-control, and competence while acclimating to the therapeutic situation. Although nonpretend play offers fewer insights into children's fantasy world, it can reveal useful information about their tolerance for frustration, attitudes toward competition, and capacity for collaboration; more importantly, the therapist's acceptance of somewhat rigid, closed activities fosters trust in the relationship and establishes the treatment as a safe environment. Over the first few months of therapy, more spontaneous and less goal-directed play frequently emerges, permitting greater access into the child's emotional life.

> Eight-year-old John was referred to treatment with Dr. Lee because of expanding anxieties and phobias that were infiltrating his various activities; for the previous several months, he had increasing trouble falling asleep alone, avoided what he described as "dark corners" of his home, and asked his parents to stay with him while he showered in case an intruder should slip into the bathroom. His parents lamented his gradual withdrawal from what struck the therapist as a dizzying array of afterschool commitments (tennis, soccer, piano, robotics); moreover, John had begun to resist leaving the house at all on weekends. The child began each session the same way, silently building a complex structure out of Lego pieces. He politely answered Dr. Lee's questions about his constructions, which he described as various types of aircraft, but showed no interest in her participation and did not use the planes for pretense; he simply built. The therapist mirrored his calm demeanor, sometimes quietly admiring the strength and impenetrable nature of his aircraft; initially, John ignored these comments, but after the first few weeks he sometimes appeared interested and followed her remarks with slight elaborations of his planes and the battles they might encounter. Dr. Lee began to shift her comments toward the pilots themselves, wondering aloud how they might feel about heading into battle. At first, John simply shrugged and continued his activity; over time, however, he responded, asserting that they were "probably scared." After many weeks, during which the two essentially focused their attention on his building and engaged in occasional, brief conversation, John suggested that Dr. Lee might wish to build her own plane. She was able to elicit his suggestions for how best to equip her construction; moreover, when Dr. Lee playfully approached his plane with her own, he proposed that her aircraft might attempt to attack his, warning her that she would likely lose the battle.

In this example, John's initial reluctance to play reflects a confluence of developmental trends and defenses (his status as a latency-age child who wishes to avoid regressive play) as well as his unique set of inhibitions and rigidities (intense desire to control situations as a way to deal with his proliferating fears). Dr. Lee begins at the level of the child's manifest comfort zone—industrious, mostly solitary, and nonimaginary play—and attempts to engage in whatever ways are possible. Her preliminary interventions include quiet attentiveness that matches John's mood, nonintrusive questions about his activity rather than the child himself, and simple attempts to add a personal touch to his constructions; these attempts at communication are guided by John's cues, with the goal of allowing him to set the pace of engagement and retain a sense of control. The therapist waits for opportunities to expand the realm of play and the potentials for mutuality.

PRINCIPLE 2

Many children spontaneously gravitate toward pretense, willingly include the therapist, and collaborate toward developing play narratives. However, when such play is limited or absent, the therapist adapts to the child's capacities and seeks other opportunities for communication and relationship building. Initial interventions may include low-keyed attentiveness, joint engagement in sensorimotor games, simple labeling or narration of the child's play, and gradual introduction of imaginary elements into the child's activities.

ESTABLISHING THE THERAPEUTIC FRAME AND MANAGING BEHAVIORAL CHALLENGES

The **therapeutic frame** refers to the consistent, ongoing structure of treatment, including concrete features, such as frequency and length of session, as well as more abstract parameters, such as the therapist's stance and the child's and therapist's modes of expression and interaction. When working with adult patients, many aspects of the frame are clarified before the start of treatment. In the case of child therapy, the parents have been engaged in conversations about these matters; however, establishing the frame with children is often a more gradual and nonverbal process that becomes manifest in the child's mind due to the consistency of routines or the therapist's responses to the child's actions. Often, children beginning treatment lack the understanding and autonomous self-regulation required for discerning and following the norms and conventions that facilitate the therapeutic process. The following three examples from Dr. Lee's growing practice illustrate common dilemmas that many therapists face when they initiate treatment with young children.

Henry, now age 7, had experienced expulsion from two preschools and a summer day camp; although typically a cheerful child with excellent cognitive skills, he could not tolerate frustrations and disappointments, often turning impulsively on his peers with angry outbursts. He approached his first therapy session with curiosity and a positive attitude, pleased to discover one of his favorite board games in Dr. Lee's closet. All went well until he encountered a streak of bad luck; his mood grew sullen and he abruptly quit the game, veering toward a Nerf ball on the floor. He initially proposed a game of catch but soon began to throw the ball harder and harder at Dr. Lee's head and body, taunting her with "It doesn't hurt; it's just a Nerf ball." Ultimately, he threw the ball at her face and it knocked off her glasses. Henry laughed loudly. Dr. Lee, who was caught off guard but not harmed, observed that sometimes people laugh when they are surprised and scared. Henry angrily denied any such feelings, insisting that it had just been "funny" when the ball hit her face. However, he was slightly more careful as they continued the game.

Four-year-old Jocelyn agreed to enter the playroom alone with Dr. Lee but soon grew restless and ran out the door. She circled the suite wildly, laughing as the therapist and then her mother appealed to her to slow down; ultimately, she burst into the office of Dr. Green, a colleague who shared the suite, compelling Dr. Lee to retrieve her physically. She soon broke away from Dr. Lee's grasp, and ran toward another child in the waiting room, demanding to know why she was there. Dr. Lee asked Jocelyn's mother to help restrain her and to escort her back to the playroom, while verbally stating that all adults and children in the therapy suite, including Jocelyn, needed their privacy.

Five-year-old Carrie was eager to engage Dr. Lee in a game of "mother and father"; she lay on the floor and invited the therapist to join her. After a few minutes of casual discussion about their imaginary children's plans for the next day, Carrie cheerfully suggested that they "do sex" and encouraged Dr. Lee to take the lead. Dr. Lee inquired about the meaning of "doing sex" and asked Carrie to explain what she had in mind. When it seemed clear that Carrie meant to lean her body on top of Dr. Lee's, the clinician pointed out that they could not touch each other in this way and suggested that they use dolls to continue the game.

In these three vignettes, Dr. Lee confronts on-the-spot decisions similar to those that often arise during the opening phase: Should a child be permitted to break toys, scribble on a therapist's walls, scream and disrupt other people's sessions, or ignore the clinician and do homework? More abstractly, is it therapeutic to adopt a permissive stance with children, such as Henry and Jocelyn, whose impulsivity and poorly regulated behavior create havoc not only in the therapist's office but also in other realms of their lives? How should a therapist respond to the child's introduction of sexual themes in play, as in the case of Carrie? In many ways, working with children forces therapists not only to confront the limits of their own theories but also to discover the perimeters of personal tolerance for anxiety, aggression, childhood sexual fantasy, chaos, and any number of other psychological challenges.

Behavioral dilemmas often arise at moments of heightened emotion, such as when the child separates from the caregiver, the play intensifies around a potentially stimulating theme, or the therapist indicates that the session is over. The child who immediately wreaks chaos when the therapist announces that it is time to leave certainly creates an inconvenient situation that may run counter to the clinician's preference for joint cleaning up, a calm departure, and an opportunity to return a composed child to the waiting caregiver. However, it is often more useful to avoid the temptation to reduce or eliminate such reactions via overly intellectualized talk (e.g., explaining the reasons for ending on time) or censorious messages (e.g., "We can't play with these toys if you won't clean up") and instead allow the child to express feelings about the end of session through action as well as words. Increased messiness as the session draws to a close, deliberate spilling of toys, frantic activity, stalling, or outright refusals to finish up and leave the room are all familiar ways in which young children communicate separation fears and protests, attempt to actualize their wish to control the session and the therapist, and seek to disavow sad or abandoned feelings through action.

In psychodynamic treatment, the main principle for handling these situations is to allow children maximum opportunity for self-expression through words, actions, and play while safeguarding their psychological and physical safety and ensuring the therapist's relative freedom to work—that is, to perform the functions of observing, absorbing the child's communications, reflecting, and responding therapeutically (Joseph 1998; Yanof 2012). When the therapist feels physically threatened, fears that the child may be injured, or anticipates disruption to a colleague's work environment, the therapist may find it impossible to maintain a focused, therapeutic stance; however, it is often preferable to work through less compelling situations, such as worries about parental reactions (e.g., if a child is yelling during a session) or annoyance and distaste due to the level of messiness created in the playroom. Achieving a balance between open expressiveness and protective parameters is an ongoing challenge—one that requires child therapists to monitor their own vulnerabilities, consider the child's developmental level, and assess the potential value or harm of the child's disorderly behaviors.

Although direct efforts to reduce the child's actions are often best avoided, helping the child modulate affective intensity, via containing functions such as labeling affects and inner states, is an essential component of the therapeutic process. Provision of developmental assistance facilitates the child's internalization of therapeutic routines, such as the timely ending of sessions that children nonetheless experience as abrupt and depriving. Such help may take the form of verbalizing the child's imagined affects and inner states, saving small artworks and constructions in a special bin, and giving reminders about the next session; these strategies can be internalized by the child and used for self-regulation, gradually reducing the need to express feelings through impulsive behavior. Some children require substantial support at times of separation, such as taking home (or borrowing) a small item from the therapist's office; in the introductory phase of treatment, this may serve the purpose of assuaging the immediate pain of departure and conveying a sense of continuity. An agreement to transport such materials back and forth between office and home can be negotiated with the child and caregiver. Other children benefit from a 5-minute warning that signals the upcoming time for departure and allows them a few moments to adjust to the upcoming transition. To accommodate a busy professional schedule, the therapist may need to begin the process of ending a few minutes early, allowing time for the child's transition back to the caregiver without undue stress over holding up the next patient. Of course, if a child persists in refusal to leave the room, it may be necessary to recruit the caregiver's assistance.

PRINCIPLE 3

The task of establishing and maintaining the frame of treatment is important and ultimately helps children develop a sense of the therapist's constancy and reliability. However, child therapists should be prepared to demonstrate flexibility during the introductory period, particularly around the child's reaction to ending sessions. Developmental assistance in multiple forms (e.g., verbalizing affects, allowing the child to take home and bring back a small item from the playroom, setting limits) may be necessary as the child learns to tolerate separation and gains confidence in the stability of the therapeutic relationship.

HANDLING SEXUAL BEHAVIORS AND CONTENTS

Certain behaviors, because of their potential for harm and overstimulation, as well as their lack of utility within the therapeutic process, are discouraged or simply disallowed altogether. Children should not be permitted to undress beyond the removal of footwear and outer garments, act toward the therapist in overtly sexualized ways (outside of pretend play), or inflict injury on themselves or the therapist. Many actions, however, fall within an ambiguous zone, and clinicians must decide to establish boundaries determined in part by their theory, the qualities and developmental status of each child, and their personal tolerance for physical closeness, stimulation, mess, and provocative acts. Moreover, the action-based nature of child treatment often results in unexpected, instantaneous behaviors: objects are thrown, the child strikes out in frustration, or an article of clothing is tossed aside without warning. Young children will inadvertently touch, brush against, or lean on the therapist, or reach out to hold hands on the way to the playroom. They may wish to create a game of doctor by using their own and the therapist's bodies, or expect to climb into the clinician's lap.

For prelatency children, normative manifestations of impulses and wishes, in combination with the limits of their self-regulatory capabilities, mean that the body and its exigencies occupy a prominent role in the children's thoughts and feelings. Moreover, very young children are apt to expect the therapist to follow the protocols of other relationships, such as those with parents, babysitters, or teachers; the children might express curiosity by asking personal questions, request help with toileting, or anticipate that the therapist is available for physical affection. Although older children can understand and tolerate the frustration engendered by certain restrictions (e.g., when the therapist, preferring to elicit the child's fantasies, declines to answer immediately direct questions about marital or parenthood status), these parameters are less meaningful and useful in the treatment of younger children, who may simply feel confused or rejected by a therapist's refusal of self-disclosure (Barish 2004; Chused 1988). The therapist should be cognizant of the possible meanings when a child attempts to satisfy curiosity through entreaties for personal revelations or when a child seeks bodily closeness. For example, it is unnecessarily rigid for a therapist to refuse a 4-year-old's request to assist with unbuttoning a sweater or retying a shoelace that has loosened; however, physical contact between therapist and child reverberates with oedipal desires, and repeated granting of such appeals may be experienced by the child as seductive and overstimulating. Requests for more elaborate physical engagement, such as help using the bathroom, are best dealt with by recruiting the child's caregiver. For this reason, it is desirable that the parents or babysitters of very young children are available as needed during the therapeutic session.

Responding therapeutically to sexualized behavior and play requires knowledge of the child's developmental level and unique environmental circumstances, consideration of the context in which these manifestations emerge, and awareness of countertransference (Cant 2002; Fabricius 1992; Holder 2000). The central role of the body in children's mental life and the normative presence of erotic feelings and fantasies during all phases of human development ensure that sexual theories, curiosities, and contents will find their way into every child treatment; the realization that even very young children experience sensual feelings and direct avid interest toward the physical lives of adults can take inexperienced clinicians by surprise, engendering discomfort and a subtle tendency to discourage the child's expressions. Of course, certain sexualized behaviors fall outside of age-expected norms; for example, when intense and compulsive sexual play materializes early in treatment, the dominance of such preoccupations may signal the child's exposure to overstimulation or maltreatment and require that the therapist pursue these concerns with the caregivers (Sherkow 1990).

In most cases, both explicit and implicit sexual contents are normative aspects of child therapy that are best handled from within the confidential therapeutic relationship. Direct attempts to touch the therapist's body, beyond expected casual or inadvertent behaviors in younger children, are best dealt with by clear limit setting ("We can play anything you like, but we aren't going to touch each other"). During the oedipal years, the child's insistence on playing doctor with the therapist's body or a child's invitation to enact a primal scene (the child's representation of parental sexual behavior) reflects efforts to actualize normal wishes and fantasies; in such cases, the therapist's tactful suggestion that they use dolls or gentle setting of limits on actual body-to-body contact is often sufficient without need for further comment (Holder 2000). Similarly, brief masturbatory behavior in prelatency children or the anxious touching of the genital region by early latency children is usually transient and yields quickly to engagement in play activities, requiring no further verbal elaboration. The older latency child, pressured by the encroachment of preadolescent development, may manifest an increase in sexual talk, joking, and erotic play themes; although it may be helpful to find tactful ways to comment on the child's escalating interest, anxiety, and excitement, the emergence of such behavior is within normal expectations.

PRINCIPLE 4

Sexual themes are a normal and inevitable component of child treatments. In general, when they arise within pretend play, they are best treated like any other contents; however, if children seek to use their own or the therapist's body, it may be necessary to redirect the play toward dolls or other substitutes. Intense, compulsive sexual play or behavior may reflect the child's exposure to overstimulating events and needs to be explored with parents.

MANAGING AGGRESSION IN THE PLAYROOM

Aggressive themes and behaviors abound in child treatments; indeed, Anna Freud (1972, p. 168) famously commented that aggression "looms larger than sex" in working with children, posing myriad challenges to the therapist's technique. When the child's hostile feelings are confined to verbal expression or conveyed within the metaphors of pretend play, the therapist generally tolerates these manifestations despite their potentially graphic, rude, or violent contents, and regardless of the inevitable countertransference reactions (discomfort, disapproval, retaliatory anger) such behavior may engender. In the opening phase of treatment, when children are especially vulnerable to overwhelming feelings of anxiety and loss of autonomy, direct angry or insulting remarks to the therapist (e.g., "I wish you would just shut up!" "You're so stupid, you can't understand anything!" "Get away from me!") represent an acceptable mode of self-expression that can crystalize the intensity and immediacy of a child's emotions. Because young children often feel frightened by the force of their aggression, fear the potential destructiveness of hostile wishes and fantasies, and worry about retribution for forbidden urges, the therapist's tolerance of angry comments, frank acknowledgment of the child's feelings, and nonpunitive response help contain anxiety and establish the sense of the therapeutic environment as safe and reliable. Indeed, the therapist's premature limit setting or overly fastidious and controlling approaches can lead to the child's inhibition of perceived unacceptable contents.

Similarly, the therapist avoids censorious comments or redirection when a child pursues aggressive contents within imaginary play, even when these involve mayhem and destruction. The child's developmental phase is an important determinant of fantasy-based aggression. For example, the play of oedipal-age children often reflects fears of bodily injury and concrete principles of justice; pretend play that centers on castration anxieties and more general physical punishments (e.g., decapitated heads or severed limbs as a consequence of mild transgressions) represents normative anxieties. By allowing full expression of such scenarios and participating in the play according to children's preferences (e.g., embodying the witch who eats up babies, or the dragon that frightens little children), the therapist helps the child express and share frightening fantasies, ultimately assuaging their intensity and immediacy by attaching them to words and narratives.

Aggressive impulses that are symbolized within the realms of language and play are therapeutically useful communications. However, the child clinician may need to limit direct expressions of hostility in the form of actions with reality-based consequences, such as injury or destruction of property. Children with limited capacity for self-regulation who lack access to language and play during states of arousal initially require the therapist's active help to avoid dangerous situations. Speaking firmly, restraining the child, restricting certain activities, removing items from the playroom, recruiting the assistance of caregivers, and even ending the session may be necessary to preserve a secure setting. Indeed, setting limits under such circumstances serves multiple developmental functions, which include protecting the child from the guilt that follows harming others; supporting the differentiation between internal and external reality; providing a sense of physical and psychological safety; containing the child's impulses; communicating that the child's feelings and fears of omnipotence and destructiveness will not be actualized; and demonstrating that the therapist can manage and is not harmed by the child's aggressive urges (Sugarman 2003; Zilberstein and Abel 2012). In addition, the therapist requires a reasonably safe atmosphere to be able to think, react, and work freely, rather than focus relentlessly on concrete issues of environmental safety. As is true in the case of sexual themes, however, a preponderance of violent imagery and persistently sadistic scenarios may reflect the child's exposure to aggression in the real world or signal self-regulatory deficits that need to be addressed through additional or substitute modes of treatment. In Chapter 13, "Play Therapy, Variations in Child Development, and More Serious Psychopathology," we discuss situations in which the usual psychodynamic approach to play therapy alone is not sufficient or optimally suited to the child's needs.

PRINCIPLE 5

When dealing with aggressive behavior, the therapist should set as few rules as possible beyond what is necessary to maintain child and adult personal safety. The goal is to allow children the greatest possible access to self-expression—via words, play, and also actions—but to protect them from actualizing hostile urges and fantasies in a way that may cause injury or make it impossible for the therapist to work freely. Aggressive themes and contents are a ubiquitous, developmentally normative component of play and should not be discouraged by the clinician. However, a preponderance of violent imagery may signal problems that require additional interventions.

SUMMARY

Initiating play therapy is a gradual process that requires adjusting to the child's developmental and emotional needs. Many children experience initial discomfort in the treatment situation; the source of their distress may include reactions to a loss of autonomy, a sense of exposure and scrutiny, worries about losing control over their intense feelings and urges, and fears that the treatment is a punishment. Often, early resistances are expressed via the child's actions, including avoidant and aggressive behaviors, but they may also take the form of overly compliant attitudes. In general, the therapist seeks to tolerate these various verbal and action-based expressions, using them to expand understanding of the child's underlying anxieties and familiar modes of reducing internal stress, while verbally acknowledging the child's internal states. Aggressive and sexual contents are normal in the play of young children; however, certain overstimulated behaviors, such as direct aggression or sexualized actions, need to be actively limited.

KEY POINTS

- Early resistances to play therapy often represent the child's sense of insecurity in an unfamiliar setting and in a new relationship; typical reactions include the resentment of being brought against one's will, fears about private matters (secrets, wishes, feelings) that might be divulged and judged as bad, and discomfort with separation from parental figures. It is most helpful when the therapist can proceed at the child's pace and not hurry the introductory phase of treatment.

- Resistances commonly take the form of actions, such as refusal to be alone with the clinician, a shift in the child's level of activity, a disruption in the play, or a need to leave the playroom. Some children may evince overly passive or compliant attitudes. Unless these initial behaviors are potentially harmful and destructive (e.g., direct expressions of aggression or sexuality), the therapist maintains an accepting and tolerant attitude while attempting to articulate the challenging aspects of the novel therapeutic environment.

- After becoming acclimated to the therapy situation, many children enter pretend play with little difficulty. However, children with limited access to imaginary fantasy or with play inhibitions will require that the therapist begin with nonpretend activities and gradually establish mutual play.

- The treatment frame serves important functions, including helping the child internalize the consistency and reliability of the therapeutic relationship. In the initial phase of therapy, young children often require flexibility and extra assistance at moments of transition, such as when the session needs to be ended.

- Aggressive and sexual themes are normal components of children's play, and the therapist may need to overcome personal discomfort to facilitate expression of the child's fantasies. A preponderance of such contents or frequent direct expressions of sexual and hostile urges may need to be further explored with the child's main caregivers.

- The therapist may need to set limits on or redirect action-based expressions of hostility or sexuality to protect the child and preserve the capacity to perform therapeutic functions.

KEY TERMS

Early resistances A patient's internal efforts to maintain a psychological status quo, and thereby sustain a sense of inner calm and control, by avoiding initial engagement in the therapeutic process. In childhood, such resistances often exist side by side with normative developmental concerns, such as separation anxiety. They tend to take the form of action-based refusals to engage with the therapist but may also manifest as overly compliant or pseudo-adult behaviors.

Later resistances A child's efforts to maintain familiar self-protective mechanisms, often due to intensification of transference and emergence of conflictual material in the play.

Therapeutic frame   The consistent, ongoing structure of treatment, including concrete features, such as frequency and length of session, as well as more abstract parameters, such as the therapist's stance and the child's and therapist's modes of expression and interaction.

Working alliance   The part of the therapeutic relationship that involves the child's basic sense of trust in the clinician, willing engagement in treatment, and beginning identifications with the therapist's curiosity, affect tolerance, and reflective stance.

REFERENCES

Barish K: The child therapist's generative use of self. J Infant Child Adolesc Psychother 3(2):270–282, 2004

Birch M: In the land of counterpane: travels in the realm of play. Psychoanal Study Child 52:57–75, 1997 9489461

Cant D: "Joined-up psychotherapy": the place of individual psychotherapy in residential therapeutic provision for children. Journal of Child Psychotherapy 28(3):267–281, 2002

Carlberg G, Thoren A, Billstrom S, et al: Children's expectations and experiences of psychodynamic child psychotherapy. Journal of Child Psychotherapy 35(2):175–193, 2009

Chused JF: The transference neurosis in child analysis. Psychoanal Study Child 43:51–81, 1988 3227088

Chused JF: Engaging the child in the therapeutic process, in The Therapeutic Alliance. Edited by Levy ST. Madison, CT, International Universities Press, 1999, pp 55–74

Fabricius J: The baby that turned into a lion, and other stories: treatment report from an under-five. Bulletin of the Anna Freud Centre 15:225–240, 1992

Freud A: Normality and Pathology in Childhood: Assessment of Development. London, Hogarth, 1966

Freud A: Comments on aggression. Int J Psychoanal 53(2):163–171, 1972 4115729

Gilmore K: Play in the psychoanalytic setting: ego capacity, ego state, and vehicle for intersubjective exchange. Psychoanal Study Child 60:213–238, 2005 16649681

Harley M: Child analysis, 1947–1984. A retrospective. Psychoanal Study Child 41:129–153, 1986 3547444

Hoffman L: Do children get better when we interpret their defenses against painful feelings? Psychoanal Study Child 62:291–313, 2007 18524096

Holder A: To touch or not to touch: that is the question. Psychoanal Inq 20(1):44–64, 2000

Joseph B: Thinking about a playroom. Journal of Child Psychotherapy 24(3):359–366, 1998

Kabcenell RJ: Some aspects of the "treatment alliance" in child analysis. Journal of Clinical Psychoanalysis 2(1):27–41, 1993

Keable H: The Freudian tradition at one hundred years through the lens of Berta Bornstein. Psychoanal Rev 98(5):723–742, 2011 22026545

Salzberger I: Resistance in treatment as a means of avoiding inner conflict. J Child Psychotherapy 1:26–34, 1963

Sandler J, Kennedy H, Tyson RL: The Technique of Child Psychoanalysis: Discussions With Anna Freud. Cambridge, MA, Harvard University Press, 1980

Sherkow SP: Evaluation and diagnosis of sexual abuse of little girls. J Am Psychoanal Assoc 38(2):347–369, 1990 2362071

Sugarman A: Dimensions of the child analyst's role as a developmental object: affect regulation and limit setting. Psychoanal Study Child 58:189–213, 2003 14982021

Yanof JA: Treating children with affect dysregulation. Discussion of Dr. Wendy Olesker's analysis of Matt. Psychoanal Study Child 66:109–121, 2012 26020994

Zilberstein K, Abel S: Holding the line: limits in child psychotherapy. J Infant Child Adolesc Psychother 11(1):21–31, 2012

10

Working With Parents Over the Course of Treatment

A school well known to Dr. Reed from her training referred 6-year-old Talicia Johnson for assessment of and cognitive-behavioral therapy (CBT) for her school refusal and phobic anxiety around bugs, which produced "meltdowns" in the spring when flies were plentiful. Mr. Johnson made the first phone call to Dr. Reed, outlining the situation in a somewhat distant and nonspecific way. Dr. Reed was immediately aware of his lack of detailed familiarity with Talicia. Given the main symptom, Dr. Reed suggested that even before she meet the parents, she would like to arrange a school visit at early morning drop-off. This was easy to schedule since she was very familiar to the school staff. Within a few days, she was able to witness first-hand a scene well described by the director: Talicia reluctantly entered the school courtyard with her mother, looking fearful and on the verge of tears. Her teacher collected the students at the entrance, gathering them in a line to enter the lobby and walk up the stairs, in what appeared to be a familiar and comfortable routine. Talicia made a few half-hearted attempts to move forward into the line, seemed to be deterred by some exchange with another student, and then began to cry and cling to her mother. It took 20 minutes and a special escort to the classroom (the assistant director) to get Talicia into what Dr. Reed felt to be a warm and welcoming classroom. Throughout this ordeal, Mrs. Johnson stood wringing her hands, looking uncertain about what to do but unwilling to separate from Talicia until the child was in the classroom. At that point, Dr. Reed introduced herself to Mrs. Johnson and confirmed their coming appointment. This 45-minute observation was very valuable to the consultation. First, it made clear to Dr. Reed that the school could be managing Talicia's entry in a way that would possibly be less socially

277

damaging to her; be more directive and supportive to her mother; be incorporated seamlessly into the established routine; and/or provide incentive for Talicia to join the class. Second, Mrs. Johnson's desperation and anxiety suggested she needed independent guidance. To address the school approach, Dr. Reed planned a meeting with the teacher, the director of the lower school, and the assistant director. Her appointment with the Johnsons was already set for the next day.

Because Mr. Johnson had made the initial contact, Dr. Reed was surprised when only Mrs. Johnson showed up, with profuse apologies for her husband, who was on an unexpected required business trip. In the interview, the topic of Talicia was often sidelined as Mrs. Johnson described how overwhelmed she was by her three children and her frequently absent husband; the live-in nanny was helpful but mostly engaged with the two younger children, both boys. She acknowledged that she herself had been quite fearful in childhood and was still a "homebody" despite having an advanced degree in social work. A second meeting scheduled with the parents was also not attended by Mr. Johnson.

Dr. Reed was concerned about Mr. Johnson's apparent relinquishment of an active role in the crisis and about Mrs. Johnson's helplessness, loneliness, and high baseline anxiety level. She was alert to what was potentially a phobic partnership between mother and daughter. She learned that they often slept in the same bed when Mr. Johnson traveled or was out late at business meetings; it was unclear whose needs were primarily served. Dr. Reed began to think that CBT with Talicia might be postponed in favor of a better behavioral program with the school and especially parent work; even though Mr. Johnson's absence was a central factor in the family's difficulties, it seemed more pragmatic to focus first on Mrs. Johnson. Dr. Reed thought a colleague from training, Ms. Hamilton, a social worker with psychodynamic training, might be able to help Mrs. Johnson in individual psychotherapy; she hoped that the referral to a smart accomplished social worker might be especially helpful as a source of potential identification. Because Ms. Hamilton's training overlapped that of the suitemates, they all knew her, so communication remained optimal. Dr. Green, a psychiatrist in the suite, said she would be available to prescribe medication, if indicated. Dr. Reed felt confident that a behavioral parenting program, achieved by working with the parents rather than the child, would be more helpful to Talicia at the moment because the parental dynamic was leaving a void in Mrs. Johnson's emotional life and needed to be addressed. She proposed this plan to Mrs. Johnson and noted that it would not really work without Mr. Johnson's participation. He was unresponsive to several attempts to bring him in, but finally he did show up for a parenting session months after his original phone call; he was attentive in the session although still somewhat dismissive of his wife. He openly insisted that her relationship with Talicia was the problem. Dr. Reed firmly disagreed with that perspective and insisted that he come to parenting meetings; surprisingly, he agreed and actually followed through, not to every session but more often than not.

The simple interventions at school, coming out of a 30-minute brainstorming meeting, were remarkably successful within 3 months. The first step was to put the assistant director in the courtyard and arrange a quick daily trade of sturdy little glass owls, taken on loan from a collection that absorbed Talicia's attention in her many visits to the director's office; she seemed to admire and even pine for these figures, making them the perfect inducement to come to school. Talicia was allowed to keep one in her pocket and take it home, knowing she must bring it back in the morning to exchange it for another one. The second step was for the teacher to assign everyone in the class a "line buddy" whose mutual responsibility was to get the other in line and ready to march upstairs. She assigned Talicia a kind, engaging, and well-liked partner in her class, a "popular" girl who was quite skilled in shepherding Talicia away from teasing and humiliating interactions with other kids. These two interventions, plus the beginning of therapy for the mother, loosened the mutual grip of mother and daughter, allowing Talicia to follow school procedure. Once the behavioral component that was interfering at school was under control, Dr. Reed felt that Talicia would be able to benefit from her own therapy and that play therapy was the treatment of choice. She made it clear to Mrs. Johnson that a gradual weaning from co-sleeping was next in a behavioral program but said that Talacia herself should signal when she was ready. A reward of a glass owl for Talacia to begin her own collection was an attractive inducement. Similarly, Mrs. Johnson's progress with Ms. Hamilton made it easier for her to support Talacia's steps toward independence. Dr. Reed referred Talicia to Dr. Lee for the play therapy.

Talicia's multipart, multistep treatment illustrates a common reality in child cases. The child's symptoms are the outcome of many interacting systems that sustain them; their interlocking can arrest forward momentum and make progress almost impossible. In this chapter, we address the central role of parents, recognizing that, as in Talicia's case, other systems, such as school and possibly a nanny, are also implicated. Nonetheless, it is usually true that parents, in addition to their role as important ancillary sources of information, are the chief therapeutic collaborators in child therapy. Because they are an intrinsic part of children's mental lives, parents figure into their conflicts and can most directly help their children through their own commitment to change.

Establishing a rapport with parents, separately or together, is a central part of the work, beginning with the first consultation. This is a delicate process for a number of reasons. First, parents are often already beleaguered by critical commentary about their child's problem; not uncommonly, they are already on the defensive about their role in creating it. Second, the parental couple's relationship is frequently strained by their child's problems and can devolve into overt hostility, blaming, or mutual avoidance. This was certainly true for Mrs. Johnson whose husband was clearly faulting her. Third, the therapist can be seen as prying, haughty, or insulting as parents struggle to maintain their confidence in their parenting and their special knowledge of their child.

Dr. Reed's choice first to see what was actually happening at school and then to pursue changes there that might calm the crisis was intuitively supportive of Mrs. Johnson, who was already overwhelmed and defeated. This line of action conveyed the message to Talicia's mother that the problem was not entirely her fault and that Dr. Reed was her ally. This became even more important over the course of consultation as Mr. Johnson's delayed in-person participation and his critical commentary underscored his very different message.

The opening phase of the consultation can be crucial in influencing the direction of the relationship between parents and therapist. Because families in trouble often have both obvious and hidden lines of alliance and antagonism, the therapist must tread carefully, especially with divided parents. Losing the support of either parent can undermine the treatment; similarly, overidentification with one parent can color the therapist's perspective and defeat any semblance of even-handedness. As in Talicia's case, there are always multiple consequential decisions to be made, almost before the process begins. An important goal for the clinician throughout a child's treatment is the sustained respectful interest in both parents' point of view, which serves as an implicit acknowledgment of their importance and the therapist's commitment to helping them help their child. This statement may seem paradoxical in regard to Mr. Johnson, whose point of view might be summed up as "not my problem; please deal with it without bothering me." From a certain perspective, the opening phase of treatment could be seen as conforming to his wishes, but, while going about the business of helping the family without him, Dr. Reed had a feeling he would eventually come in of his own accord. Despite signs to the contrary, she saw him as committed to the marriage and Talicia.

OVERVIEW OF PARENT WORK

It is not uncommon to hear child clinicians lament the obligation to work with parents, even while recognizing that the parents' goodwill is fundamental to the therapeutic task. Parents are usually deeply distressed by the time they arrive at the therapist's office; their discouragement, feelings of inadequacy, and self- and mutual recriminations heighten their defensiveness and their mistrust of the clinician. The parents' experience and the circumstances surrounding the consultation undoubtedly contribute to child therapists' experience of parent meetings as problematic, with the tone ranging from combative to derisive to desperate. Of course, therapists' attitudes are never purely reactive; their countertransferences are frequently informed by their own childhood suffering, competitive feelings, and anger at their own parents' perceived destructiveness. Frankiel (1985) observed that wishes to "steal" (and sometimes thereby to "rescue") children are universal fantasies that are ubiquitous in our culture; such stories are seen in myths (e.g., the Oedipus story), beloved fairy tales (*Rumpelstiltskin*), and biblical legends (Moses). In addition to their own conflicts, then, child clinicians also may harbor intensified versions of these universal fantasies and struggle with the conviction that they could parent their patients better than the parents can.

The problem of working with parents can be traced back to the origins of child psychoanalysis and its struggle to establish itself on a par with the analysis of adults. Novick and Novick (2000) suggest that pioneers in the field, such as Anna Freud, faced a psychoanalytic culture that viewed work with children as a lesser form of treatment: as patients, children did not verbalize their inner lives and did not free associate, and their transferences were diluted by the ongoing, availability of primary objects (parents). These critiques, combined with the emphasis on the pathogenic potential of unconscious fantasy over environmental factors, supported the tendency to view parents as interferences in work with the child. Although Anna Freud certainly recognized the parents as active agents in the child's mental life and, according to the Novicks, did parent work as part of all her child treatments, she did not elaborate the technique of parent work in her many discussions of child analysis.

Child therapists' ambivalence about privileging parent work, as well as their preferred psychoanalytic approach that consigned contact with parents to information gathering without intervention or guidance, unfortunately went unchallenged for decades; work with parents remained an amorphous modality without clear theoretical or conceptual underpinnings. The family in reality was not felt to bear a meaningful relationship to the family as represented in the child's mind, shaped by the child's cognitive capacity and unconscious fantasy. Indeed, the real family was likely to be distracting: "the more the real family is excluded from the analytic situation, the more frequently do the transitional and transference families make their appearance" (Anthony 1980, p. 25). That is to say, children are more likely to produce their internal models in play or transference and elaborate their projections onto the clinician if the actual parents are not in constant attendance.

Parent work was relegated to a minor role for decades, until it was officially revived as a critical ancillary support of child psychotherapy and psychoanalysis by the Furmans, especially Erna Furman, in their work at the Hanna Perkins Center for Child Development. Erna Furman proposed a theory of parent–child relationships that conceptualized the parent–child dynamic as "a complex overdetermined interaction in which two closely interwoven personalities complement each other in various ever-changing unconscious ways" (Furman 1995, quoted in Novick and Novick 2000, p. 61). The baton then was taken up by Jack and Kelly Novick, who champion the importance of work with parents during child treatment (Novick and Novick 2000, 2002a, 2002b, 2002c, 2005, 2011). In their view, the goal of treatment delineated by Anna Freud as "restoring the child to the path of normal development" has been matched by another goal, that of "a restoration of the parent-child relationship to its potential as a lifelong positive resource for both" (Novick and Novick 2000, p. 61).

There are still psychodynamic clinicians who see the merit of limited contact with parents in some cases (e.g., see Chused 2000), perhaps especially in circumstances where the child is relatively high functioning, the parents usually act in the child's best interest, and the therapist believes that the parents will tolerate minimal contact. Nevertheless, sensitive parent work is an essential skill for child clinicians that is still undertheorized and has not earned its rightful place in training. Despite the inclusion of family therapy in child residency curricula, training programs rarely focus directly on the ancillary work with parents as a distinct therapeutic entity. Clinic time is not carved out for parent work independent of the child's therapy; therefore, to give parents any attention, the therapist is compelled to sacrifice the child's time. In private practice or in situations where the therapist can determine the nature of parent visits, there is opportunity to see parents regularly and to engage them in their child's process. How the clinician conceptualizes the parents' role (and possibly other family members' roles) in treatment sets the stage for ongoing relationships that potentially sustain and even amplify the benefits of therapy; at the very least, regular contact can foster a cooperative atmosphere and mitigate divisiveness. Because the premise of therapy poses a threat to the status quo, however maladaptive, that the family and child have established, anyone in the family can experience the therapist as an adversary or as allied with "the others."

SYSTEMS THINKING

Work with parents requires special skills to negotiate a position of relative neutrality and avoid common problems. Examples of problems include treatment of parents as patients; overidentification with one or both; and avoidance of parent contact because it is viewed as a drain on time, an unpleasant and futile exercise, or an extraneous intrusion into the work with the child (Novick and Novick 2005). The child assessment and recommendation period will establish foundational principles for the work: mutual respect and a collaborative relationship between parents and therapist, the right of their child to independent personhood, and the relinquishment of the parents' tendency to determine causality and blame. This last-mentioned tendency, which Novick and Novick (2005) identify as a major manifestation of the defense of **externalization**, is also the mainstay of a young child's limited defensive repertoire. Parents unwittingly reinforce and augment this defense via a misguided search for a single causal agent. Needless to say, there are circumstances in which change in a particularly problematic aspect of the child's environment is not contraindicated if it is deemed potentially helpful to the child's well-being; changing something like a school, a nanny, a sleeping arrangement, or a pattern of caretaking that regularly produces conflict can diminish rising tensions and reinforce progress.

We find that approaching the child's world from a complex **systems perspective** serves to orient the clinician away from a search for ultimate "causes" (Gilmore and Meersand 2014); rather, this approach looks to characterize the multiple nested systems that maintain maladaptive patterns, most often because of stasis in their self-organizing potential produced by their interaction or a single stalled component that prevents further transformation (Thelen 2005). For example, in a situation where a child holds the family hostage by demanding an elaborate ritual around toileting, the family's compliance is a pivotal factor in perpetuating this behavior. Similarly, in households where a highly fraught homework battle occurs nightly, the parents' refusal to obtain a psychoeducational evaluation, proper remediation, or simply a homework helper can be tantamount to a commitment to the behavior's persistence. To be able to help, the clinician needs to be conversant not only with the presenting problems but also with the child's cognitive profile, fantasy, conflicts, defenses, and developmental pace, and contextualize these in regard to the parents' own histories, the family dynamics, the child's (and possibly the parents') school life, nannies (relationships, losses, and changes), afterschool activities, subcultural traditions, and so on. Work with parents alongside the individual child work, supplemented by meeting with other family members (siblings, grandparents), nannies (Scheftel 2012), and school staff as needed, is almost always indicated with a young child in treatment. Depending on whether the parents are themselves in therapy and how they understand their child's current difficulties, parents may need regular weekly, biweekly, or monthly sessions. The recommendation may evolve over time; scheduling can be an open question as the therapist gets to know the child and family situation. It is usually advisable, however, to frame parent involvement as an intrinsic part of the work and to avoid relying on "crisis sessions." Because parent work is so often challenging and even onerous, it can rapidly slide into a pattern of erratic meetings called to avert imminent catastrophes. The therapist can confidently advise parents that parent work is an ongoing essential adjunct to the child's treatment, even if it may wax and wane in importance and regularity; such a statement prepares the parents for the reality that therapy may extend across developmental phases and that their parenting challenges and tasks will change over time, requiring reconsideration and revisions.

UNDERLYING PRINCIPLES OF PARENT WORK

Drawing from our own experience, work on **resilience** (Cicchetti and Curtis 2007), the reflective functioning model (Fonagy et al. 2002; Slade 2006; Slade et al. 2005), the psychodynamic parenthood therapy model (Oren 2012), and the work of Novick and Novick (2005), we offer some fundamentals of parent work, understanding that these ideas inform an infinitely modifiable process that is firmly "nested" in the multiple systems surrounding the child (Newland 2015).

At consultation, the therapist has to make a crucial clinical decision that determines the initial approach: Is the presenting problem best addressed through treatment of the child; of the couple; of both parents, individually or together; or of the family? In Talicia's case, although parenting work with the couple was urgently needed, it had to wait until Mr. Johnson agreed to participate. Dr. Reed was willing to meet with Mrs. Johnson alone at first, especially because her individual therapy was beginning simultaneously. Dr. Reed had the sense that psychotherapy and medication might make enough of a change in Mrs. Johnson's state to shake up the status quo; the problematic relationship between mother and daughter was embedded in the currently problematic relationship between husband and wife. Although she could not be sure, Dr. Reed thought that either Mrs. Johnson's or Talicia's improvement would get Mr. Johnson in the office.

PRINCIPLE 1

Not all presentations of young children are best treated by individual play therapy; sometimes a crucial part of the work is to help parents, through parent guidance, parenthood psychotherapy, couple counseling, or individual treatment. These therapies can be undertaken in tandem with or precede the child work.

The following is a corollary of this principle: The child's therapist cannot be the couple's counselor or the individual therapist for a parent, in either name or function. If marital problems cannot be managed with the parents' development of a fuller appreciation of the child's conflicts, they need a referral for couple therapy. If the parents' individual problems are interfering with the child's progression, this too requires referral to an adult clinician. Finally, if the family system is sufficiently maladaptive and/or the parents require behavioral training, they may require referral to appropriate professionals.

With practical modifications, the most basic assumption is that the child's treatment (especially the young child's treatment) can succeed only to the extent that the parents participate and are able to reflect on both their child's mind and their own (Novick and Novick 2011; Slade 2006). Some parents need a broad focus that leads to greater self-awareness of their parenting approach and to recognition of conflicts about their self-representations as parents, whereas other parents have more specific challenges that pertain to their child's current difficulties. Of course, parents do not function as a united front, nor should they; their differences are important for their children's appreciation of complexity and for their potential mutual compensation for each other's weaknesses. Trouble ensues from deep fault lines in their approaches to a range of issues; an example is when one parent makes the relatively innocuous demand for politeness while the other parent shows vicarious delight in the child's precocious mastery of swear words. At the very least, the shared understanding of how the parents disagree, how their disagreements may be confusing or subject to manipulation, and how they plan to compromise when necessary is hugely beneficial to parenting. In cases of separation and divorce, such disagreements can become a destructive source of strain and tension for the child. Parents who recognize and address disagreements help their child manage the culture clash of different households. When parents are truly at war, as in Becky Singer's case (introduced in the section "Unstanding Moments of Referral" in Chapter 8, "The Logistics"), it not only is a source of anxiety for the child but also seriously compromises the possibility of an effective treatment (Downey 1988).

PRINCIPLE 2

Parent work is an essential part of child mental health because parents are an essential part of their child's development and inner life. The parents' willingness to work together, even if divorced, is in and of itself salutary.

This fundamental principle may seem self-evident, but it was slow to be formally acknowledged in the history of psychoanalysis. As discussed by Gilmore (2012), Sigmund Freud's discovery of unconscious fantasy eclipsed Freud's earlier focus on trauma; to his credit and despite accusations to the contrary, he never discounted the impact of environmental trauma, even as it diminished in importance in his theorizing. Unfortunately, the role of the environment was underemphasized within psychoanalysis for decades. This neglect has been definitively corrected, and contemporary dynamic thinkers evince a detailed and nuanced appreciation of the role of outside impingements, with trauma representing only one extreme of a wide continuum of influence. Of course, this is particularly important in regard to family life and the profound role of parents in influencing children's mental lives.

The shift is evident in the contemporary rapprochement among attachment theorists, developmental researchers, systems theorists, contemporary psychoanalytic developmental thinkers, and others. John Bowlby, the father of attachment theory, asserted that children, like immature members of other altricial species, are biologically driven to form attachments with the caregiver(s) that guarantee survival and provide a base for future development, whether secure or insecure. The primary caregiver's sensitive ministrations to the infant shepherds the child's developmental trajectory in optimal directions (Weil 1970). In contrast, parental mental illness, abuse, and neglect deform a child's developmental progression. Between extremes are many gradations of care and "goodness of fit" between parents and children, especially because both are in continuous process of change and may be more or less well matched in a given phase. For instance, this variability may be manifested in the parents' attitudes toward their child in different developmental phases; a father who is warm and loving to his son in early childhood may experience deep disappointment when the boy enters grade school and shows no athletic talent. Such a feeling is likely to be communicated, overtly or covertly, and thereby heightens the boy's sense of failure in relation to his athletic peers, his performance in school sports, and his overall status in school.

The parent–child relationship is a crucial shaper of childhood adaptation and developmental outcome; the relationship determines past and future flexibility both within the child and the system and can aid or hamper the child's progression. The observation that some children possess the capacity to adapt to a range of environmental variations and can resist the deleterious impact of adversity especially if they are supported by appropriate caregiving (Jaffee 2007; Weil 1985) led to the conceptualization and study of resilience (Cicchetti and Curtis 2007; Masten and Obradovic 2006; Rutter 2006). Since its introduction in 1970, resilience research has evolved in waves, yielding a more complex conceptualization that is multidimensional and does not single out parental psychology and parenting skill over genetics or vice versa; every wave of study has identified the importance of human relationships in the child's capacity to manage stress and to maintain a maximal level of adaptation (Masten and Obradovic 2006). Current views suggest that resilience is not a "trait" but rather a highly variable and changing dynamic outcome of the myriad environmental, genetic, and experiential systems in which the child is embedded (Masten 2014); even prior adversity can prove to have a "steeling" effect (Rutter 2012).

PRINCIPLE 3

From the perspective of systems thinking, the child is understood to evolve from the dynamic interplay of his or her endowment with the specific human environment in which he or she develops (the nested systems of family, subculture, larger culture, and historical context). Change is only possible if the system has potential to reequilibrate at a higher level; inevitably, parents are a constraint on that potential and must be willing to tolerate a destabilization of the status quo. Their commitment to helping their child should ideally transcend their own personal and interpersonal conflicts and mobilize their united efforts.

This principle seems commonsensical and may be "obvious" to parents, who nonetheless balk at changes in their child in the course of treatment. In the case of the Johnson family, both Talicia and her mother began to manifest changes due to their own therapies and parenting work. Mr. Johnson came into the fold when both Mrs. Johnson and Talicia showed signs of change and demanded more of him.

After over a year of individual therapies for mother and daughter, Mrs. Johnson began to make some significant changes in her situation. Her anxiety was rapidly responsive to support and a selective serotonin reuptake inhibitor; her phobic avoidance and retreat were greatly diminished, and she reconnected with her professional colleagues after a 7-year hiatus. She realized that she could leverage her assets for a good cause: she was a professional black woman with a social work degree, and, through her husband, she had access to a network of influential, socially conscious and affluent colleagues. She decided to assume a more active role in an organization that both she and Talicia loved, one that supported African girls and women artisans. She and Talicia obtained permission for a fund-raising drive to support girls in a crafts collective who created appealing woven totes. Both mother and daughter achieved a different kind of status at school with this project.

In treatment, Talicia's play progressed as follows: for many months, she played with the doctor kit, baby doll, and stroller, assigning Dr. Lee the role of the mom while she played the pediatrician who was trying to diagnose and help the baby. Dr. Lee as the mother was instructed to act very worried but was always making one mistake after another in her care. Talicia indicated that the mother should misunderstand most of what the doctor told her, forcing her to return daily to the doctor's office in a state of confusion. Talicia as doctor was very stern, scolding the mother and making her feel very bad about how dumb she was. This play gradually yielded to a shift to the smaller play sets of a family with five children, in which the oldest girl was clearly in charge; she was dismissive of the mother and managed the cooking, cleaning, doctoring as needed, schooling, and child care. A father, never before encountered in her play, would come and go randomly; he appeared to be ignorant of his daughter's domestic superpowers, and sometimes tried to correct the little girl's tone and advise the mother on how to run the household.

Dr. Lee felt that Talicia's play progression was an advance; from this new plot development, she extrapolated Talicia's greater tolerance of her aggression and competitive feelings, which Dr. Lee described in general terms to the parents. She linked these changes to some behaviors that were decidedly new at home: Talicia's willingness to criticize her mother and her growing demand that the father engage with her. Talicia struggled to extricate herself from the mutual clinging with her mother by careening between the old dependency and her new defiance; the cosleeping continued intermittently, often temporally connected to arguments between mother and daughter. Talicia was also more insistent on getting her father's full attention. She complained directly to him about his absence, was sullen when he arrived home only in time to kiss her good-night, and became agitated every time he used his cell phone in her presence, which, according to her, was "always." Mr. Johnson reached out to Dr. Lee to register his displeasure at this turn of events. She seized the opportunity to point out to him that in order for one thing to change in a family, everything had to change a little, and everyone would have to participate in it. She invited him in to see her for a parenting session and also urged him to attend *all* the parent-training sessions with Dr. Reed.

Whenever a child is identified as the patient, there is a family involved that undoubtedly plays a role in the disturbance. This concept can and should be introduced to the parents from the first contact, because it is fundamental to the success of treatment. However, it is not always possible to engage both parents or convince them of their importance to their child's mental health. In Talicia's case, Mr. Johnson was not initially prepared to involve himself; Dr. Reed nonetheless proceeded because she took a long view of Talicia's treatment as a sequence of interventions, involving different members of the family at different times. After a number of overtures, she felt prepared to wait, hoping that Mr. Johnson would eventually recognize his importance or that Talicia would force the issue by virtue of the changes emerging in play therapy.

Attempts to engage the parents as a couple and/or as individuals can run aground for a number of reasons: one or both parents may fault the child or each other and absolve themselves of any role in the trouble; the parents may be unwilling to discuss with their child's therapist any "private matters" concerning their relationship; one parent may be keeping secrets—for example, a love affair, financial problems, or imminent legal action—that they have no intention to disclose; and parents may together be keeping a secret of a pending separation or illness. The therapist may need to gain the parents' confidence and allow the time necessary for their recognition of their importance and their willingness to trust the therapist. Whatever the sequence of the approach, the process ideally will involve the whole family in a transformation that permits and supports the child's change.

The contemporary systems approach stands in contrast to the traditional model in psychoanalytic child work, where meetings with the parents were intended to provide information for the therapist, as described in a classic paper by Chused (1988). She suggested there that guidance to parents should be kept to a minimum, since weighing in on major parental decisions regarding the child may prove "hazardous" (Chused 1988, p. 67) to the child's treatment. Even with the trend toward more active intervention, therapists may still need to tactfully refuse a major decision-making role urgently requested by parents. Offering them the opportunity to think things through in the consulting room, where the child's needs can be represented by the therapist, is often adequate. Hopefully, the major benefit to parents will be that they understand their child better and can shoulder the responsibility for decisions, even painful ones, whether or not these gratify or distress the child. Complex issues about which the parents vociferously disagree are more challenging still; the therapist's role is not to cast the deciding vote but to investigate sources of disagreement, to work with the parents to achieve greater self-awareness, and to help parents recognize the inevitable externalizations directed at the child. Such a situation may merit preliminary couple or parent counseling, or a combined approach. The latter might also prove fruitful if the parents are collaborating to keep secrets, a situation that inevitably obstructs the child's treatment. Even family secrets that do not directly involve the children may nonetheless affect their development. Reiteration of the clinician's approach to confidentiality may be important when he or she senses this kind of reluctance; if the parents are concerned that the secret would be revealed to the child, this needs to be addressed.

In the case of Ellie Park (who was referred by the school psychologist for impulsive aggression directed at her peers, as discussed throughout Chapter 8), Dr. Green's initial concern that the parents were holding something back persisted. Dr. Green was as up-front as possible given her uncertainty about where this feeling was coming from. In that both parents were Korean American, Dr. Green wondered if there was still an undisclosed cultural issue to which she was not privy. She was determined to keep the topic open, although she remained uncertain about its relevance.

> Over the course of her work with Ellie, Dr. Green worked openly with potential cultural differences, specifically addressing the issue of the paternal grandparents' disapproval of Mrs. Park's professional commitments described in their second meeting. In a meeting that Mr. Park was unable to attend, Mrs. Park seemed willing to extend the conver-

sation about the conflict with her in-laws and her feelings about working; she offered that her own mother was professional and had struggled
against traditional attitudes expressed by the entire extended family
about working women. This issue highlighted a source of ongoing tension between the two sets of grandparents, one first-generation Americans (father's) and the other second-generation Americans (mother's).
Mrs. Park eventually returned to the visit to the grandparents that
occurred just before Ellie became symptomatic. In great shame, she
acknowledged that there had been some harsh words exchanged between herself and her mother-in-law that had reduced her to tears.
She noted that any displays of anger and/or distress were not very common in Ellie's experience. She knew that Ellie heard some of the argument and certainly saw her mother crying, but Mrs. Park was not
sure about how much her daughter understood of the exchange, which
was in Korean.

Mrs. Park had withheld this particular precipitant to the outbreak
of Ellie's symptoms for months; as noted, Dr. Green was aware of something lurking beneath the surface and was relieved about the triviality
of this event, although she recognized that it was not trivial to Mrs.
Park. Dr. Green knew that her cultural awareness was imperfect and discussed the issue with Dr. Lee, who recommended some literature and
gave her a cursory summation: it was indeed a big deal that there was
open conflict with in-laws, and this in turn may have shocked Ellie,
who had never before been exposed to raised voices and her mother's
tears. Dr. Lee felt it was no accident that Mrs. Park revealed this information when Mr. Park was absent and suggested that Dr. Green would
need to await Mrs. Park's signal to have it discussed openly with him. Dr.
Green was able to make use of this input to augment her appreciation
of Mrs. Park's willingness to be open and move her toward a three-
way conversation. She had no particular theory about the role that
this event played in Ellie's symptoms but she felt it enlightened her
about how distressing Ellie's aggression must have been to the Parks
and alerted her to Mrs. Park's guilt about the possibility that she was
responsible for Ellie's "breakdown."

PRINCIPLE 4

Parent work is a fundamental component of child therapy, requiring
commitment from both parents and therapist and the establishment of
a working alliance.

At the most fundamental and pragmatic level, then, there is no change possible without the caregivers' participation. No play therapy can even be initiated without parental support; they must make and sustain financial, logistical, and emotional commitments (Baldwin 2014). The considerable demand on the family to simply sustain the routine of psychotherapy for a child, who must be accompanied to the therapist's office from one to four times per week, should not be underestimated. Siblings, geographic challenges, and complex after-school schedules all complicate the process.

Beyond this basic level of commitment, the parents are an essential part of treatment proper; a therapeutic collaboration between parents and between parents and therapist are the best predictors of a successful outcome. This is no small challenge, because referrals are often generated by parental discord or separation; even when the parental couple is functioning relatively well, they are often on the defensive in regard to their child. In such circumstances, parents have often lost sight of how important they are, not only for comforting and protecting their child, but also in their primary contribution to the child's optimal development. The therapist must mobilize the parents' best instincts and their strained capacities to identify and empathize.

Despite their differences in theoretical persuasion, scholars have converged on essential features of parenting that promote child development in general and children's success in treatment. Parents, by virtue of their capacity to identify with their child's state, provide the child the experience of "containment, regulation, and modulation" (Slade 2002, p. 2). By demonstrating a capacity to think about the child's mind and to bear the child's intense emotion, the parent helps the child do likewise, while simultaneously providing comfort and support. From the vantage point of attachment research, Fonagy and his collaborators (Fonagy 1999; Fonagy and Target 2002; Fonagy et al. 1991) introduced the concept of self-reflective function or **mentalization**, a parent capacity that is associated with secure attachment in the child. The capacity of the parent to grant the child independent subjectivity and to seek to understand it ultimately stimulates the child's **theory of mind**—that is, the developmental capacity to understand another's subjectivity.

Novick and Novick (2011) use the broader term **emotional muscle** to capture a set of qualities, with some points of convergence with self-reflective function; they feel that this term appeals especially to children who like the idea of "muscles" as a marker of strength, and who can be motivated to get through difficult moments by joining in with the parents' "hard work." The Novicks' elaboration of the concept of emotional muscle includes working on the family's acceptance of conflict, struggles, and independent subjectivities; it also conveys the reassuring notion that everyone's life has its ups and downs and that these can be managed and understood.

When a couple is divorced, the challenge for the therapist is magnified. Parents' refusal to meet together with the therapist has the potential to foment misunderstandings and to jeopardize the child's treatment (Downey 1988). It sometimes helps when the clinician highlights the importance of parents' collaboration as a signal to children that devotion to their care overrides the parents' disagreements and that parental authority remains united.

More challenging still is a situation in which one parent is keeping secrets from the other (e.g., a planned separation, an affair, a financial setback). These are circumstances that may jeopardize the treatment on many levels: withdrawal of funds; an atmosphere of detachment; frequent missed parent sessions by the parent with the secret; or a lack of warmth or affection in the family that may only add to the child's distress and potentially heighten the value of the symptomatology, with the idea that this forces parental unity or its fragmentation under the child's control. Even something that may seem trivial to a given clinician, like Dr. Green's initial understanding of Mrs. Park's fight with her mother-in-law, must be considered in regard to cultural traditions and acknowledged in terms of its cultural gravitas (in Mrs. Park's case, as a source of shame).

In cases where one parent is planning a separation but has not yet disclosed this to the other parent or the child, the therapist's dilemma is considerable. If it is a "secret" and yet obvious to the therapist, he or she has to consider whether to invite such a disclosure and maintain its confidentiality. Clinicians can explain that hearing secrets involving potential changes, as yet unknown to the child or the other parent, may hamper the ability to stay at the level of the child's awareness and to continue the parent work for the couple. These circumstances are often resistant to modification because the parent wishing to separate is afraid and ambivalent. Such an impending yet unrealized change of marital status is highly detrimental to the child's therapy because it creates tension and even desperation in the parents, but remains unnamed. Because any therapy, including play therapy, seeks to find words for feelings and to examine the fears and fantasies that accompany an imminent change, this kind of situation is countertherapeutic. It is helpful to remember the basic premise that a prepared ego is able to withstand the deleterious impact of events more successfully than a surprised one; in the case of a parent's covert plan and surprise announcement, the opportunity to manage the trauma in gradual increments is denied and the therapist is rendered helpless.

Thus, extreme marital discord, secrets, and unannounced plans to separate make serious collaborative parent work difficult. In addition, severe parental pathology or doctrinaire attitudes toward child rearing that are resistant to mentalization can prove resistant to parent work and can obstruct the child's progress. Strong-armed parent training may be helpful and necessary if the therapist feels that the family system is so maladaptive that it requires a direct focus: it is usually best to suggest other specialists in that case to supplement the work. Sometimes such systems are very difficult to modulate.

> Dr. Lee had been seeing Becky Singer for concerns over bedtime anxiety and distractibility at school after her parents divorced (as first discussed in Chapter 8) for several months in twice-weekly play therapy. Becky had been showing gradual improvements in her level of anxiety and lack of focus. Based on the child's play narratives (e.g., "The mommies and daddies don't get out of bed!" or "There's no food in this house!") and occasional direct comments, Dr. Lee realized that Becky perceived both adults as lonely, depressed, and unable to fulfill their usual functions. Without divulging the contents of the child's sessions, she found ways to direct parent meetings toward Becky's keen awareness of her parents' moods and changes in their own routines: the mother acknowledged that she had been sleeping more than usual, to the point that Becky had been late for school on a couple of occasions, and Mr. Singer spontaneously described that he was more irritable and less playful than in the past, and sometimes forgot to stock up on Becky's favorite snacks. However, the situation continued to deteriorate as both parents and their respective attorneys moved to sort out a contentious visitation schedule. To maintain the therapeutic relationship with Becky, Dr. Lee clearly stated that she would not participate in these proceedings, citing the need for Becky's trust and sense of confidentiality in regard to the vacillations in her feelings. Despite the parents' manifest agreement with these principles and their

expressed delight with their daughter's improved mood, monthly joint parent meetings soon devolved into accusations and arguments. Dr. Lee agreed to their demand for separate parent meetings; each used these sessions to press her to see his or her side of things, delivering scathing reports of the other's ineptness and insensitivity and inviting Dr. Lee to pass judgment on the other parent's behavior. After repeatedly clarifying that she would listen to anything they had to say but not choose sides, they agreed to attempt another joint meeting.

In Becky's case, a promising collaborative effort unfortunately devolved over time; in such hostile circumstances, it may be impossible to champion the goal of unity. Dr. Lee was able to get some traction when she spent time alone with each parent and ultimately succeeded in bringing them back to work together. It sometimes helps to remind the parents of the platitude that they are the most important people in their child's world, because in difficult times, they can lose sight of the obvious. The therapist can further point out that the parents' ability to work together delivers a number of important messages to their child: it is possible to overcome conflict, to work as a team to maintain parental authority despite differences of opinion (see Principle 6 below), and to recognize that well-intentioned people can have different lifestyles and rules.

PRINCIPLE 5

Parent work is a distinct but multidimensional therapeutic modality that aims to facilitate the parents' optimal parenting, including emotion regulation and loving acceptance of their child.

"Working with parents" is a nonspecific term that may refer to a number of therapeutic modalities, including fostering mentalization, addressing problematic self-representations and personal meanings associated with parenting, and promoting parental understanding and management of the child. In this discussion, the term does not encompass couple therapy or manualized behavioral parent training. Instead, it refers to the examination of the relationships between the child and each parent, on the parents' self-image as parents, both individually and together, and on the relationship between the child and the parental couple (Herzog 2005). Working with parents is aimed at enhancing mentalization and emotional muscle, addressing how the parents conceptualize and optimize the child's internal representation of adult relationships, and exploring how they in turn conceptualize the role and meanings of being a parent. Even in child cases involving divorce, such as Becky's, the parents' capacity to come together to help their child is key; antagonistic and mutually contradictory parents can create insurmountable obstacles to their child's progress. Inevitably, successful child therapy involves a *transformation of the parent–child relationship* (Novick and Novick 2005) (see Principle 9 below) and enhanced self-reflectiveness in parents and child (Slade 2006). In most presentations of a child to a therapist, the child's internal conflicts and defenses are the primary focus, but these are embedded in a family that has developed its own way of managing the child's difficulties, usually at considerable cost. Because the family system may incorporate many other individuals besides parents, it is important to keep in mind that the designated patient in a family comes to serve purposes for everyone. Therefore, the clinician may need to work with various permutations of caretakers and family members.

The working alliance with parents is a long-term project that must weather crises in the child's life, parental dissension, the child's fluctuating attitudes toward therapy, and many other tests. It is sometimes helpful to give parents a picture of the ups and downs of therapy and to advise them that a child's feelings about therapy are changeable; there are likely to be times when the parents will have to stand firm, such as with a little girl who is happy to attend at first because she loves the therapist's collection of the latest popular dolls, but who refuses at a later date. Preparation is not necessarily a guarantee of optimal management of the crises ahead, but it can help parents manage expectations and provide some reassurance that these changes are expected rather than indications that the treatment is not working.

The main thrust of work with parents is to facilitate their capacity to appreciate the subjective experience of everyone in the family, especially the child in question. Because any conversation can be construed as a search for causes and blame in the context of a child in trouble, it is important for the therapist to preface parent meetings with an explanation that the families who work best are those who accept complexity; who tolerate each other's different ways of seeing things, including different values and priorities; and who look for ways to relieve suffering rather than seeking its causes. The fact is that there is never a singular causality for any human problem; time together is better spent understanding and attempting to address the child's state. This task is greatly aided by the therapist turning that same open-minded and nonjudgmental curiosity toward the parents, with the goal of becoming better acquainted with each parent as an individual with his or her own psychology and personal history. Sometimes this is best to do individually, but at other times the couple benefits most when each partner sits quietly and listens to the other tell his or her story. This gives the therapist an opportunity to deliver a message that bears repeating: it is important to listen and to try to understand whatever is being said, without raising objections, becoming defensive, or dismissing a viewpoint out of hand. Each parent's take on the problem, thoughts about the path to the consulting room, and description of his or her relationship to the child and role in the family dynamics can be remarkably illuminating and can be deepened by the examination of each parent's childhood experience. This work is practice for what the clinician hopes parents will develop in relation to the child—that is, a more attuned ear to what the child is saying or what his or her actions are saying, because actions are communications in early childhood and indeed in much of the first two decades of life.

PRINCIPLE 6

The child should be privy to the nature of this "team" approach and to the idea that communication between parents and therapist is open.

The "open" communication between parents and therapist is, in fact, not completely open. The flow from parents to therapist about the child should be understood to be free; the therapist is considered part of the team, and the parents should neither "threaten to tell the doctor" or agree to the child's demand that they withhold information. This transparent stance is intended to reassure the child patient that important and helpful information will be shared for the purpose of helping the treatment. In contrast, the therapist must be clear to child and parents that the confidentiality of the treatment relationship is maintained: the therapist is not obligated to share information from either the child or the parents without both a therapeutic indication and permission. It is inevitable that communications deemed confidential by parents to the therapist pose significant challenges, complicating the therapeutic goals of remaining at the level of the child's awareness and not over- or underinterpreting events in the treatment that seem to reflect the child's unconscious knowledge. The child's communications to the therapist remain confidential to the extent that the child's safety is not at risk.

> Eight-year-old Jeremy McAlvin (introduced at the beginning of Chapter 9, "Getting Started, Creating an Alliance, and Facilitating Play"), who had resisted therapy from the beginning, told his parents that he wasn't going to talk to Dr. Vargas and "you better not either!" He repeated this demand every time his controlling behavior led his parents to remark, "This is why we want you to see Dr. Vargas," to which he yelled, "Don't tell him; it's just for our family!" In parent meetings, Dr. Vargas acknowledged how hard it is to open the family system up to a stranger, and harder still when Jeremy seemed so desperate to keep many of his rituals secret. Jeremy made it clear that he felt his parents were betraying him by talking to the therapist. Dr. Vargas also commented to the parents that when a child is brought to therapy for behavioral problems, there is an inevitable tendency to position the therapy as punishment. He emphasized Jeremy's suffering and his helplessness in the face of inner pressure. Dr. Vargas was concerned that Jeremy's parents were indeed using the therapy as a reprimand; he also worried that they heard his comments as criticism of their parenting. The McAlvins were growing discouraged at every turn as the struggle escalated.

Dr. Vargas hoped to develop an alliance with the McAlvins while not isolating Jeremy. This is a typical challenge in work with parents, especially in the opening phase of treatment before the child is engaged. A child can experience and express a deep sense of betrayal beginning with the first consultation, questioning how the parents could tell a stranger the child's secrets. This can become an intractable resistance if the parents use the therapy or disclosure to the therapist as a threat or a punishment. Despite its patently counterproductive effect, this dynamic frequently emerges: the parents "tell on" the child to the therapist; the child begins to see the therapist as an unwelcome interloper, a parental tool, and a higher judge. Such an impasse should raise a question in the therapist's mind about the parents' loss of confidence in their authority—that is, it implies that the parents have assumed a sibling position "telling on" the child to the therapist–parent. A similar dilemma is created when parents intrude into and violate the sanctity of the child's therapy session in order to "tell on" their child. Certainly, parents may demand part of the child's session if they feel they have no other means to inform the therapist of recent events or ongoing struggles; this situation is especially common in clinic settings where parents do not get regular meetings. Other means of communicating with the clinician, such as dedicated patient portals, can be offered but may require explicit restrictions. For example, a parent who leaves endless messages on the electronic medical record can stretch the clinician's capacity to respond; limitations to once-daily or even once-weekly messages may need to be imposed.

The concept of the "child's team" is helpful in addressing the child's potential for divisiveness, although this too requires a firm foundation in parental trust. When the child "tells on" the therapist, for example, by repeating a version of an interpretation that parents find disturbing, rifts may occur in the parent–therapist rapport; it may be helpful for the therapist to forewarn the parents of such possibilities, especially when the child is already divisive at home. At the same time, it is important to underscore that such behavior usually stems from the child's anxiety that the status quo is crumbling and change is imminent.

PRINCIPLE 7

If the clinician or the field at large is divided about how to handle a clinical problem, then it is important to acknowledge the uncertainty and/or controversy to the parents. This allows for a more genuine process of discovery and for meaningful collaboration between parents and therapist.

From the beginning of his work with Beno (introduced in section "Consultation Around Gender Dysphoria" in Chapter 8), Dr. Vargas knew that the Greenhills wanted him to give them answers about why Beno was so unhappy being a boy and how they could help him. Dr. Vargas was apprehensive about these questions for a number of reasons: 1) he didn't know the answers; 2) he wanted Beno to feel free to express his feelings in the play therapy and would not want to restrict the child's behavior in any way; 3) he knew that he could not make a prediction about Beno's development, which could go in a number of different directions, at least according to the literature (although the literature was not objective or purely scientific either— to wit, the many "expert" errors in surgically treating congenital or traumatic ambiguous genitalia, as described by Diamond [2009]); and 4) he knew that the continuity of transgender feelings in Beno's future was dependent not only on his own psychological development but also on the hard road ahead—in terms of his peer group, his family, and his own struggle with the body he had. Dr. Vargas was certain that the Greenhills were likely to have doubts, questions, and possible disagreements about how to guide their son. Beno's perception of his father's disappointment was accurate up to a point, but of course recruited for his own purposes.

Dr. Vargas decided that his best approach to the Greenhills would be to lay out these issues: his own uncertainty, the lack of clear guidance in the literature, and the likelihood that Beno would be challenged and confused about his development going forward. He wanted to make clear that he was committed to helping Beno deal with his dilemma. This meant he wasn't going to direct him or resist the play that enacted Beno's female identification. He noted that while he wanted to respect the parents' feelings, he also wanted them to be aware that suppressing Beno's desires was counterproductive. He knew he would have to help Beno grapple with everyone's reactions; he especially acknowledged that Beno's father was experiencing a lot of distress and that he was prepared to work on that with him as well. Dr. Vargas told them that if they all took the position of trying to help Beno understand and come to terms with the painful contradiction between identity and anatomy, this would allow Beno to find his own path. Although Dr. Vargas was in favor of regular meetings with the parents, he also recommended a number of books for them to read, in particular those written by parents of transgender kids.

Gender dysphoria may represent the most challenging request for "answers" in the field today, and child therapists are inevitably faced with questions about "what to do" about a symptomatic child. Parents ask questions about whether to consider a school change, whether the child is safe walking home from school alone, whether to hold the child back a grade, whether to allow the child to dress as the preferred gender, and so on. Most therapists prefer not to be active agents in the patient's real life for various reasons. One reason is that although a therapist may help parents consider important decisions and will sometimes play the role of the child's advocate, the parents' preferences and ultimately their choices have to be honored in the treatment, as in the child's life. In the rare event that, following lengthy exploration, the therapist really cannot embrace a parental decision of significant gravitas, the therapy is unlikely to proceed. A second reason is that the therapist's role is to help the child understand and come to terms with the decisions made by the adults around him or her. Having a direct role in such decisions makes it difficult indeed to be a neutral party who can encourage exploration of the full gamut of the child's feelings. Too much investment in any course, whether in concert with parents or in opposition to them, may make it difficult for the therapist to remain attuned to the child's feelings.

The parents' own conflicts and ambivalence can also enter into a conflictual dynamic with the child's treatment. Because the parents are likely to be part of the dysfunctional system, with their own motives for maintaining it, they may sabotage the treatment before it gets off the ground; in this dynamic, which has been termed a *negative therapeutic motivation* (Novick 1980; Novick and Novick 2005), the child's therapy must fail in order to satisfy unconscious needs of one or both parents. There are many variations of this motivation, including one parent's use of the treatment to vilify the other parent through keeping the child ill; attempts to prejudice the therapist against the other parent or the child, making productive work impossible; or grilling the child after sessions and implicating the therapist in consequences. Such reactions can arise from the affront to parental narcissism that does not tolerate a therapist's "success" with the child in the context of parental "failure." In the following vignette, a productive treatment was disrupted by the intrusion of an angry and possibly psychiatrically disturbed parent who was determined to demean the very capable clinician working with his 4-year-old son, in order to externalize blame for the child's enormous anxiety and exonerate himself. In this situation the clinician made good use of a senior colleague both as consultant and for support.

> Mr. Ling, a nurse-practitioner clinician, saw patients in the office of a pediatrician who was a well-known expert in foreign adoptions and adoption in general. Another member of this team was a senior psychiatrist named Dr. Lowe, who collaborated with Mr. Ling on a number of cases. Mr. Ling asked for Dr. Lowe's help in the following

situation: He had been working for about 2 years with a now 4-year-old adopted boy named Hudson. Hudson's parents, the Sullivans, separated when Hudson was 6 months old and his mother obtained sole custody: Dr. Sullivan (the father, who was a pain management specialist) was minimally involved and did not contribute to Hudson's support. Hudson was brought to treatment for severe separation anxiety, which his mother dated to the violent altercation between parents that led to their physical separation. Hudson was very much in the middle of that argument and was physically pulled back and forth between the agitated and shouting parents. Dr. Sullivan essentially disappeared following this fight and had nothing to do with Hudson for over 3 years. Then he suddenly stormed back into the mother's and son's lives, demanding regular contact with his son, including visitation and weekly sleepovers. Up to that point he had not taken any responsibility for Hudson, claiming initially that the adoption occurred "against his will"; he had thoroughly abandoned mother and son physically, emotionally, and financially. Now, however, he insisted that he was prepared to reconcile with Mrs. Sullivan and Hudson whenever they were ready and take charge of the family. Mrs. Sullivan, who was aware that her husband had no legal rights, did begin to have conversations with him and allowed him to play with Hudson in her home; she wanted Hudson to have a relationship with his father. As Dr. Sullivan learned what had transpired during his absence, he became incensed that Hudson was in therapy; from his point of view, this violation was made worse by the fact that the therapist was a nurse, which he insisted constituted an attempt to "stab him in the back." He refused to see or speak to Mr. Ling.

Mr. Ling was concerned that he was being drawn into an unmanageable family battle that would make it impossible to work productively with Hudson. He asked Dr. Lowe to comment, when he had a sense of the situation, on whether it would be best for him to step aside entirely. Mr. Ling also wanted another opinion in regard to Dr. Sullivan's psychiatric condition, because he was irritable, hostile, and impulsive; in Mr. Ling's opinion, the father was either in a hypomanic state or using drugs.

Dr. Lowe met with the parents. Dr. Sullivan was less agitated in this meeting, but Dr. Lowe agreed that he was unstable. Dr. Sullivan was accusatory about Mr. Ling, controlling with Mrs. Sullivan, and slightly paranoid. Dr. Lowe had the strong impression that Dr. Sullivan was hostile toward Hudson's treatment and therapist and was determined to end treatment. Dr. Lowe offered regular consultations in an attempt to avoid such an outcome, but both the meetings with Dr. Lowe and the therapy with Mr. Ling came to a premature end within a period of months.

The sense of teamwork is clearly fragile, subject to the inner state of the parents, the larger family dynamics, and the ups and downs of any therapy. The possibility of disruptions in the context of divorcing or divorced parents is particularly high, as the child's well-being is often sidelined by parental power struggles. Premature termination of therapy is unfortunately common in situations of contentious divorce. In such polarized situations, the clinician's transparency is usually helpful but is not so easy to manage when complex custodial arrangements, prickliness about "private" information, and ongoing tensions between parents impose time-consuming and emotionally draining demands on the therapist. Providing both parents with the same clear information and regular communications about their child may diminish the likelihood of a treatment unilaterally interrupted by one parent or the parents united against therapy. Even with the best intentions, knotty problems (e.g., about whom to address in e-mails: both parents, stepparents, the remarried spouse's partner but not the stable live-in partner, the stepparent when the other parent has remained single, etc.) are often insoluble and exhausting to the busy clinician. The required deliberations consume time and highlight the potential for wrong turns and impossible choices, because there is rarely a "right way" that will please everyone involved.

PRINCIPLE 8

Parent work involves a range of interventions, including seeing each parent individually and/or meeting with a variety of dyads or groups. Interventions may involve psychoeducation and guidance; explication and clarification of the child's developmental needs and intrapsychic challenges; interpretation of parents' defenses and distortions, and explanation of their impact on their child; and some translational work from play to feelings so that parents get to know their child's inner life, at least in broad strokes. The importance of both parents to a child's mental life is worth repeating, especially in circumstances of divorce.

SESSIONS OR MEETINGS WITH OTHER INVOLVED PARTIES

It is sometimes useful to meet with other combinations of family members. Mother–child, father–child, sibling–child, or any combination of these may be deemed helpful. The sibling dynamic has been historically underestimated in psychoanalysis and is often a crucial contributor to the child's disturbance (Mitchell 2003; Vivona 2007, 2010). The sibling is clearly not the therapist's patient and should not be approached as such, but working with this dyad can be experienced as extremely affirming to the child who suffers from an unrecognized or an undersupervised problematic relationship with a sibling. The therapist's observations may convince the parents that a logistical change is needed, such as a different plan for after-school activity, a more authoritative babysitter, or playdates outside the home. Also, having met with patient and sibling may help the therapist convey information to the parents about the role of the sibling relationship in the designated patient's problem and lead to a shift in their management. Moreover, the therapist may discern important transference paradigms that were not previously understood. The sibling relationship is a primary shaper of the transference and of relationships in general (Graham 1988) and has a profound influence on personality development (Mitchell 2003; Vivona 2010). Through this work, the child therapist has an opportunity to see developmental distortions *in statu nascendi* and can hopefully direct the parents toward family therapy or other measures that can change the child's course of development via environmental modification.

When the original referral came from the child's school or was at the school's behest, it is crucial that the clinician reach out periodically to school personnel (e.g., teachers, principal, school psychologist, special educational staff) during ongoing therapy, meeting with them periodically or arranging phone conferences as indicated. In these instances, maintaining rapport with parents should be taken into account, either by including them in such meetings or providing feedback. A meeting called at the child's school may serve multiple purposes if the school's agenda involves the parents directly, as for example, in situations where a parent's behavior causes concern. A skilled therapist can simultaneously establish his or her commitment to the family and also demonstrate to the school a willingness to understand and, if necessary, help communicate the school's point of view. This is especially important if the school has plans to counsel the child outside of the school; in such cases, the therapist may be helpful to both school and parents, ensuring that guidance is provided in regard to planning next steps.

WORKING WITH INVOLVED THERAPISTS, TUTORS, OCCUPATIONAL THERAPISTS, AND OTHERS

Work with parents as part of their child's treatment is independent of the parents' own treatment or couple treatment. Even though some parents may complain of "too much therapy," their participation in their child's therapy remains an essential part of the work. Parents' attitudes about communication between their own and their child's therapists vary. Some parents object to communication on the grounds that their own treatment is entirely unrelated or irrelevant to their child's problems. Although that is unlikely, it may be true that such communication is not necessarily useful and may be experienced as an intrusion.

Within the parent–therapist relationship, the therapist may choose from a variety of therapeutic interventions. Among these, psychoeducation is a tool that is vastly underrated and underutilized. Parents are often quite ignorant of developmental transformation, phase-related needs, resources in the community, and other helpful programs that can help them understand parenting better. There are times when explanation goes a long way toward repositioning a parent's attitudes. More specific suggestions may be directed toward a particular couple's barriers to understanding their child's symptoms and to the parents' resistance to recognizing certain problems. For example, high-powered parents may struggle aggressively against recognizing their child's cognitive limitations. For some parents in this position, a child with an average or lower IQ is intolerable and may lead to therapist shopping to find someone who will refrain from psychoeducational testing or is willing to frame testing results as psychogenic. To such parents, neurotic inhibition is far preferable to intellectual weakness relative to the family standards.

> Mary was adopted at age 10 months from an orphanage in eastern Asia and had a very stormy early adjustment, with sleeplessness, inconsolable crying, and outbursts of screaming and hitting. With patience and dedication, her mother, Mrs. Quagliari, worked to build an attachment and by age 36 months, Mary was far more pliant, affectionate, and stable. Although her adoption was part of a few conversations

with Mary very early on, when she queried her mother after hearing a story about pregnancy and observing pregnant mothers, it was never otherwise mentioned or explained. Her mother, who had taken a protracted maternity leave for the adoption and postadoption phase, finally returned to work when Mary was 3½ years old. Her father always traveled extensively and, although involved with Mary, could not be counted on to fill gaps in her caretaking schedule. Mary's care was divided between her nanny, mother, and grandmother. At age 3 years 10 months, Mary began preschool and had a severe reaction to separating from her mother, who was already prepared for a full phasing-in but was shocked and disappointed, first by Mary's regression and then by her lack of progress over the 2 weeks allotted to this process by the school. Both her parents were surprised and dismayed because they felt they were "finally out of the woods" when Mary reached age 3. Mary's behavior at bedtime also regressed. This went on for 3 months until the Quagliaris became desperate.

They were referred to Dr. Vargas by the director of the infancy training program. Due to an unresolvable scheduling conflict, he proposed that the parents meet with Mr. Ling, the nurse-practitioner clinician, who had vast experience helping families with foreign adoptees. The Quagliaris were immediately troubled by this referral to an adoption specialist and sought counsel with the training director; in their opinion, the adoption was a closed chapter in Mary's development. They were also apprehensive that referring them to a Chinese American clinician would complicate their situation, possibly confusing Mary and disenfranchising them. They were urged to meet with Mr. Ling with an open mind, because he was well liked by most families and was able to work with the inevitable mixed feelings involved in talking about adoption. The Quagliaris met with him for six sessions before bringing Mary to see him.

In the first parent meeting, Mr. Ling was forthcoming about his conversation with the program director, noting that their many feelings about Mary's adoption were important and he hoped that they would be able to discuss those feelings with him; he also wanted them to feel free to discuss his heritage in whatever way it affected them. After another meeting devoted to Mary's early adaptation, the parents began to describe their road to the adoption: their attempts to get pregnant, their fertility workup, its impact on their sexual life, conflicts about adoption, and anxieties about Mary's birth history. This exploration allowed them to verbalize some of the intense feelings around Mary's arrival that they had previously suppressed for fear of hurting each other or their little daughter. Mr. Ling encouraged the parents to attend some lectures by his colleague and mentor, an adoption specialist/pediatrician, and directed them toward an organization for parents of Chinese adoptees which offered support groups, play groups for the children, organized exposure to Chinese culture, and an anonymous forum in which adoptive parents were able to write about painful feelings such as ambivalence. He was careful to say that some parents and/or children do not benefit from the approach embraced by this organization but he wanted to make them aware that it was one of several that had helped other families.

To himself, Mr. Ling wondered about the fact that this couple was not aware of any of these groups, even though many had been featured in the newspapers; in general, he was struck by how little research they had done about Chinese adoptees. He felt as if any acknowledgment of Mary's "difference" from them was tantamount to a rejection. He wondered if his Chinese heritage further squelched their attempts to look into the vast number of services and information available about Chinese adoptees and Chinese culture, since now they felt they were confronted by an "expert." He assured them that his own education began in his late 30s when he got involved in this specialty; he had no exposure growing up in an established, successful, and thoroughly assimilated Chinese-American, family, but working in the adoption field gradually educated him. He felt compelled to say, at least once per month, that as far as he was concerned (and surely as far as Mary was concerned), the Quagliaris were and would always be her parents. However, both her ethnic heritage and her adoption were undeniable aspects of her identity, and her parents had a huge role in helping her come to terms with those facts. As part of a psychoeducational approach, he explained that while there were likely many contributions to Mary's current state, her unverbalized and unverbalizable fears of abandonment, unconsciously linked to the adoption, were undoubtedly reinvoked by her mother's return to work and the start of preschool. The opportunity to observe many children who looked more like their parents and, worse yet, who looked more like her own parents may also have heightened her anxiety.

The process that Mr. Ling initiated was woven into work with Mary and her family over the 3 years they worked together. The parents' growing tolerance of and preparation for Mary's difficulties with transitions, separations of all types, and other challenges facilitated the child's capacity to verbalize her feelings and communicate them in words, keeping pace with her growing vocabulary and cognitive skills. The play therapy often involved themes of loss. In the first year the recurrent story was about a child or baby animal being given away or stolen. This evolved into a story that occupied her attention for the next year or more: a child or baby animal was always getting into trouble for misbehaving in increasingly serious ways, ranging from not doing homework to telling parents all kinds of lies about what happened when they were out. Some of these stories ended with the child running away from home. Mr. Ling abstracted these themes and explained their counterphobic purpose to Mary's parents. The Quagliaris, in turn, became increasingly attuned to the presence of adoption themes in books and movies encountered in daily life. They were increasingly able to address these themes directly, creating openings for Mary's questions and opportunities to respond in a gentle and measured way. When Mary was 5½ years old, she had a cooking class in school and requested a Chinese-Italian night, to which she invited some of her Chinese American friends who were also adopted.

Another intervention, almost always requiring collaboration with a colleague, is parent coaching directly in the family's home. If the child's therapist feels that the parents are unable to develop a new approach to problematic behavior through better understanding, it is often helpful to partner with a behavioral therapist willing to go to the home. Psychodynamically informed behavioral guidance differs from Parent-Child Interaction Training (PCIT) developed by Sheila Eyberg (1988; Eyberg and Bussing 2010) and other evidence-based programs teaching concrete parent management techniques most typically in a clinic setting. In contrast, an in-home visit by a sensitive behavioral colleague guides the development of a tailor-made approach for behavioral interventions while gathering data about the level of the household organization, consistency, and routines. The two clinicians have invaluable information to share: the behaviorist supplies details unlikely to be learned from parent sessions, and the play therapist provides psychodynamic knowledge of the child. Their ongoing dialogue ultimately enriches both treatments. An in-home intervention requires tact and skill, because parents can feel invaded, and the threat to the status quo is immediate and direct. Nonetheless, such visits, if handled in a spirit of support, interest, and working together, can help the parents feel understood "in the trenches."

In Talicia Johnson's case, the use of an in-home behaviorist was determined by Dr Green's sense that Talicia's symptom was creating a roadblock:

> The various members of the Johnsons' "team" felt that their progress was significant, but Dr. Reed continued to worry about the fact that Talicia, despite her feistiness, ended up in her mother's bed 3–4 nights per

week. Even though there were already four professionals involved, Dr. Reed encouraged Mrs. Johnson to contact another colleague, Mrs. Dixon, a pediatric nurse who had developed a specialty in working with sleep disturbances. This referral proved to be a turning point. Mrs. Dixon took a careful history of Talicia's sleep problems and then slept in Talicia's room for 4 nights, talking her through staying in her bed and providing expert reassurance and a special "sleepy treat" (warm milk and honey). She got to know Talicia's interests and instituted a reward system for the nights Talicia stayed in her room. With these inducements, Talicia finally gave up going to her mother's bed.

As a clinician develops a larger network, he or she is likely to gain knowledge and contacts that will provide brief interventions and much needed services to children and families. The clinician can recommend books, social skills groups, summer programs, and the like. For example, parents of a young child, especially parents who have full-time jobs and little opportunity to exchange information with other parents, are often uninformed about available community resources and shared arrangements for activities among parents in a given school. The parents may persist in patterns of care that compound their child's inhibition or other problematic behavior. Of course, there may be significant psychological contributions to their lack of awareness, and these will have to be addressed. For example, the Quagliaris' relative ignorance of very visible and vocal groups of adoptive parents was not framed as a choice; they simply "didn't know anything about it." Mr. Ling came to feel that their obliviousness was defensive; they needed the opportunity to discuss their ambivalence more than simply get recommendations about available services and organizations.

PRINCIPLE 9

A central aim of children's treatment is transformation of the parent–child relationships. The parents themselves undergo a process of transformation over the course of their child's treatment and ideally welcome and support the evolution of their relationships.

This principle is the cornerstone of Novick and Novick's (2005) approach to parent work and underscores its central role in child therapy. It is worth noting that relational transformation is a natural process in childhood development and the key challenge to parenting; throughout development, the parents must calibrate their approach to meet the rapidly evolving developmental needs of their child and renegotiate their role. This necessitates a high level of attunement, the ability to tolerate their child's growing autonomy, and the recognition of and flexibility to meet new challenges. Any or all of these adjustments may stir up a parent's own conflicts and disrupt the parent's personality organization, in addition to yielding quantum shifts in the mental organization of the child. Failure to transform simultaneously is ubiquitous and inevitable in parent–child relationships, but ideally after some detours and hiccups any snag is organically corrected. This process is especially visible and challenging in adolescent development, where the child's push for autonomy and demand for agency may be premature in terms of the teen's actual developmental capacity, eliciting parental alarm and attempts to exert excessive control. Unevenness between children's drive to "grow up," their readiness, and their parents' level of anxiety arises earlier in childhood as well but is played out on a smaller scale. The child cannot change without changes in the system and without parental recognition of the need for a new approach, even if limited to their acknowledgment that the child is straining to move forward. Of course this is a hugely complex process, in that the presence of multiple siblings and the evolution of the parents and their relationship each has its own trajectory. The more openness there is to variation in the family system, the more flexibly the system accommodates change in order to achieve a new state of equilibrium. It is sometimes helpful to remind parents of this fundamental challenge of child rearing; because development is so rapid from early to middle childhood, parents are required to adapt to their child's transforming needs, new tensions in sibling dynamics, and the multiple changing demands on them as parents.

SUMMARY

Parent work has been definitively recognized as a key component of child psychotherapy. Especially in work with young children, where therapeutic action occurs mostly in play, regular communication with parents benefits all parties. Therapists can clarify vital developments in family life and in the child's unconscious mind (often containing unmetabolized elements of parents' history), ongoing strain trauma, and myriad other unforeseen aspects of the child's daily experience; parents can come to understand and appreciate their child's inner life, dilemmas, unconscious conflicts, and pain; and children have the confidence that the therapy is a secure and parent-approved setting in which their conflicts, impulses, hates, and desires can be expressed and understood. We hasten to add that this notion of teamwork does not erode confidentiality; information to parents need not be specific and detailed. Parents may require extensive psychoeducation to understand that play is communication and will usually accept a version of the developments in therapy that is true but generalized and nonrevealing of secrets. The therapist's aim in meeting with parents is primarily to help them understand and appreciate the child that they have, their own contribution to that child's problems, and ways to correct those problems.

KEY POINTS

- Not all child referrals identify the party most in need of treatment. The preliminary visits provide a child clinician with an important decision point about whether psychotherapy is indicated and, if so, what kind, for whom, and in what order. Children are embedded in multiple interacting systems whose parsing for purposes of formulating an approach takes considerable time and sensitivity.

- Parents are part of their child's development and health or illness. This truism does not imply causality but simply highlights the importance of parents in working toward the child's well-being.

- As the pioneers in the recent emphasis on parent work in child psychotherapy, Novick and Novick (2005) assert that truly effective child therapy transforms the parent–child relationship. Parents need to be engaged in their children's treatment, participate in the change process, and become acquainted with the methodology of therapy. This involvement is especially important in the treatment of young children in play therapy, because many parents do not understand that play is the premiere expressive medium of childhood and the way in which children make meaning out of their experience (Slade 2002).

KEY TERMS

Emotional muscle   Term coined by Novick and Novick (2010, 2011) to denote parenting based on an understanding of children's developmental needs and challenges. The concept encourages parents to consider good parenting as a process that demands practice and effort, often requiring them to stretch beyond their own reflexive responses to help their children grow their own emotional muscle. This may require a willingness to hear children out when they may seem irrationally angry, to collaborate with them to understand everyone's reaction to a crisis, and to reflect on their own and their children's mental lives.

Externalization   The attribution of one's own impulses, capacities, or weakness to another person or thing. In the context of parent work, this often has to do with attributing responsibility for problems onto other individuals, agencies, or forces (e.g., "It's the school's fault" or "It's our child's aggression").

Mentalization   The developmental capacity to perceive and imagine behavior—one's own and others'—as a reflection of intentional mental states; "holding mind in mind" (Bateman and Fonagy 2012 quoted in Freeman 2016).

Resilience   The "reduced vulnerability to environmental risk experiences," which is inferred from variations in outcome (Rutter 2012, p. 336). Contemporary views suggest that differences in outcome may be due not only to the complex and changing interface between positive and negative influences in the environment (including family, school, cultural institutions, etc.), genetics, and culture, but also to the "steeling effect" of exposure to stress, "turning points" that can produce quantum shifts, the meanings attached to experience, and the plasticity of the human brain (Rutter 2012, pp. 341–342).

Systems perspective   The schematic, nonmathematical application of *general systems theory* or *nonlinear dynamic systems theory*. This theory suggests that biological organisms must be studied as "wholes," each with its own organizing potentials. Important for the theory's application to developmental science is the idea that organisms are open systems that maintain themselves in nonequilibrium steady state through interaction with the environment (i.e., other open systems), tending to reorganize into new "attractor states" as the various interacting systems evolve (Hammond 2010).

Theory of mind   A developmental capacity that allows children to form complex attributions of unverbalized mental states to themselves and others. Theory of mind requires a range of capacities based on mentalization and, in turn, is felt to be foundational for reflective functioning. According to Mayes and Cohen (1996, p. 121), the achievement of theory of mind has the following prerequisites: 1) the ability to substitute one thing (object, person) to represent another; 2) the ability to understand that one thing (object, situation, or person) can simultaneously be experienced differently by different minds; and 3) the ability to "hold in mind" other people's mental or representational world, recognizing that their actions and words are determined by their feelings, beliefs, wishes, and memories. These elements are also essential for the capacity for pretend play.

REFERENCES

Anthony EJ: The family and the psychoanalytic process in children. Psychoanal Study Child 35:3–34, 1980 7433585

Baldwin E: Recognizing guilt and shame: therapeutic ruptures with parents of children in psychotherapy. Psychoanalytic Social Work 21(1–2):2–18, 2014

Bateman AW, Fonagy P (eds): Handbook of Mentalizing in Mental Health Practice. Arlington, VA, American Psychiatric Publishing, 2012

Chused JF: The transference neurosis in child analysis. Psychoanal Study Child 43:51–81, 1988 3227088

Chused JF: Discussion: a clinician's view of attachment theory. J Am Psychoanal Assoc 48:1175–1187, 2000

Cicchetti D, Curtis WJ: Multilevel perspectives on pathways to resilient functioning. Dev Psychopathol 19(3):627–629, 2007 17972420

Diamond M: Clinical implications of the organizational and activational effects of hormones. Homones Behav 55: 621–632, 2009

Downey TW: The disavowal of authority in a child of divorce. Psychoanal Study Child 43:279–289, 1988 3227077

Eyberg SM: Parent-child interaction therapy: integration of traditional and behavioral concerns. Child and Family Behavior Therapy 10(1):33–46, 1988

Eyberg SM, Bussing R: Parent-child interaction therapy for preschool children with conduct problems, in Clinical Handbook of Assessing and Treating Conduct Problems in Youth. Edited by Murrihy RC, Kidman AD, Ollendick TH. New York, Springer, 2010, pp 139–162

Fonagy P: Psychoanalytic theory from viewpoint of attachment theory and research, in Handbook of Attachment: Theory, Research, and Clinical Applications. Edited by Cassidy J, Shaver PR. New York, Guilford, 1999, pp 595–624

Fonagy P, Target M: Early intervention and the development of self-regulation. Psychoanal Inq 22(3):307–335, 2002

Fonagy P, Steele M, Steele H, et al: The capacity for understanding mental states: the reflective self in parent and child and its significance for security of attachment. Infant Ment Health J 12(3):201–218, 1991

Fonagy P, Cottrell D, Phillips J, et al: What Works for Whom? A Critical Review of Treatments for Children and Adolescents, 2nd Edition. New York, Guilford, 2002

Frankiel RV: The stolen child: a fantasy, a wish, a source of countertransference. Int Rev Psychoanal 12(4):417–430, 1985

Freeman C: What is mentalizing? An overview. Br J Psychother 32(2):189–201, 2016

Furman E: Working with and through the parents. Child Analysis 6:21–42, 1995

Gilmore K: Pretend play and development in early childhood (with implications for the oedipal phase). J Am Psychoanal Assoc 59(6):1157–1182, 2011 22080503

Gilmore K: Childhood experiences and the adult world, in The American Psychiatric Publishing Textbook of Psychoanalysis, 2nd Edition. Edited by Gabbard GO, Litowitz BE, Williams P. Washington, DC, American Psychiatric Publishing, 2012, pp 117–131

Gilmore K, Meersand P: Normal child and adolescent development, in The American Psychiatric Publishing Textbook of Psychiatry, 6th Edition. Edited by Hales RE, Yudofsky SC, Roberts LW. Washington, DC, American Psychiatric Publishing, 2014, pp 139–173

Graham I: The sibling object and its transferences: alternate organizer of the middle field. Psychoanal Inq 8(1):88–107, 1988

Hammond D: The Science of Synthesis: Exploring the Social Implications of General Systems Theory. Boulder, CO, University of Colorado Press, 2010

Herzog JM: Triadic reality and the capacity to love. Psychoanal Q 74(4):1029–1052, 2005 16355717

Jaffee SR: Sensitive, stimulating caregiving predicts cognitive and behavioral resilience in neurodevelopmentally at-risk infants. Dev Psychopathol 19(3):631–647, 2007 17705896

Masten AS: Global perspectives on resilience in children and youth. Child Dev 85:6–20, 2014

Masten AS, Obradovic J: Competence and resilience in development. Ann NY. Acad Sci 1094:13–27, 2006 17347338

Mayes LC, Cohen DJ: Children's developing theory of mind. J Am Psychoanal Assoc 44(1):117–142, 1996 8717481

Mitchell J: Siblings: Sex and Violence. Cambridge, UK, Polity Press, 2003

Newland L: Family well-being, parenting, and child well-being: pathways to healthy adjustment. Clin Psychol 19(1):3–14, 2015

Novick J: Negative therapeutic motivation and negative therapeutic alliance. Psychoanal Study Child 35:299–320, 1980 7433584

Novick J, Novick KK: Parent work in analysis: children, adolescents, and adults. Part one: the evaluation phase. J Infant Child Adolesc Psychother 1(4):55–77, 2000

Novick J, Novick KK: Parent work in analysis: children, adolescents, and adults. Part two: recommendation, beginning, and middle phases of treatment. J Infant Child Adolesc Psychother 2(1):1–27, 2002a

Novick J, Novick KK: Parent work in analysis: children, adolescents, and adults. Part three: middle and pretermination phases. J Infant Child Adolesc Psychother 2(2):17–41, 2002b

Novick J, Novick KK: Parent work in analysis: children, adolescents, and adults. Part four: termination and post-termination phases. J Infant Child Adolesc Psychother 2(2):45–55, 2002c

Novick KK, Novick J: Working with Parents Makes Therapy Work. Plymouth, UK, Rowman & Littlefield, 2005

Novick KK, Novick J: Emotional Muscle: Strong Parents, Strong Children. Bloomington, IN, Xlibris, 2010

Novick KK, Novick J: Building emotional muscle in children and parents. Psychoanal Study Child 65:131–151, 2011 26027142

Oren D: Psychodynamic Parenthood Therapy: a model for therapeutic work with parents and parenthood. Clin Child Psychol Psychiatry 17(4):553–570, 2012 22084417

Rutter M: Implications of resilience concepts for scientific understanding. Ann N Y Acad Sci 1094:1–12, 2006 17347337

Rutter M: Resilience as a dynamic concept. Dev Psychopathol 24(2):335–344, 2012 22559117

Scheftel S: Why aren't we curious about nannies? Psychoanal Study Child 66:251–278, 2012 26021001

Slade A: Moments of regulation and the development of self-narratives. J Infant Child Adolesc Psychother 2(4):1–10, 2002

Slade A: Reflective parenting programs: theory and development. Psychoanal Inq 26(4):640–657, 2006

Slade A, Sadler L, De Dios-Kenn C, et al: Minding the baby a reflective parenting program. Psychoanal Study Child 60:74–100, 2005 16649676

Thelen E: Dynamic systems theory and the complexity of change. Psychoanal Dialogues 15(2):255–283, 2005

Vivona JM: Sibling differentiation, identity development, and the lateral dimension of psychic life. J Am Psychoanal Assoc 55(4):1191–1215, 2007 18246759

Vivona JM: Siblings, transference, and the lateral dimension of psychic life. Psychoanal Psychol 27(1):8–26, 2010

Weil AP: The basic core. Psychoanal Study Child 25:442–460, 1970 5532125

Weil AP: Thoughts about early pathology. J Am Psychoanal Assoc 33(2):335–352, 1985 4020027

RECOMMENDED READING FOR PARENTS

Benedetto N: My favorite color is pink. CreateSpace Independent Publishing Platform, 2015

Hall M: Red: A Crayon's Story. New York, Greenwillow Books, 2015

Miller SA: Parenting and Theory of Mind. New York, Oxford University Press, 2016

Newton R, Schore A: The Attachment Connection: Parenting a Secure and Confident Child Using the Science of Attachment Theory. Oakland, CA, New Harbinger, 2008

Novick KK, Novick J: Emotional Muscle: Strong Parents, Strong Children. Bloomington, IN, Xlibris, 2010

Solomon A: Far From the Tree: Parents, Children and the Search for Identity. New York, Scribner, 2012

11

Deepening Play Therapy

Verbalizing Inner States, Expanding Narratives, and Working With Transference and Defense

Six-year-old Ellie Park (who has been discussed in earlier chapters) attended twice-weekly therapy with Dr. Green for several months. Ellie no longer required her mother's presence in the playroom and she followed Dr. Green confidently from the waiting area, embracing play therapy with intense focus but not a great deal of pleasure. Her withdrawn, irritable demeanor at school had abated slightly, and she manifested greater interest in her peers and classroom activities. Her parents met regularly with Dr. Green, working to understand their daughter's somewhat inhibited style, accept her jealous feelings about her baby sister, and realize the impact of their own busy lives and attitudes on Ellie's experience of family life. In addition, they were coming to terms with how sensitive Ellie was to events around her: months after a dispute between Ellie's mother and grandmother, the 6-year-old still tensed up whenever she learned that the grandparents were coming to visit.

Despite her very adequate verbal development, Ellie's play narratives impressed Dr. Green as limited and unelaborated. Using small dolls and furniture, Ellie repeatedly arranged family scenarios that centered on a baby who lay in bed with her parents while a big sister slept alone in another room, or a mealtime during which the older sister was similarly left to her own devices while parents fussed over the infant. Ellie provided little accompanying narration beyond her indications that Dr. Green should play the role of the excluded older sister. Ellie reserved for herself the triad of parents and baby but did not

319

spontaneously enliven her characters other than with the exchange of superficial pleasantries (e.g., "What would you like for breakfast today, baby? How about some yummy cereal?"). Occasionally, grandparents entered the play at breakfast time; when this happened, Ellie quickly removed the parent dolls and hurried them off to their offices. She ignored Dr. Green's verbalized observation that the two grown-up couples were never in the same space.

In general, Dr. Green matched Ellie's muted emotional tone, but she also supplied more affect-laden material in the play; although these contributions were partly thought out, based on Dr. Green's reflections on Ellie's possible underlying feelings and her knowledge of the child's situation, they often flowed from more immediate and less conscious origins. From her vantage point as the outcast sister, Dr. Green spoke mournfully about how hard it was to sleep or enjoy her breakfast while feeling sad and alone; once or twice, remembering Ellie's earlier school observation (described in Chapter 8), Dr. Green included in her monologue how difficult it was to look forward to having fun at school when she was feeling so left out of things at home. Ellie listened attentively to Dr. Green's comments, and even encouraged the therapist toward more elaborate monologues, but did not further animate her own play roles.

In forming a hypothesis about Ellie's rather sparse, inhibited play, Dr. Green took into account her growing understanding of the Park parents and their emotional reserve, their discomfort with displays of negative emotion (including the tensions with Ellie's grandmother), and their emphasis on Ellie's very substantial cognitive developmental achievements. From her experience playing with Ellie, Dr. Green sensed that the child felt threatened by the spontaneity of pretense and by the potential for intense affects to find expression; while happy enough with Dr. Green's more lively depictions, Ellie seemed to fear her own play characters' outpouring of feelings. In addition, the distress of having witnessed her mother and grandmother's argument seemed clear: in play, the child simply ensured that the generations were never present together.

On one occasion, after Ellie indicated that they should pretend it was nighttime and switched off the playroom light, Dr. Green played that the older sister lay awake in the dark. She embarked on a soft-spoken monologue, commenting on how life had changed since the baby was born: there was less attention from Mother and Father; the baby did so many things wrong and never got scolded; the grandparents were always exclaiming over everything the baby did, even if it was just to coo. Ellie smiled and added, with uncharacteristic warmth, "Or just to pee and poop! Or drink a bottle!" For a while, they took turns labeling the absurdly simple things that babies did and that everyone seemed to admire. Suddenly, Ellie assumed a mock frightened expression, looked directly at Dr. Green, and whispered "Shhhh! The mommy might hear!" "What would happen if Mommy heard?" asked Dr. Green, matching the child's whispering tone. Ellie declined to answer and turned her face away. After a few moments, she focused her attention back to the dolls and began to rouse the mother from sleep. "Uh oh," whispered Dr. Green, "I better keep these feelings to myself so Mommy won't be angry." Ellie nodded sagely and commented, "You have to just love the baby." At this moment, it was unclear whether Ellie was speaking as the pretend mother or as herself. Dr. Green responded in a way that related to but was at a slight distance from the play: "I think the big sister is having some big feelings. She loves Mommy and Daddy but she isn't sure she always loves this baby." Back in play character, Ellie as the mother doll sighed in exasperation: "Big sisters just love their baby brothers and sisters. Everybody loves babies." "But then who loves me?" asked Dr. Green, as the big sister. The mother responded, "Nobody. You are just a mean old big sister." Dr. Green felt enormous internal pressure to provide a corrective to this displaced version of Ellie's self-perception and hastily considered various reassuring comments. However, she also realized that the affects and self-feelings in the room, including Ellie's sense of herself as bad and unlovable, needed to be expressed and not covered up with niceties. Dr. Green noted that her sense of pressure to turn Ellie's unhappy, worried feelings into more palpable versions reflected countertransference but also might parallel Ellie's perceived interpersonal experience at home.

As treatment progresses, the therapist works through the medium of play to facilitate exploration of conflicts, defenses, and relational patterns that contribute to disruption of a child's developmental progression. Their relationship deepens as the dyad continues to play on a regular basis, achieving greater narrative complexity and sharing new meanings as they enrich pretend scenarios and roles. While following the child's lead, the clinician finds opportunities to expand storylines, clarify affects, and connect characters' internal states to outward behaviors; these interventions are guided by the child's play creations, by the therapist's knowledge (of the child's developmental needs and tendencies, personal history, current circumstances, and psychological dynamics), and by the dyad's less conscious, emotional responses to the evolving play.

Although a child's spontaneous depictions of family constellations and animation of play characters represent central perceptions of self and others, the clinician needs to keep in mind that children's play creations never simply embody a direct representation of reality-based experience. Rather, they reflect the child's highly subjective *psychic reality*—that is, interpretations of real-life events that are immediately suffused with fantasies, distortions, needs, and wishes that derive from the child's development phase. During childhood, such perceptions are powerfully shaped by naïve cognition that limits the child's ability to grasp fully complex family dynamics and hold in mind multiple individuals' perspectives. The various metaphors of pretense serve manifold functions and represent diverse aspects of the child's inner world (Mahon 2004); as symbols and themes emerge into the ongoing play, the therapist's tasks include maintaining openness to shifting meanings, avoiding imposing significances that detract from the child's subjective communications, and resisting investment in specific narratives. Receptivity to the child's narrative preferences and emotional signals requires a continuous process of clinician self-awareness; opportunities for reflection and self-monitoring, often impossible during the rapidly unfolding action of play, may arise during talks with colleagues, supervisors, or a personal psychotherapist or psychoanalyst.

In the opening vignette, Ellie's play constructions of family scenes wherein an older sister is painfully ignored are highly subjective renderings of imagined and actual events. Dr. Green quickly recognizes a blending of wishful and reality-based elements in Ellie's narratives: the therapist knows the Parks's home situation includes a toddler as well as parents who work full time and are rarely present for either of their children's meals. Ellie's play scenarios, while vividly conveying her painful sense of exclusion when the full family is present, are also designed to protect her from the daily experience of parental absence; in pretense, at least the parents are home and focused on one of their daughters. Moreover, the child's representations of prolonged periods alone, with the parents and baby huddled together over meals and in bed, potently indicate Ellie's affects and fantasized alliances, but should not be taken as literal signs of family behavior. Like many children in the oedipal phase of development, Ellie is wrestling with the feelings that accompany a deeper realization of triadic relationships (jealousy, exclusion) and is struggling to integrate hostile and loving urges toward important figures; in addition, she endeavors to make sense of unique family dynamics and complex interactions, including the unsettling re-

cent argument between her mother and grandmother. Ellie's perceptions are further shaped by her parents' attachment histories and by their
ready sense of shame about negative affects; these intergenerational
qualities, and her experience of them, are observable in her low-keyed
manner of play, her somewhat joyless approach (that nonetheless quickly
falls away to reveal a more mischievous, lively potential), and her authoritative pronouncements about love and hate ("You have to just
love the baby").

Conscious and unconscious aspects of the clinician's mental life also
contribute to evolving play scenarios. Achieving a **mutual playing
state** requires the therapist's immediate and whole-hearted immersion
in the child's imaginary fantasy; while the clinician sustains receptive-
ness to the child's intense affects, action-oriented tendencies, and rapidly emerging play narratives, access to sustained reflection is severely
constrained (Galatzer-Levy 2008). Dr. Green's spontaneous responsiveness to Ellie's play, and to the child's other verbal and nonverbal signals,
captures elements of her own early memories, unresolved conflicts, and
fantasies. During a quieter moment, she becomes conscious of certain
countertransference pressures and recognizes her urge to provide reassurance when Ellie's painful feelings are vividly portrayed through play;
at the same time, Dr. Green realizes that deepening the play requires
their mutual tolerance and gradual exploration of Ellie's negative affects. Such emotional and relational information is useful, as it also
alerts Dr. Green to possible parallels with important figures in Ellie's life;
she wonders if the Park parents, who have always maintained that their
daughter's behavior at home is unproblematic, have tended to handle
Ellie's expressions of painful feelings by quickly subduing them.

WORKING WITHIN THE PLAY

Young children's freedom of self-expression and their tolerance for affects are heightened when therapeutic work is conducted through the
safe displacement of play; indeed, when the child is playing fluidly, it
is both unnecessary and undesirable for the clinician to speak about
pretend scenarios as potential representations of the child's inner life
(Birch 1997; Bornstein 1945; Joyce 2011; Mayes and Cohen 1993). In
the chapter's opening vignette, deepening of the ongoing treatment is
served best by Dr. Green's work within the play itself and by her avoidance of direct comments about Ellie's personal life; such remarks would

likely lead to inhibition of Ellie's creativity and expression, to a closing down rather than an expansion of the play, and to the child's increased self-consciousness and shame in the presence of the therapist. In fact, even their brief face-to-face exchange about the play proves slightly too threatening to Ellie: after Dr. Green inquires "What would happen if Mommy heard [the older sister's complaints]?" Ellie breaks off eye contact and turns away, needing a moment to regroup before resuming. This very brief disruption does not derail the narrative; they return to play, and from within her pretend roles Dr. Green addresses central issues in a way that maintains Ellie's trust and security while conveying the important message that emotions can be named and understood. As a result, Ellie's curiosity about sisterly feelings is increased, and her emerging ego capacities (affect tolerance, self-regulation, and self-reflection) are strengthened.

As play treatments progress, opportunities for more direct comments about the child–therapist relationship and the child's defensive patterns often emerge; they may stem from children's directly expressed curiosities (e.g., questions about other patients in the therapist's practice, queries about the clinician's personal life), may be reactions to the therapist's behavior (e.g., limit setting, taking of a vacation), or may arise when the child momentarily shifts out of the playing state to negotiate storylines or reflect on characters and plots. With older children, the increased presence of verbal interactions (e.g., relating a story from the school day, complaining about a teacher's unfairness) leads to more direct conversation. In all cases, the therapist's task is to target interventions at the level of the child's current and most comfortable self-expression, avoiding comments or play actions that might disrupt the flow of pretense or talk, or that might prematurely expose inner states that remain hidden from the child's conscious awareness.

PRINCIPLE 1

When the child is playing freely, and co-creation of narratives is proceeding well, the therapist's interventions are designed to maintain the flow of affective expression and avoid disruptions to play. Interpretations within the play, rather than remarks directed at the child, serve the treatment best under these circumstances.

VERBALIZING AFFECTS AND INNER STATES

Among the therapist's key functions are naming and delineating the child's previously unlabeled, poorly tolerated affects and inner states as they appear in the play, often via disavowed roles that are assigned to the clinician. These unwanted characters offer hints as to feelings, urges, and wishes that arise within important relationships but that the child considers potentially overwhelming, destructive, and punishable, and that therefore need to be repudiated. Children's efforts to circumvent uncomfortable, anxiety-arousing inner states may involve inflexible patterns of avoidance; such rigidly enforced defenses are key components of disruptions to developmental progression. Within the mutual state of play, such feelings are differentiated, labeled, and jointly reflected upon; the therapist's verbalization of affects and split off inner states helps the child integrate disowned emotions, bringing them in contact with evolving ego capacities and leading to more modulated and tolerated emotional states, as well as to enhanced ego control (Gilmore 2005; Katan 1961).

For Ellie, strong affective states (anger and jealousy, but also desire and excitement) elicit anxiety and imagined condemnation; this sense of emotional life was perceived as validated when she witnessed an upsetting argument between her mother and grandmother, an event in which the mutual expression of feelings led to her mother's considerable upset, as well as to increased interpersonal tensions and estrangement. Although positive affects are not specifically implicated in this scenario, Ellie's inhibitions lead to a general dampening of arousal, including avoidance of pleasure and withdrawal from exciting activities. In the vignette above, Dr. Green maintains the integrity of the playing state and begins to highlight affectively meaningful moments. She accepts Ellie's assignment as the older sister and enters into the role in a low-keyed manner, initially matching the child's rather slow pace and down-regulated emotional expression; gradually, however, she introduces imaginary elements with potential to move the story forward in relevant ways. Dr. Green has noticed that Ellie attends to and takes increasing pleasure in therapist-led verbalized mental riffs, so she creates an older sister monologue that incorporates feelings and perspectives she envisions as reflecting Ellie's disowned affective states.

This action by Dr. Green leads to a clarifying but also precarious few moments, in which Ellie more freely expresses feared punishments—

namely, maternal anger and rejection—for emotional expression. She reveals her perception that negative feelings, especially those toward a younger sibling, are unacceptable; the mother will be angry if she knows. Ellie communicates a sense of morality rooted not only in her parents' strictures and her serendipitous exposure to mother–grandmother tensions, but also in the young child's naïve cognition and fantasy: right and wrong are perceived as rigid, categorical constructs. Within this system of ethics, "wrong" feelings are condemned as manifestations of badness; if Dr. Green's older sister character does not evince pure love for the baby, she is "just a mean old big sister." This point in the play seems precarious because it clearly arouses Ellie's anxiety. Indeed, the direct dialogue about the play has become too threatening, so Ellie abruptly turns her face away from Dr. Green and then falls silent for a minute before being able to reengage with the dolls and return to the play narrative. Dr. Green follows her lead, and makes her comment about Mommy's angry reaction through her play character, not directly to Ellie.

PRINCIPLE 2

A key therapeutic function involves naming affects and inner states that have previously been unlabeled and disavowed so that the child can reintegrate more modulated versions of split-off aspects of self. The clinician speaks about emotions, fantasies, and interpersonal experience from the safe vantage point of play, using roles that the child has assigned and that often reflect disowned feelings and fantasies.

WORKING WITH TRANSFERENCE AND DEFENSE IN PLAY THERAPY

All manifestations of feelings about the clinician, both directly expressed and more hidden within play narratives, are important sources of information about the child's relational patterns; the clinician is particularly attuned to children's communications about feelings, perceptions, and fantasies of self and others. As discussed in Chapter 5, "Basic Psychodynamic Concepts and Their Use in Play Therapy," the child–clinician relationship encompasses their here-and-now interactions, the child's

identifications with therapist functions that support the forward progression of development, and representations of past attachments; the
latter reflects the child's transference-based use of the clinician to re-
vive old wishes and conflicts that originally arose within the parent–
child bond (Abrams et al. 1999). Transference does not appear as a
"pure" entity but is always embedded with multiple components of the
therapeutic relationship, including the dyad's intersubjective exchanges,
the child's reactions to the clinician's behaviors and interventions, the
nature of the **working alliance**, the vagaries of countertransference, and
the therapist's function as a **new object** who facilitates completion of
developmental tasks.

Despite the complexities, we view the gradual elucidation of transference themes as a central feature of deepening play therapy; use of
the clinician to re-create outmoded relational paradigms, with the goal
of reintegrating them in more mature and healthy ways, contributes
to the child's increased tolerance of emotions, softens fears about the
potential consequences of wishes and fantasies, and ultimately leads
to greater freedom within relationships both new and old (Abrams and
Solnit 1998). Manifestations of transference may appear in overt ways,
such as in immediate, affective reactions to the therapist's here-and-
now behavior (e.g., angry reactions to the clinician's remarks or limit
setting); often, however, they are more oblique, masked within the
layered themes of the play itself, and unlikely to present themselves as
direct replicas of the child's past experiences (Yanof 1996a, 1996b).

The child's transference and defensive patterns are inextricably linked;
indeed, working with transference requires the therapist's close attention to young children's difficulty tolerating the uncomfortable feelings that arise within the therapeutic relationship. Children often react
with avoidance (e.g., a sudden need to leave the room) or more active
forms of **protest** in connection with surging emotions toward the therapist; a previously safe playing environment may suddenly appear
threatening as the child experiences increasingly intense affective states
(e.g., anger, jealousy, feelings of deprivation, strong dependency urges)
and fears their actualization within the playroom (Sugarman 2003).
Under the pressure of strong emotions, and without access to mature
levels of reality testing and self-regulation, transference-based projections take on frightening ramifications: expectations of the therapist's
punitive responses or hostile urges toward the clinician feel real and

immediate to the child and are not perceived as mental projections from former relationships. Moreover, young children struggle with abstract concepts, such as hypothesized connections between current reactions and the distant past.

These various cognitive and emotional immaturities limit children's grasp of the "as if" nature of transference and guide the therapist's use of interventions that can meaningfully elucidate relational experience. Complex verbal formulations about prior events and their impact on current interactions (e.g., "I think you stopped playing because you felt hurt when I suggested you move out of my lap, and it reminded you of when your mother's lap was always occupied by the baby") are often undesirable in play therapy; despite being potentially accurate and useful for the clinician's private understanding, such comments may lack meaning and relevance for the child. More typically, work with transference themes and defensive patterns is embedded within the play itself.

Ellie's level of engagement in school activities continued to grow, although she persistently manifested an unpleasant and sometimes downright hostile attitude toward one girl; on a couple of occasions, the teachers had noticed Ellie refusing to give this classmate a turn on the playground slide, and once she pushed the child when she thought nobody was looking. At home, her parents reported that Ellie was more relaxed and cooperative, and that the intensity of her jealousy toward her younger sibling was less directly evident although she sometimes teased the baby or withheld toys she knew the younger child desired.

In her play with Dr. Green, Ellie began to create a narrative in which Big Sister, a role still inhabited by the therapist, waited at home with an aunt while Mother and Father went to the hospital to "get" a new baby. Based on Ellie's suggestions, Dr. Green emphasized the older sister's anticipatory excitement, her intense curiosity about "where the baby comes from," and her acute sense of missing her parents while they lingered at the hospital and were focused only on the new infant. Ellie played Auntie, a calm and helpful figure who reassured the child that the parents would soon return, and reminded her about how much fun it would be to dress and feed a baby. Dr. Green recognized that the aunt represented a way in which Ellie experienced the therapist; she did not communicate this hypothesis to Ellie, instead choosing to speak from within her sister role about how hard it was to wait when she was missing her parents so much, and by asking if Auntie knew what she was feeling. Auntie responded sagely, indicating that Big Sister would feel better when everyone returned home. Meanwhile, she would cook them both a lovely dish of rice and vegetables. When Big Sister responded that she did not know if she could eat, because of the intensity of her feelings, Auntie's tolerance declined; with severity, she reminded her niece that "You have to be good, and calm down, and eat your food that I make for you." Responding to the sudden change in Ellie's character's responsiveness, Dr. Green used her role to verbalize Big Sister's worries and frustrations: "Are you mad at me, Auntie? I was just wanting to tell you that I'm feeling really upset right now." "Shush," responded Auntie, with firmness.

Ellie then enacted the scene in which the parents ceremoniously arrived home, carrying the infant. Speaking directly to Dr. Green, Ellie suggested that they place the baby's crib very close to an open window in the dollhouse; somewhat excitedly, Ellie pretended that the wind was strong that night, the window blew open, and the baby was blown away "in a whoosh." Then, she hesitated, looked uncomfortable, and quickly revised the story: the baby would get very close to the window, but the Aunt, who was sleeping in a part of the house separate from the children and parents, heard the commotion caused by the gusts, raced to the crib, and shut the window before any harm could come. Dr. Green commented quietly on Ellie's shift in affect: "You looked a little nervous for a moment." "I was just worried about the baby," answered Ellie. "But Auntie knew what to do. Mommy and Daddy never even woke up." "What about the big sister?" asked Dr. Green. Ellie responded, "She's the one who woke up Auntie! She heard the wind first!" "So she and Auntie saved the baby together," remarked the therapist. Ellie looked pleased, and suggested that there might be more dangers awaiting the baby. "But don't worry," she added. "Auntie is moving into the house so she and Big Sister will always be there."

In this interaction, Dr. Green attends to affective states that reflect both transference and defense; through her selection of interventions, she underscores both Ellie's manifestations of feelings about the therapist and elements of her self-protective style. From outside sources, Dr. Green is made aware of Ellie's aggression toward a particular classmate, a likely displacement of resentment toward her younger sibling. In play, however, the therapist does not attempt to make conscious Ellie's underlying sibling hostility, her wish to harm the baby, or her inevitable anger at the parental figures who have left their child at home; direct interpretation of unconscious aggression would likely cause the girl to feel exposed and intruded upon, eliciting further defensiveness and **resistance** rather than opening up affects and themes. Instead, Dr. Green stays within the play scenarios and addresses some of the painful emotions that are closer to the surface, namely Big Sister's loneliness and sense of exclusion during the parents' stay at the hospital. She recognizes play depictions of herself and of the therapeutic relationship (Auntie's calm reassurance and reflection, Auntie and Big Sister's joint thinking about feelings, and their mutual planning of solutions to apparent dangers of which nobody else is aware). Indeed, Ellie's embodiment of Auntie's role suggests an active, ongoing identification with the clinician's interest in mental states and her nonjudgmental acceptance of affects; the child's expanding emotional resourcefulness is also captured in her representations of solutions to affective dilemmas (the sister will feel better when everyone arrives back home) and hidden, emotional menaces such as rage and destructive impulses (Auntie and Big Sister will handle these threats together). However, transference-based shading of Auntie is also present: even though the older woman is kindly and helpful, she grows annoyed when affects are too forcefully expressed. In this play scenario, Dr. Green is able to vocalize a version of Ellie's long-standing relational experience: the sense that she must keep hidden aspects of herself that will be judged as bad and unlovable.

Dr. Green notes Ellie's anxiety-laden response to the themes of play at a point when the narrative has grown very dramatic (the new infant, placed close to the window as per Ellie's suggestion, is victim to the hostile forces of nature), and the play is nearly disrupted; at this moment, the imaginative scenario too closely approximates disavowed wishes and impulses that threaten to emerge into the child's conscious awareness. Dr. Green comments on Ellie's abrupt emotional change but allows the child to handle the remark in her own way, without insisting on a "correct" response or a return to the original storyline (i.e., she does not press the child toward linking the play with her own unconscious wishes, and does not veer the play back toward the infant's imminent demise). Ellie registers the therapist's observing, interested stance without feeling pressured toward discomfort or exposure. In this way, she is free to identify with Dr. Green's reflective attitude and mark the importance of internal signals; ultimately, the continued elaboration of feelings about self and others and the gradual connecting of uncomfortable affective states with defensive avoidance lead to greater affect tolerance, awareness of self-protective strategies, and softening of habitual interpersonal and defensive patterns (Hoffman 2014; Sugarman 2008).

PRINCIPLE 3

Working with transference and defense is critical to deepening play therapy. The child's use of characters and narratives yields important clues to feelings about the therapist, including distortions based on past relationships, as well as to habitual self-protective mechanisms. Momentary disruptions in play, due to the child's anxiety, are especially indicative of affects perceived as dangerous or unacceptable. The therapist uses play roles, often assigned by the child, to vocalize aspects of relational experience and to highlight ways in which the child protects the self from unwanted feelings.

WORKING WITH COUNTERTRANSFERENCE

Five-year-old Brandon Smith was referred to Dr. Green by a social worker at a children's hospital, where the boy's 9-year-old brother was a patient with leukemia. The social worker provided ongoing support for the parents and the boys but felt that Brandon needed his own therapist separate from the hospital environment. She had encountered Dr. Green at a local conference on childhood bereavement and had been impressed with the young psychiatrist's empathy and dedication. Although Brandon's brother was responding well to treatment, the initial manifestations of illness had led to numerous emergency room visits. During one particularly frightening late-night episode, Brandon's father was traveling for business; 5-year-old Brandon had needed to accompany his mother and brother as they rushed to the local emergency room, where he witnessed his mother crying and overheard her whispered comments to the pediatric resident about fears that her ill son would die. At various points that night, before the maternal grandmother was able to get to the hospital and stay with Brandon, his mother was forced to leave him alone in a waiting area for several minutes at a time while she attended to her other son.

Mrs. Smith tearfully recounted these events to Dr. Green, noting that she found it uncharacteristic that Brandon never asked her about what he heard or demanded to know about his brother's illness; generally, Brandon was an avidly curious child who loved science and reveled in facts about the body, space, oceans, and other natural matters. In addition, he had been fascinated by a previous visit to the Children's Museum where he was entranced by child-friendly depictions of germs and antibodies that presented them as warring entities.

However, there was total silence following the hospital visit; even after his brother's illness was properly diagnosed and treated, and family life began to return to normal, Brandon continued to appear shut-down and remote, refusing to talk about the medical situation and becoming angry and tearful if anyone even mentioned the words "leukemia" or "cancer." In addition, he had begun to refuse to go to school. The parents' sense of grief over their older son's suffering and their guilt about the impact on Brandon were palpable: both were tearful and seemed overwhelmed, although they referenced the progress they had made in sessions with their social worker, who had helped them find better ways to cope with their situation.

Brandon was happy to separate from his mother and join Dr. Green in the playroom. Although he enjoyed pretend play and eagerly gravitated toward her toys, he always began his sessions by bringing in his latest science-based magazine; after a cursory greeting, he typically ignored Dr. Green for about 10 minutes while looking at the pictures. Then, he would locate an interesting picture, often involving the eating habits of an animal or insect, and present it to Dr. Green for her response. Initially, she sought to reduce his solitary reading time by commenting on the page, seeking to establish common interests and rapport. However, Brandon was not especially responsive to her interventions. He continued his preferred pattern, controlling the selection of pictures that were then offered up for discussion. After a while, he transitioned comfortably into pretend play with Legos wherein the main theme involved space travel.

Five months into treatment, Dr. Green felt that Brandon's play narratives were somewhat redundant, lacking in richness and spontaneity; although this made sense, given her knowledge about trauma and its potential to inhibit and make repetitive certain aspects of children's play, she felt uncertain about how to proceed. Almost always, once he had finished his reading, Brandon assumed the role of a solitary astronaut, represented by a Lego figure and a rocket ship constructed out of paper, who floated above the earth and visited various planets. He did not name the figure or create other characters and did not initiate a role for Dr. Green; however, he talked excitedly to her as his astronaut journeyed from planet to planet, exclaiming over the various challenges and needed protections of planetary life ("He's freezing on Pluto! Good thing he brought his special suit!" or "He could burn up on Mercury! But don't worry, he has a fireman's suit for that!"). Dr. Green found herself drawn to questioning the astronaut about his solitary status; she asked whether he missed his family during his lengthy travels, or whether he ever invited friends to join him. She realized she felt moved by what she initially perceived as Brandon's loneliness and helplessness. In her mind a question formed: How could she reach this child, who appeared to her suspended precariously above the world, deprived of human protection and companionship? For a brief period, she increased her efforts to populate Brandon's space world; however, the astronaut was not particularly responsive to her play, and rejected her creation of an astronaut friend he might encounter on the planet Mars.

One day, as she and her colleague Dr. Lee were closing up the office for the night, Dr. Green mentioned her frustration over a young boy's play. As she talked, she associated to her own memories of being left alone in hospital waiting rooms while her mother attended to an elderly aunt with terminal illness; in fact, she had recently explored these memories with her own analyst and become more aware of their impact on her physician identity.

Children provide necessary corrections to the therapist's interventions, requiring that the clinician remain attuned to children's verbal and nonverbal cues. In this instance, Brandon resists Dr. Green's attempts to remediate his solitary stance, efforts that not only reflect her knowledge of the boy's real-life experience but also assuage her deep identification with Brandon's isolation and her wish to rescue both this lonely boy and her childhood self. As she becomes more aware of countertransference pressures, she is better able to recognize that her previous contributions to the play (focusing exclusively on the astronaut's aloneness and attempting to induce a less isolated state for the play character) are not opening up and deepening the pretense, and are not leading toward greater mutuality. Such self-awareness sometimes dawns during play itself but more often emerges into the clinician's consciousness only after the session, when there is time for reverie, such as during one's personal analysis or therapy, talks with supervisors, or discussions with colleagues. Indeed, one key benefit of shared space with other child practitioners is the opportunity for informal exchanging of ideas and experiences that often lead to greater insight about the child and the self.

Once Dr. Green achieves conscious awareness of countertransference-driven **enactments** in the playroom, her receptivity to Brandon's signals is less hampered. She experiences greater internal freedom for accessing the multiple meanings of Brandon's play, and then for seeking effective ways to extend his scenarios. Her evoked fantasies and memories serve as an invaluable, indirect source of information about Brandon, once she is able to reflect on them and begin to use her empathic responses to name and elucidate rather than oppose his affective states.

In addition to Brandon's sense of aloneness and his painful exclusion from the intense mother-father-ill brother triad, Dr. Green becomes conscious of other ways to think about his narrative: she considers his use of outer space as an escape from the scary, incomprehensible, and overstimulating events of Earth; she reflects on the story of the brave, resourceful, and heroic astronaut as an oedipal tale, perhaps representing a wished-for role vis-à-vis the mother in the face of her intense distress during a time of his father's notable absence; and she realizes that the astronaut may represent Brandon's brother, who has endured so much alone as the sole ill member of the family. Recalling her own early hospital experience as she awaited news of her aunt's fate, she envisions space travel as Brandon's attempt to grasp death, which might seem to a small boy as akin to floating out in the sky forever, alone and unable to return home. Moreover, she is better able to integrate these feelings and fantasies with her knowledge of normative oedipal-phase pressures and vulnerabilities. She realizes that Brandon's inevitable conflicts over desire, possessiveness, exclusion, and jealousy, as well as his fears of bodily punishment and injury, have been exacerbated by the perceived actualization of normal fantasies in real life; key competitors are actually vanquished (absent father, ill brother), and his brother's disease appears to embody a cautionary tale of what can happen to boys with bad thoughts. In addition, being alone with his overwhelmed mother in the hospital only makes him feel more small, frightened, and helpless than ever.

With a greater sense of mental freedom, Dr. Green is better equipped to follow Brandon's signals and expand the play without introducing unnecessary elements that detract from his meanings.

> Once Dr. Green resisted attempting to counter the solitary nature of Brandon's astronaut, she discovered other opportunities to work toward greater mutuality and exploration of the boy's self-protective stances. He announced a new mission to Saturn and enthusiastically described the astronaut's need to protect himself from the planet's "poisonous rings." "There are so many unexpected dangers in space!" exclaimed Dr. Green. Brandon soberly agreed, beginning to focus on the details of the special suit he would construct in order to survive. Dr. Green remarked on the courage and self-reliance of the astronaut, wondering aloud if he perhaps sometimes acted braver than he actually felt, or if he ever wished he could just stay on Earth and play without having to go on difficult adventures. "But that's what astronauts

do. They have to act brave," responded Brandon. Dr. Green suggested that acting might be different from feeling; maybe the character sometimes acted tough when he was feeling scared. Brandon smiled and answered, "You know what's the scariest place of all in space? A black hole! He's gonna go super close and maybe get sucked in!" Together, they exclaimed over the scariness of black holes and the uncertainty of the space traveler's fate. Their shared excitement over his close calls put them on the same page, affectively speaking, during the play. For the first time, Brandon suggested that Dr. Green might come along in a supportive role, such as a spaceship mechanic or someone who could repair ruptures in the astronaut's suit. Their joint adventures were expanded: they continued to travel into space, but also sometimes under the ocean, still as astronauts. Always, they were invincible and ventured into places other humans did not ordinarily occupy.

Although Dr. Green now accompanied the astronaut, he often scooted ahead of her, discovered something amazing ("This crater is bigger than anything people have ever seen!" "You won't believe this rainbow fish!"), then looked back and impatiently beckoned for her to catch up. However, her character was sometimes frustrated as the astronaut might change his mind and decide that there was not time for her to take a close look. As they were wrapping up a session, placing Legos into Brandon's bin, he playfully pushed past Dr. Green so he could position his toys first, while remarking, "The astronaut always gets to places first!" Dr. Green responded, "I've noticed that! He gets to be the one who sees amazing things first. It reminds me of when you first come in to the playroom, you like to bring a magazine and go places reading alone, and then sometimes you tell me about one of the exciting things. I think it's how you let me know what it feels like to have to wait, to be shut out of exciting and important things." "And also scary things," added Brandon enthusiastically. "Like when Mommy and Daddy are talking about Jason being sick, and they think I don't hear them." Referencing his scary night at the hospital directly for the first time, Dr. Green suggested, "And also like when you were in the hospital, and lots of scary things were happening." Brandon continued, "Did you know I had to wait alone before my Grandma came?" "Yes, your parents told me about that part." Both remained silent together for the last few moments as the session ended.

PRINCIPLE 4

Countertransference and enactments are essential, indirect ways of knowing about the child. It is important to find opportunities to reflect on private reactions (by talking with colleagues, supervisors, or a personal psychotherapist or psychoanalyst) in order to grasp fully and enable use of this emotional knowledge, and to avoid subtly detracting from the child's meanings or missing opportunities to deepen the therapeutic relationship and the play narratives.

WORKING FROM INSIDE, NEAR, AND OUTSIDE THE PLAY

In general, the therapist seeks to encourage and maintain the flow of the child's self-expression via the continuous interweaving of action and verbal narration. Potential disruptions are kept to a minimum, which requires that the therapist stay close to the child's communications and meanings, avoid premature or overly exposing verbal interpretations (e.g., pausing while in the midst of a play scenario to make direct links to the child's life), and evince an accepting and tolerant attitude toward evolving narratives, themes, and contents. However, opportunities arise in which more direct remarks are useful to elucidate the child's self-protective mechanisms or clarify transference-based wishes and perceptions. Such openings proceed most organically when they are initiated by the child, who indicates a moment of curiosity or awareness about the self or about a play character. Often, they arise first in the midst of play when children, without display of uncomfortable affect or disruption, simply sit back momentarily and comment on characters or narratives, or they might evolve while child and therapist plan storylines or when the play session is coming to an end. In the example of Brandon, above, a window for direct discourse opens when he makes observations about the play characters as he and Dr. Green are cleaning up ("The astronaut always gets to places first!"), and she responds at a similar level of reflection. These interactions are not technically "inside" the play itself; they arise from the ongoing action and narration but involve a level of reflection that is positioned just outside immersion in the playing state.

At other times, the therapist might take the lead in child-directed comments, intervening in order to help make meaning of sudden urges and reduce the immediacy and intensity of affective states. These opportunities occur at varying points in the session, such as during the opening minutes, when the therapist may notice a change in the child's usual presentation or the child may relate an experience at school or home; during the session, when a shift in affect and activity disrupts play narratives and signals that the child is experiencing an internal discomfort; or at the end of a session, when the child's behavior suggests difficulty with separation. In these cases, the therapist verbally notes the change (in focus, facial expression, or action), links it to a hypothesized affect, and speculates aloud about the potential source (a play theme, the therapist's announcement of the end of session). Such interventions function best when they draw the child's attention to his or her behaviors and attribute underlying meanings, but leave within the child's control how the child will respond. If the therapist's invitation to self-reflection or proposed meaning is rejected, there is no value in insisting or disputing the child's dismissal; this will only increase resistance and cause the child to feel unheard and misunderstood. At a later point in time, the child might manifest signs that the therapist's comments have been absorbed, via a less negative reaction to subsequent interventions or an incorporation of new themes into the play.

The following brief example in the treatment of Becky Singer, seen by Dr. Lee in the midst of a contentious parental separation (as discussed beginning in Chapter 8), illustrates how a more direct discussion of the child's internal states might develop.

> After several months in twice-weekly treatment with Dr. Lee, Becky Singer continued to create play narratives that involved a child named Gina traveling back and forth between houses; the clear links to Becky's personal situation had never been articulated, although both child and therapist spoke openly about Gina's confusion over the visitation schedule. On one occasion, after indicating that Gina could not accept a friend's invitation for a play date because she did not know which parent to ask, Becky looked directly at Dr. Lee and commented about the character: "She's having a very hard time today. Just sad about you-know-what." Dr. Lee said, "You seem like you know a lot about how she's feeling." Becky replied, with sadder affect, "I sometimes feel that way when I have to remember that it's almost three o'clock because the teacher says 'time to get your backpacks,' and I have to go see one parent and not the other." Dr. Lee commented, "You have fun during the day, but then when it's time to go home, you remember about the sad things." Both sat silently for a couple of minutes, and then Becky suggested a change in the play: they would have Gina go on a play date after all so that she could feel happy.

In this instance, Becky herself briefly departs from her absorption in play—a moment likely stimulated by the affects arising from play narratives that have run extremely close to her reality-based situation—to reflect on the Gina character she has created. Dr. Lee responds in a way that reaches slightly beyond Becky's manifest communication but does not specifically reference the child's personal experience with "you-know-what." In this way, Becky is free either to expand the conversation or go in another direction entirely. Once she has endorsed identification with the play character, and Dr. Lee has elaborated her feelings and the difficulties of dismissal time at school, Becky devises a solution within the play. There is no need to continue to work outside of the pretense at this point; the successful arc of these verbal exchanges will open up future possibilities for direct discussions of Becky's personal experience. The definitions of "you-know-what" have been implied, but it is not necessary for the therapist to name it as "divorce" or "separation." Dr. Lee has followed Becky's lead and allowed the child a sense of control, but also implemented a meaningful elaboration of the child's initial comments.

At other times, the child's direct behavior toward the therapist signals underlying discomforts that can be addressed by verbally linking overt action with internal states. As described in Chapter 9, "Getting Started, Creating an Alliance, and Facilitating Play," early resistances to treatment may yield to verbal interpretations of the child's underlying sense of exposure, resentment about feeling coerced to see an unfamiliar adult, and worries about separation from parents. At later points in therapy, sudden shifts in the child's interpersonal behavior may represent intensification of transference feelings (e.g., increased sense of dependency or deprivation), connect to developmental pressures (e.g., an internal push toward autonomy), and reflect the child's experience of age-salient demands (e.g., teacher's and parents' expectations).

In the following example, Dr. Vargas continues his work with 8-year-old Jeremy (introduced at the beginning of Chapter 9), who engages in controlling, oppositional behaviors with his parents to ward off his intense states of anxiety. The therapeutic relationship evolves slowly; joint play is established very gradually but eventually yields a greater sense of mutuality and provides the child with a venue to begin expressing his wishes for strength and bravery. The child's serendipitous encounter with an age-mate in the waiting room leads to an intensification of transference and self-protective feelings, but also provides an opportunity for greater openness in the treatment.

> Dr. Vargas had been treating 8-year-old Jeremy McAlvin for several months, tolerating the boy's ongoing (although diminishing) rants against the stupidity of adults who imagined that he needed help; during Jeremy's stony silences, Dr. Vargas continued to verbalize what he imagined as the child's sense of betrayal and outrage about having his private behaviors—rituals at night and refusals to cooperate with parental limits—exposed and discussed by adults. Although many sessions continued to feel combative and frustrating to Dr. Vargas, he realized on reflection that there were small but meaningful changes in the relationship. For example, Jeremy occasionally briefly referenced his presleep regimens (always referred to as "my own business" and accompanied by adamant insistence that they were not a problem); at these times, Dr. Vargas commented that the behaviors, which he called "sleep routines" to use Jeremy's labels, sounded necessary and important, and that Jeremy might wish to protect them from scrutiny and interference. He did not address the potential meanings of the rituals, including the ways in which they kept his parents in close proximity and protected Jeremy from anxiety. In addition, Jeremy had begun to indicate interest in a bin of toy soldiers that he recognized from his own collection at home; during occasional sessions when he and Dr. Vargas battled in play displacement, conducting wars that Jeremy's troops inevitably won, the child relaxed considerably and revealed his intense interest in the soldiers' various forms of self-protection (weaponry, tough attitudes), their bravery, and their determination to follow a "chain of command" and a set of rules.
>
> Meanwhile, Dr. Vargas worked regularly with Jeremy's parents to help them understand the importance of their consistency and support for the treatment. Parent sessions focused on helping the adults perceive the level of Jeremy's anxiety, the link between anxious inner states and their son's efforts at controlling the external environment, and the way in which the parents' responses (anger, giving in, avoidance) ratcheted up the boy's worries by convincing Jeremy of his badness, destructiveness, and power within the family. In addition, Dr. Vargas pointed out that frequent parental punishments for rude and uncooperative behavior were counterproductive, as they relieved Jeremy from developing a sense of internal responsibility for himself. Currently, his provocative actions at home were followed not by inner guilt but by external judgments, which then led him to further rail against the unfairness of others. To everyone's relief, the parents observed that Jeremy's protests about coming to therapy had significantly abated after his initial stormy refusals.

A change in Dr. Vargas's scheduling led to a waiting room encounter between Jeremy and another boy about his age; although there were several practitioners in the suite, Jeremy heard the other boy's mother say Dr. Vargas's name. Upon entering the playroom, Jeremy imperiously demanded to know why the other boy came to see him, what they did together, and how the child "survived" his sessions. "I guess you are torturing him, too!" he declared when Dr. Vargas acknowledged that kids often wonder about each other in such circumstances. Dr. Vargas did not interpret Jeremy's underlying emotional states (his sense of curiosity about what goes on behind closed doors; feelings of exclusion and jealousy), because he expected this would have elicited shame and rage and thereby shut down any nascent opportunities for communication.

Jeremy gestured toward the bin of soldiers and commented casually that they could look at them again if Dr. Vargas wanted to. The therapist evinced enthusiasm, recalling their previous battle. Together, they removed each figure and, as in prior sessions, commented on the soldiers' uniforms and guns before initiating a battle in which Jeremy forcefully swept the opposing troops away. However, Jeremy soon returned to complaints: "You didn't answer my question about what the other kid plays with. Does he like these soldiers or not?" Dr. Vargas responded, "Lots of kids like them and play with them." He realized that his answer frustrated Jeremy and quickly added," I know you were asking specifically about that boy, but if another kid asked about you, I wouldn't tell what we do or discuss. It's private." Jeremy looked scornful, but considered this and responded, "It's a good thing. The kids would think I'm a loser if they knew what you know, that I still need my parents to sit with me at night." He looked ashamed, but then almost instantly resumed his imperious tone: "You have to get some stuff in this stupid room that kids actually like, not baby toys. That other kid probably likes your stuff and doesn't know any better." Dr. Vargas remarked that he was realizing Jeremy sometimes acted tough and scoffed at babyish ways when he was feeling badly about himself, like about being scared at night. Jeremy looked as if he was about to embark on one of his habitual protests, but he stopped and suggested that next time, he could bring some of his figures from home so they could "have a real battle."

In this case, play functions as a source of mutuality and relationship building, as well as a safe, displaced setting within which Jeremy can battle with adults and reveal his inner worries and sense of inadequacy, but also as a backdrop to more purely verbal interactions between child and therapist. As a mid-latency child, for whom pretense retains importance but who also uses additional tools for self-expression, Jeremy benefits from a sensitive balance between play and direct conversation with Dr. Vargas.

PRINCIPLE 5

The clinician should avoid transgressing the child's play material. Although it is important to stay as close as possible to the child's play themes and characters, the clinician also needs to be alert to opportunities in which more direct interventions might help to elucidate the child's personal experience and inner states. These opportunities arise in different ways, including when children momentarily depart from their full immersion in the playing state to comment on characters or scenarios.

SUMMARY

Deepening play therapy involves the gradual expansion of play narratives and characters so that the child's affects, fantasies, modes of relating, and self-protective mechanisms are meaningfully verbalized and connections are made between feelings. This work requires careful attention to the child's verbal and nonverbal signals, as well as the therapist's awareness of potential countertransference pressures that can limit internal freedom and receptivity. When child and therapist are fully immersed in play, the therapist should avoid transgressing the play material by making direct comments about the child; however, other opportunities arise in the here-and-now interactions for the therapist to utilize interventions such as elaborations of the child's relationships and defenses against painful emotions.

KEY POINTS

- Deepening play treatment involves sustaining and solidifying the child's sense of the therapist as consistent and trustworthy. When play is progressing well, the therapist aims to maintain the mutual state of play and avoid transgressions of the material that might lead to disruptions and inhibitions.

- Naming the child's inner states and linking affects to meaningful play narratives serve to render previously disavowed, poorly tolerated emotions more bearable, more knowable, and less overwhelming.

- Gradual elaboration of transference feelings and the self-protective mechanisms that the child employs to avoid them is a major way to deepen play treatments and lead to better tolerance for affects, reduced fears about the consequences of wishes and fantasies, and overall greater freedom within new and old relationships.

- Countertransference information is an indirect, potentially invaluable, and unique way to deepen the therapist's knowledge of a child and his or her play meanings. Gaining full benefit from personal reactions to the child requires the opportunity for reflection and reverie, via talking with colleagues, supervisors, or a personal psychotherapist or psychoanalyst.

- As treatment progresses, opportunities arise for work that is slightly removed from the play (e.g., talking about play characters, negotiating narratives) or that deals directly with shifts in the child's affects and behaviors. The therapist seeks to make links between internal states and outward signs, and draws attention to the child's self-protective patterns.

KEY TERMS

Enactments Symbolic therapist–patient interactions wherein their mutual unconscious conflicts and fantasies are actualized in the treatment.

Mutual playing state The child–clinician shared special consciousness or ego state that accompanies play during which reality is mutually suspended and the dyad is fully engrossed in pretense.

New object The therapist's functions as a potential figure for identifications that serve the child's developmental progression, such as use of the clinician's affect tolerance and reflective stance to scaffold emerging capacities.

Resistance The patient's self-protective tendencies that may at times oppose the therapeutic process in order to maintain a psychological status quo.

Working alliance   Also referred to as "therapeutic alliance." A component of the child–clinician relationship that allows the work to go forward, even during moments of discomfort and distress. It refers to the child's capacity to trust in the therapist's essential benevolence and willingness to participate in treatment.

———●————————————————●———

REFERENCES

Abrams S, Solnit AJ: Coordinating developmental and psychoanalytic processes: conceptualizing technique. J Am Psychoanal Assoc 46(1):85–103, 1998 9565900

Abrams S, Neubauer PB, Solnit AJ: Coordinating the developmental and psychoanalytic processes: three case reports. Introduction (discussion). Psychoanal Study Child 54:19–24, discussion 87–90, 1999 10748626

Birch M: In the land of counterpane: travels in the realm of play. Psychoanal Study Child 52:57–75, 1997 9489461

Bornstein B: Clinical notes on child analysis. Psychoanal Study Child 1:151–166, 1945 21004307

Galatzer-Levy RM: The nuts and bolts of child psychoanalysis. Annual of Psychoanalysis 36:189–202, 2008

Gilmore K: Play in the psychoanalytic setting: ego capacity, ego state, and vehicle for intersubjective exchange. Psychoanal Study Child 60:213–238, 2005 16649681

Hoffman L: Berta Bornstein's "Frankie": the contemporary relevance of a classic to the treatment of children with disruptive symptoms. Psychoanal Study Child 68:152–176, 2014 26173332

Joyce AF: Interpretation and play: some aspects of the process of child analysis. Psychoanal Study Child 65:152–168, 2011 26027143

Katan A: Some thoughts about the role of verbalization in early childhood. Psychoanal Study Child 16:184–188, 1961

Mahon EJ: Playing and working through: a neglected analogy. Psychoanal Q 73(2):379–413, 2004 15108405

Mayes LC, Cohen DJ: Playing and therapeutic action in child analysis. Int J Psychoanal 74(Pt 6):1235–1244, 1993 8138367

Sugarman A: Dimensions of the child analyst's role as a developmental object: affect regulation and limit setting. Psychoanal Study Child 58:189–213, 2003 14982021

Sugarman A: The use of play to promote insightfulness in the analysis of children suffering from cumulative trauma. Psychoanal Q 77(3):799–833, 2008 18686791

Yanof J: Language, communication and transference in child analysis, I: selective mutism: the medium is the message. J Am Psychoanal Assoc 44(1): 79–100, 1996a 8717479

Yanof J: Language, communication, and transference in child analysis, II: is child analysis really analysis? J Am Psychoanal Assoc 44(1):100–116, 1996b 8717480

12

Ending Play Therapy and the Process of Termination

Dr. Green had been treating Ellie Park, who was now nearly 8 years old, in twice-weekly play therapy for 2½ years. The child's transition to second grade was uneventful. Ellie was firmly established in the social milieu at her school and had developed close friendships with a couple of girls; moreover, teachers reported that she was performing well academically, even excelling in reading, and engaging content-edly in classroom activities. Her parents observed that Ellie's mood was far less negative and noted her increased ability to verbalize frustrations and disappointments, rather than sulking and withdrawing from challenging situations.

In therapy, Ellie still favored pretend play but had also begun to manifest keen interest in board games; in addition, she often wanted to tell Dr. Green about an event in school, show her the latest homework, demonstrate a recently acquired skill, or describe how her friend group met online to play popular digital games. In Dr. Green's conceptualization, Ellie demonstrated clear signs of latency-phase development, including improved capacities for self-expression and self-regulation, a cooperative stance and industrious attitude, and a decisive pivot toward peer connections; her play themes sometimes now reflected her 7-year-old perception of adolescent life, often revolving around a teenage girl having exciting weekend adventures. Recently, Ellie had begun to question how long they would continue to play together. At first, when Dr. Green attempted to elicit the child's thoughts and feelings about the possibility of ending treatment, Ellie feigned disinterest and either changed the subject or returned to play. Gradually, however, Dr. Green noted that she appeared more open to the topic and better able to express ambivalence: Ellie acknowledged that she liked to come and play but also that she wished she had more time for play dates and practicing for gymnastics meets.

Dr. Green was aware of her own ambivalence about ending the treatment. She enjoyed seeing Ellie and felt the therapy had progressed well; moreover, Ellie was one of her most verbal child patients, well able to engage in a fair amount of insight-oriented work. In addition, her relationship with the parents had deepened significantly over the years; despite their initial reticence and the disapproval they had incurred from their extended family members, who had not supported Ellie's treatment, the Parks had persevered. Their trust in Dr. Green factored importantly in their creation of a more growth-promoting atmosphere at home, one in which they were able to tolerate Ellie's occasional bouts of negativity and encourage her to vocalize dissatisfactions, even when these were difficult to hear. At times, however, Dr. Green became aware of an underlying urge to protect Ellie and to continue to function as her confidante and advocate, knowing that the parents still struggled to verbalize their own and their daughter's inner states.

Ellie's parents had not raised the issue of termination, despite their daughter's developmental gains. Dr. Green decided to broach the topic in a monthly parent meeting, reporting that the idea of ending was already on Ellie's mind as well as her own. She was met with the Parks's anxious questions: "How do we know she's ready to handle things on her own? What if she gets worse again?" As if to contradict Dr. Green's remarks about their daughter's improved mood, reduced symptoms, and developmental progress, they provided recent evidence of Ellie's ongoing jealous feelings toward her sibling. Dr. Green reassured them that they would talk again before making any final decisions together. In addition, she pointed out that the goal of treatment was not the abolishment of negative emotions, such as sibling resentment. She reminded them that Ellie had gained sufficient self-control to contain her feelings and pointed out that Ellie's newfound interests (gymnastics, reading, digital games with social components) and friendships provided her with extensive opportunities for the channeling and sublimation of strong emotions. At the same time, Dr. Green acknowledged that there is often a period of adjustment both during and immediately after termination, and that Ellie might even experience a transient regression with a brief reintensification of symptoms. The Parks proposed a compromise: "Can't we just cut back to once a week and see how she does, and then reassess?" Dr. Green explained that she was reluctant to change fundamental aspects of the treatment, and recommended that they remain at twice per week and continue to discuss termination. The parents had additional questions about the post-termination period: Could they contact her to discuss how Ellie was doing? Could Ellie come back in the future if there were problems?

Could they schedule "check-ins" even if there were no compelling issues, just to stay in touch? Dr. Green responded favorably to these requests for continued contact, letting the Parks know that there were no absolute rules and that she would continue to be available if needed.

The following month, the adults met again and agreed to set a tentative date for Ellie's final session (4 months in the future, in the middle of the academic year), which could be confirmed once Ellie's reaction had been factored into the plan. "How should we tell her?" was the parents' next question. Dr. Green asked how they preferred to handle telling Ellie, and both responded that they had hoped Dr. Green would initiate the conversation with Ellie and they would then follow up with their own discussion. A few days later, as Ellie and Dr. Green were setting up their usual pretend play materials, the child excitedly described a conversation with her best friend at school in which they had discussed a much-anticipated sleepover party at a third girl's house. Dr. Green commented on how much fun Ellie was having with friends this year and how sleepovers had become a highly enjoyable social event. Ellie looked thoughtful and then agreed that she no longer worried about what her parents and her younger sibling were doing while she was out of the house. Dr. Green mentioned that in the most recent parent meetings, the adults had discussed how Ellie was now very busy with school, friends, and activities and might be ready to stop coming for therapy. "I think it has been on your mind, as well," Dr. Green remarked, referencing the girl's recent questions about their future together. Ellie looked surprised, then quietly asked if they could resume playing their game.

Termination represents a universal outcome of therapy; many writers have referenced the inevitable but somewhat ironic treatment situation wherein the intimate therapeutic relationship is established only to foster its own dissolution (Bergmann 1988; Craige 2009; Pinsky 2002). Ideally, termination embodies a process that arises organically as an outgrowth of patients' improved functioning and fuller engagement with life. Often, however, the end of treatment is precipitated by reality-based exigencies (the patient relocates, the therapist's training at a particular site has come to an end) or hastened by intensification of resistance during a particular phase of the therapy (Loewald 1988). In child treatments, endings that are premature (at least by the therapist's standards) are frequently precipitated by parental reactions (Deakin et al. 2012; Midgley and Navridi 2006); however, they are also initiated

by young people themselves, reflecting their drive for autonomy and aspirations for greater social, academic, and extracurricular immersion.
Indeed, children's desires to terminate, even when embedded with more
complex motivations, may represent real gains in the treatment that cor-
respond with restored developmental momentum: a previously sepa-
ration-anxious teen can finally leave home to attend boarding school
or university, or a school-age child, formerly too conflicted or inhibited to enjoy after-school activities, now wants greater involvement in
the world of peers and seeks age-appropriate outlets. Ellie's dawning interest in termination partly reflects an increasing investment in and capacity for age-salient tasks such as peer socialization (play dates) and
mastery of skills (gymnastics); time spent with Dr. Green now poses a
conflict, as it detracts from these other exciting and pleasurable activities in the outside world.

Like every other stage in the referral and treatment of children, ending therapy involves multiple individuals and their points of view: the
child, the therapist, and at least one parent or guardian contribute their
subjective sense of the child's readiness for termination. In addition,
the opinions of teachers, tutors, and daytime caregivers are often so-
licited to assess children's social, academic, and self-regulatory progress
in settings outside of home and therapy. These potentially divergent
perspectives derive from conscious considerations of the child's current functioning, the child's and parents' emotional responses to the
experience of treatment, and a range of unconscious pressures that include transference and countertransference reactions.

Children's feelings about ending treatment reflect the trends and pressures of their developmental phase, attachment to the therapist, sense
of parental attitudes toward treatment, perception of treatment goals,
and reactions to a particular period in the therapy.[1] As termination looms,
children might feel excitement and relief at the prospect of more free
time and less adult scrutiny, combined with a sense of impending loss

---

[1]We are distinguishing these responses from the more abrupt, urgently experienced desires to flee that often arise during treatment as specific themes,
wishes, and impulses emerge in play; such transient psychological resistances
are discussed more fully in Chapters 9, "Getting Started, Creating an Alliance,
and Facilitating Play," and 11, "Deepening Play Therapy: Verbalizing Inner
States, Expanding Narratives, and Working With Transference and Defense."

(Bernstein and Glenn 1988); such ambivalence is illustrated in Ellie's raising and then avoiding the topic of termination, and in her genuine surprise when Dr. Green remarks, "I think it has been on your mind, as well." Similarly, the therapist's sense of the patient's readiness for termination is subject to conscious conceptualizations about the treatment (e.g., Dr. Green's intellectual awareness of Ellie's developmental gains and entry into the latency phase of development) but also aspects of countertransference (e.g., Dr. Green's pleasure in the therapy, her reluctance to lose a valued connection with Ellie and the family, and her sense of protectiveness toward the girl) (Fabricius and Green 1995). Finally, parental attitudes toward termination are affected by feelings about and reliance on the clinician, tolerance for the ongoing time and money burdens of maintaining the child's treatment, and a sense of what has been accomplished in therapy. The Parks demonstrate an intellectual awareness of Ellie's social and emotional gains, but their reluctance to terminate derives from their dependence on Dr. Green and insecurity about their parenting competence, which reflect feelings and self-perceptions that originate in their own past relationships as well as in the more recent challenges they have faced with their children.

The child clinician's awareness of and attention to these complex reactions are key to facilitating a termination process that continues the work of treatment, maintains as much as possible a positive connection with the child and parents, and fosters the family's ability to sustain therapeutic benefits once the treatment has drawn to a close. In the case of Ellie, despite consensus about the child's developmental gains, Dr. Green must attend to the emotional surround, including the child's attachment to her and to their mutual play, the parents' intense anxiety about losing her support in the face of future uncertainties, and her own investment in the therapy. Despite the clinician's careful planning and preparation, and the sensitive work with the family, a sense of abruptness, arbitrariness, and loss is unavoidable as treatment comes to an end (Bergmann 1988). In the minds of many psychoanalytic writers, painful and bereaved feelings are an essential part of the termination process.

THE PHASES OF TERMINATION IN PLAY THERAPY

Within psychoanalytic literature, the process of termination is often divided into phases; although these phases are not rigidly distinct from each other, each reflects specific therapeutic tasks (Novick and Novick 2002). The **pretermination phase** refers to a period in the treatment when major goals have been achieved (e.g., diminishment of symptoms, restoration of developmental functioning) and winding down appears as a looming possibility in the mind of the therapist, and often in the mind of the patient as well. A mutual discussion of ending is initiated, allowing for further assessment of the patient's readiness without the immediate pressure of an impending date. The **termination phase**, which involves coming to terms with the meaning and imminent loss of the therapeutic relationship, covers the time between when an end date is set and when the final day arrives; this period is often of several months' duration and may encompass a retrospective of the treatment. The **posttermination phase** is not a part of treatment per se, as it occurs after therapist and patient have ceased to meet; this period is marked by the patient's reaction to the loss of the treatment relationship and the ongoing consolidation of the therapist's and patient's previously shared explorations and reflective functions (Conway 1999; Craige 2002).

Inevitably, termination involves an experience of loss for therapist and patient, as both must relinquish a highly valued, long-standing bond marked by shared work (and play) and the intense emotional involvement that accompanies mutual exploration of the unconscious (Blatt and Behrends 1987; Craige 2009; Kantrowitz 1997; Novick and Novick 2001). In psychoanalytic theory, *mourning* represents a process that follows a bereavement, during which an important lost relationship is gradually internalized; after termination, unique shared aspects of the therapeutic bond are carried on alone, via the patient's inner dialogue and self-reflection, and continue to impact subsequent experience (Bonovitz 2007; Loewald 1988). However, the immediate posttermination process is not always one of steady adjustment and fond memories of the therapist, and does not always reflect positive aspects of the therapeutic relationship. Individuals with histories of traumatic loss may experience particular difficulty during termination, because separation from the therapist revives earlier abandonments and a concomitant sense of helplessness (Craige 2009). Even without such vulnerabilities, adults and children may not sustain a positive representation of the therapist; some individuals experience a return of symptomatology or a regression in development (Bergmann 1988; Karush 2014).

Although the three phases and the associated process of mourning are useful in conceptualizing child terminations, children's experience of and participation in the ending of treatment are powerfully shaped by the nature of their developing relational and ego capacities (Novick 1990). Emerging abilities for verbal expression and interaction, insight, abstraction, and reflection, as well as an ongoing attachment to and dependency on parental figures, impact all aspects of termination. Although transference feelings achieve significant intensity in child treatments, parents remain the central focus of the young child's love and security; therefore, resolution of transference, which is a prominent aspect of adult termination, is often less conspicuous in play therapy. Adults tend to retain an inner awareness of the therapist's voice and their mutual past conversations; many young children, like Ellie in the vignette, experience the attachment to and loss of the therapist primarily through feelings about and memories of the routines of treatment and their shared play. The child's sense of missing the therapist is not necessarily articulated but may be demonstrated in a transient regression after treatment ends, including a tendency to seek action-based outlets for affective states.

During the termination phase, children do not necessarily engage in verbal retrospectives or speak about the therapeutic relationship. Ellie's brief comment about her newfound independence and sociability, as she remarks on her pleasure in sleepovers, represents an important moment of self-reflection and insight, but it will not necessarily lead to further discussion with Dr. Green about her past problems. With her developmental momentum restored, Ellie is avidly focused on the here-and-now, as well as on the future: she envisions the excitement of her next play date, fantasizes about success at her next gymnastics meet, and has begun to imagine her adolescent self.

PRINCIPLE 1

The process of termination is often conceived in three phases: pretermination, termination, and posttermination. The pretermination phase includes assessment of the patient's readiness and initiates preparation for loss of the therapeutic relationship, whereas the posttermination phase encompasses the work of mourning and internalization of the patient's and therapist's previously shared reflective functions. Although the end of treatment elicits feelings of bereavement, children's developmental status and attachment to parents impacts how they experience and react to loss of the therapist.

CRITERIA FOR TERMINATION

Therapists' beliefs about their patients' readiness for termination are closely tied to conceptualizations of treatment goals. Psychoanalytic writers variously emphasize such indicators as increased awareness of unconscious forces; capacity for insight and autonomous self-reflection (i.e., self-analysis); softening of harsh superego standards; less conflictual and more satisfying interpersonal relationships; greater preparedness to pursue personal goals and achieve them according to potentialities; reduction in painful, debilitating symptoms; and development and resolution of a full transference relationship with the therapist (Gabbard 2009; Kogan 1996; Ticho 1972). Many theorists suggest that the main deciding factor for termination is having attained a good overall outcome for the patient rather than having solved an exhaustive range of identifiable problems and conflicts (Bernstein 2001; Freud 1937; Gabbard 2009; Glucksman 2011; Shane 2009).

In child treatments, termination is foreseeable when the forward progression of development has been restored, meaning that there has been satisfactory resolution of the inhibitions, anxieties, and rigid modes of relating that blocked the child's capacity for age-appropriate pursuits, positive family bonds, deepened social connections, and expected levels of emotional and behavioral self-regulation (Ablon 1988; Chazan 1997; Freud 1971). The reinstatement of developmental momentum represents improved balance between normative defenses and affective openness, between progressive and regressive forces, and between the normative use of fantasy and the child's engagement in reality-based experience; the child is better able to handle a wide range of developmental tasks with increased autonomy and more stable self-esteem (Abrams 1992; Bernstein 1975; Novick 1990; Shane and Shane 1984). In Ellie's case, a reduction in symptoms (irritability, withdrawal, avoidance) and significant developmental gains (improved self-expression and emotional self-regulation, deeper engagement in social life, immersion in the life of the classroom and beyond) signal that the main goals of therapy have been satisfactorily achieved.

The therapist rarely gauges a child's readiness for termination without input from parents and other adults. How a child presents within the therapeutic environment is not necessarily a complete or fully accurate indicator. Some children, positively impacted by the attentive, accepting, and containing attitude of the therapist, manifest a reduction in difficult behaviors that other adults, such as classroom teachers, may still be struggling to help the child control; in other instances, the intensity of transference may lead the child to behave in overstimulated ways that are not representative of outside conduct. Moreover, parents', teachers', and the therapist's assessments of a child's overall functioning are not always in sync and may reflect highly subjective experiences of the child. For example, a parent may feel strongly about a child's lingering occasional aggression or distractibility and advocate for additional time in treatment, or a therapist's concern over a child's lack of joy and enthusiasm, even in the presence of vastly improved behavior, may not be shared by parents and teachers whose treatment goals centered on a reduction in disruptive outbursts. Indeed, the therapist's dawning sense of termination readiness sometimes reflects aspects of the unique therapeutic situation, such as a realization that play themes and contents have grown repetitive, and that narratives are no longer expanding and deepening; although these are significant clinical indicators, they are understandably less meaningful in the eyes of nonclinicians. Realities in the child's environment, including the parents' ability to help sustain developmental gains in the absence of treatment, also factor into any assessment for termination (Novick 1990). If parents demonstrate vulnerability to certain interpersonal patterns, such as a child's provocative bids for attention, termination might be postponed while the adults strengthen and consolidate their emotional resources, even if the child's development is back on track.

In termination considerations, the child's likely capacity to navigate challenges in the near future is part of the overall assessment. Some writers (e.g., Abrams 1992) suggest that treatment continue until the child has entered the next developmental phase to ensure that forward progression is established. However, it is important to realize that child treatments do not necessarily reach into the far future; a successful therapy equips the child for current developmental tasks but neither guarantees the smooth negotiation of subsequent phases nor "inoculates" the child against serendipitous events, discontinuities in maturation, and future problems (Freud 1971). Children often return for one or more additional courses of therapy (sometimes referred to as **serial treatments**) during later periods of growth as they encounter new obstacles neither predicted nor warded off in their previous treatment (Beiser 1995).

PRINCIPLE 2

When a therapist is assessing a child's readiness for termination, the main standard is the restoration of developmental momentum so that the child can engage fully in age-salient tasks (adjustment to school, establishment of peer relations, pursuit of interests and activities). However, in setting a date for ending treatment, the therapist must integrate potentially divergent perspectives from parents and other adults in the child's outside life, and remain sensitive to the needs of the family.

PREPARING FOR TERMINATION AND POSTTERMINATION CONTACT

After the termination date had been set, Dr. Green arranged a few extra meetings with Ellie's parents to help resolve their remaining concerns (sibling fights, the stresses of her beloved gymnastics as the sport grew more serious and competitive), to address the possibility of future meetings (the Parks pressed for a scheduled parent meeting, around 2 months after termination, rather than taking a wait-and-see approach), and to discuss Ellie's potential posttermination reactions. The parents were very reassured by Dr. Green's agreement to a scheduled posttermination meeting, and by her reiteration that she would remain a resource for them and for their daughter in the future. They reviewed several times the multiple areas of Ellie's growth, including her happier mood and the shifts in her openness to school and friendships, but also the parents' increased skill at reading her signs, supporting her newfound adventurousness, and helping her identify and verbalize emotional states before sulkiness and avoidance set in.

There were 3 weeks and six play therapy meetings left. Although Ellie was a highly verbal child, she initiated few direct comments about the upcoming termination. When Dr. Green asked about her reaction to ending treatment, Ellie acknowledged, "I'm so used to coming here after school, it'll feel weird to go straight home." She also said, "Here I get to play whatever I want. You don't always grab the best characters for yourself!" However, she also mentioned that the extra time would allow her to pursue an after-school class that her gymnastics friends were attending. Looking directly at the therapist, she asked, "How do *you* feel about this ending?" Dr. Green answered that she felt sad when she thought about losing the special time they spent playing and talking together, and that she would miss their relationship, but she was pleased to think that Ellie would be having fun with friends. She questioned whether this mixed set of feelings was similar to what Ellie was describing. Ellie nodded and returned her attention to a game in which she and the therapist made predictions about each other's futures based on lists of categories that were written down on paper; the lists included such contents as "places you wish to live," "jobs you want," and "people you hope to marry." There were set rules: each individual could select three choices, but the other player made the final decision about her fate. The game was derived from one that Ellie and her friends played avidly at school, with modifications that Ellie made for herself and Dr. Green. As the session was coming to a close, Ellie suddenly returned to the topic of termination. She pointed to a bin of dolls that she and Dr. Green had not used for a while and declared, "I'm gonna miss those dolls. I don't have them at my house. Maybe I could come back and see you sometimes. Like maybe if I have a problem at school or something." Dr. Green agreed that it would be very nice to see each other in the future and to work on problems together again. Although her responses to Ellie were spontaneous and, in the moment, felt resonant with the child's emotional state, Dr. Green found herself wondering later whether she had perhaps inserted too much of her own termination experience: was she, more than Ellie, feeling sad and ambivalent about their impending separation?

About a month after termination, Dr. Green received a worried call from the Parks about a sudden increase in Ellie's old obstinate and sulky behaviors. They recalled that Dr. Green had prepared them for a possible return of old problems and wondered whether this sounded serious enough to require a session with Ellie. Dr. Green resisted an urge to encourage them to come in sooner, realizing that the impulse was based more on her desire to hear about Ellie than a sense of urgency about the child's behavior. As they talked more by phone, the adults concurred that Ellie's behaviors were mild and intermittent; the Parks acknowledged that they were feeling insecure about handling her and that their day-to-day behavior likely reflected a certain hesitancy that had always exacerbated their daughter's overreactions in the past. They reached a mutual decision to wait until the scheduled meeting, a month later, to review more fully how things were going posttermination.

Once a child's readiness for termination has been determined, the therapist allows adequate time to facilitate the ending process with the child and parents. The therapeutic tasks of this period are highly dependent on the child's developmental capacities and on the parents' attitude toward the treatment but often include elements of the following:

- Enabling the child's self-expression, via talk and play, of feelings, conflicts, and anxieties related to termination
- Eliciting, according to the child's capacities, more general reflections on the therapeutic relationship and experience
- Helping the parents prepare for typical posttermination reactions, such as the child's sense of loss, or brief regressions and reintensification of old behaviors
- Allowing the parents to express their own sense of the ending, including their positive and negative reflections on the child's therapy
- Eliciting the needs, wishes, and fantasies of all parties about posttherapeutic contact
- Arriving at a mutually satisfying protocol for future communication

In the case of Ellie, the girl mostly describes her experience of termination in the context of losing routines and shared play ("I'm so used to coming here after school, it'll feel weird to go straight home" and "I'm gonna miss those dolls. I don't have them at my house"). Within this framework, she references the unique aspects of the therapeutic relationship, acknowledging that playing with Dr. Green is different than with other people ("You don't always grab the best characters for yourself!"). She solicits the therapist's response to termination ("How do *you* feel about this ending?") as an indirect means of self-expression, to avoid ownership of her uncomfortable feelings and to deflect exposure, but also as a genuine seeking of validation for their mutual experience.

In responding, Dr. Green is reminded that her own feelings about termination run deep, and she reflects on the need to avoid dominating, diverting, or unduly shaping Ellie's reactions. The therapist's self-awareness is key during the termination process in order to monitor a personal tendency to prolong the treatment, misgauge others' sense of loss, or terminate too quickly to avoid painful emotions. Reactions to the loss of a child patient may include parent-like worries about future challenges, as well as regrets that one will not witness the child's subsequent development (Fabricius and Green 1995).

Often, the child's perception of therapy termination is represented indirectly through play, where themes of loss, change, or striking out on one's own may emerge; some children reveal feelings of betrayal or abandonment, or a sense of being discarded (Abrams 1992). Ellie's preferred termination game, which integrates elements of pretend play (imaginary jobs, husbands, futures) with latency-phase tendencies (categories, rules), reflects her future-oriented leanings, her wishes and fantasies about what her life might be, her fear about the unknown, and her desire that the therapist be involved in making choices for her in the forthcoming phases of her life.

Contemporary notions about the guidelines for posttherapy contact have shifted toward a more flexible and varied stance. Traditionally, psychoanalysts advocated a strict no-contact policy in order to facilitate the patient's interior termination process. The physical absence of the clinician was considered necessary for the patient to work through the procedure of mourning, fully experience the attendant feelings (sadness, anger, loss, and gratitude), deal with the realities of the separation, and further develop autonomous functions in the areas of previously shared self-observation and self-reflection (Lanyado 1999). A number of contemporary writers point out that the no-contact rule reflects inherent and unnecessary theoretical biases, such as privileging separation and autonomy over attachment and mutuality (Craige 2002). Moreover, they caution that such rigid tenets have the effect of pathologizing people's natural desire for continuing an important relationship, while denying patients potentially beneficial meetings with the therapist (Frank 2009). Indeed, some authors suggest that the word *termination* itself might best be replaced with *ending*, a label not quite so harsh and reminiscent of morbidity (Fosshage and Hershberg 2009).

In regard to child terminations, protocols have always tended toward greater flexibility, reflecting the expectation for more varied posttreatment outcomes; no contact, one or a few subsequent sessions with parents or with the child, and eventual serial treatments wherein the child is seen again for a new course of therapy are all commonplace (Beiser

1995). Parents' levels of anxiety and sense of loss may exceed the child's (Karush 2014); many child therapists look favorably on the use of post-termination sessions to assuage parental insecurity, help the adults maintain their child's treatment progress, and deal with the very real possibility of unexpected developmental and situational challenges that arise in the child's life after therapy has ended. Pretermination meetings with the parents are often used to clarify the therapist's potential role as an ongoing resource, while also supporting parental autonomy; the latter function includes reviewing the gains made in collateral parent meetings, underscoring improved parenting skills and empathic understanding of the child and reminding parents that these newfound capacities will help them as they negotiate any future problems (Novick and Novick 2002).

Many writers advocate an open approach to the logistics of initiating termination and determining the date; in this view, any party involved in the treatment (child, parent, or therapist) can introduce the idea of ending, and the length of the termination process is adjusted to accommodate the child's and adults' needs and preferences (Chazan 1997; Fabricius and Green 1995). The therapist may believe that it is ideal to maintain the usual frequency of sessions until the very end so that the fundamental nature of the treatment and the relationship are not altered, but an empathic and accepting attitude toward the child's or parents' wishes to cut back gradually may supersede such preferences; often, members of the family feel very strongly about reducing from multiple sessions to once per week, insisting that a gradual decline in intensity will be easier and allow for the child's adjustment (Karush 2014). In these instances, the therapist can freely voice concerns over the change in treatment frame but ultimately might deem it best to allow the child or parents to retain a sense of control and autonomy over the particulars of the termination process (Abrams 1992; Poynton 2012). Another area that often elicits parent and child reactions is the time of year set for termination. Some authors (e.g., Abrams 1992) suggest that the therapist avoid selecting June as a natural ending point, although this timing is often preferred by families due to its familiar status as the ending of the school year; however, stopping treatment in June tends to conflate these various endings, so that the child's feelings about termination are masked behind reactions to leaving teachers and friends, and transitioning to summer activities.

PRINCIPLE 3

When it comes to determining the specifics of the termination process and making decisions about posttermination contact, therapists should be guided by their beliefs about what is best for the child, but also by the patient's and family's unique needs and preferences. Although it is helpful for the therapist to conceive a general framework for termination, maintaining an attentive and accepting attitude toward children's and parents' wishes is often a more important principle.

ABRUPT TERMINATIONS AND INCOMPLETE TREATMENTS

Premature termination is generally defined as withdrawal from treatment after the initial period of assessment but before stated goals and objectives, as defined by parents and therapist, have been achieved. Proportions of untimely endings are extremely high in the treatment of children and adolescents, ranging between 40% and 60% of cases (Deakin et al. 2012; Midgley and Navridi 2006). Whereas adolescents themselves drive up the frequency of their incomplete treatments, often due to developmental pressures (the need to avoid adult scrutiny and closeness; the drive to assert self-determination; a desire for action to counter fears of passivity and dependency), terminations for younger children are generally precipitated by parents. High dropout rates for younger groups often reflect highly subjective parental perceptions, such as their level of shame about their child's need for therapy, their past negative experiences with therapeutic services, or their sense that the therapist poses a threat to their relationship with the child or to the family system as a whole (Midgley and Navridi 2006). In addition, premature child terminations are linked to broader social and economic conditions, such as families' financial concerns (including pressure from insurance companies to limit sessions) and overall cultural attitudes that favor a quick fix over the slower pace and lengthier commitment that are hallmarks of psychodynamic treatments (Deakin et al. 2012).

These findings about treatment terminations suggest that establishing an initial solid therapeutic alliance with parents plays an important role in avoiding treatment disruptions, as does ongoing parent work. Important parts of building and sustaining parent relationships include the following: an initial open discussion about financial arrangements that realistically reflect parents' resources; preparing them for what lies ahead, such as the potential for the child's resistance to intensify or the possibility that the treatment might proceed slowly; returning to these topics as the course of treatment is further clarified; and working to achieve a sense of shared treatment goals, which may shift as the therapy proceeds, necessitating further discussion. See Chapter 10, "Working With Parents Over the Course of Treatment," for a more detailed description of parent work and its impact on the child's treatment.

Even when parents and therapist have a solid working alliance, they may find themselves diverging in how they view the continued benefits of therapy. Once symptomatic relief is achieved and the child's behavior is less distressing to adults, parents often declare themselves satisfied and begin to talk about withdrawing the child. Unexpected events, such as a change in a parent's job, an illness in the family, or problems with a sibling, may impact the way in which the child's family balances needs for treatment with other pressing concerns. In cases of parental divorce, as demonstrated in the following continuation of Becky Singer's case (which has been discussed since Chapter 8, "The Logistics"), the parents' anger and blaming urges may be played out in the context of the therapeutic relationship, leading to divisive attitudes and arguments over the child's ongoing involvement in therapy. In other instances, the initial therapeutic alliance with the parents is a somewhat tenuous one: the inevitable ups and downs of treatment, such as a transient phase of the child's regression, a stalemate, or a period in which the child's resistance and protests are heightened, may burden the fragile parent–therapist relationship and lead the parent toward premature termination.

> Dr. Lee had been treating 6-year-old Becky Singer in twice-weekly play therapy for about 8 months. Play themes and narratives continued to expand and deepen; they often involved scenes in which bad and unlovable children were banished from their homes and sent to forage on their own in deep forests and other dangerous environments. Over time, Becky felt more comfortable speaking directly with Dr. Lee about her family situation. She would mention the disruption of transitioning between her parents' homes, witnessing one side of an angry phone call, or sharing her parents' attention with other adults (both mother and father had established new relationships). Becky had entered

first grade and her teacher reported that she was doing well; compared with the previous year, she was more focused and less anxious about who would be picking her up after school and where she would be spending the night.

Dr. Lee felt that her alliance with the Singers, who had finalized their divorce, was not entirely solid. Although both parents had initially agreed to the therapy, disagreements and blaming erupted fairly frequently, including conflicts over who should pay for parent meetings. At times, the couple resisted attending together and came to separate sessions; both used this private time to try to sway Dr. Lee's opinion against the absent parent. Moreover, Dr. Lee was aware that they had both resented her neutral stance vis-à-vis their custody and visitation battles.

Dr. Lee continued to appeal to their sense of common cause over helping their daughter, but this approach was no longer as effective once Becky's behavior improved at school. Indeed, each parent recruited the girl's fairly rapid symptomatic relief as evidence that she was inherently fine and that the only source of difficulty was the other parent. In her meetings with the parents, Dr. Lee described her concerns about Becky's sense of the divorce; without quoting the child's comments or directly divulging play narratives, she explained how therapy would address the girl's distorted sense of responsibility for the parents' failed marriage, her deep belief that she was an unlovable child, and her ongoing fears of parental abandonment. To work on the Singers's resistance to the treatment, Dr. Lee decided to address directly her suspicion that each of them felt let down when she did not actively support anyone's visitation plans. Both parents denied any negative reactions to Dr. Lee and professed concern for what the therapist described as Becky's ongoing fragility of self-esteem and security. However, they were not swayed to continue the treatment; in fact, the Singers informed Dr. Lee that they had already selected a date for termination 2 weeks away. Financial worries were prominent, they insisted, and the cost of therapy was a major stress; they refused Dr. Lee's offer to alter the cost of the remaining weeks in order to prolong the termination phase. Dr. Lee realized that their minds were made up, and intuited that they would not be receptive to exploratory work around their felt need for an abrupt termination, such as examination of their own difficulties with endings and separations. She decided to focus her remaining efforts on maintaining a positive working alliance with the Singers. Keeping her significant personal disappointment and concern to herself, she accepted the proposed date for the final session; in her remaining meeting with the parents, she focused on the positive changes they had both made for Becky's benefit (better preparing her for the twice-weekly transitions between houses, refraining from openly criticizing each other in the child's presence) and assured them that she would be available for consultations in the future.

In cases like Becky's, where adults' conflicts and resistances threaten the child's treatment, the therapist's main objective is to advocate for the child's needs while maintaining the best possible working relationship with the parents. Dr. Lee clearly states her position, acknowledging Becky's symptomatic improvements but making it clear that she recommends continuing treatment and explaining why. However, there is nothing to be gained from allowing a contentious treatment relationship to develop. Once she realizes that the parents are fixed in their decision to terminate, Dr. Lee defers to their wishes, hoping to support the gains of the therapy and leave the door open for future contact. Parents will not return to a treatment setting wherein they feel misunderstood, accused, or disrespected; moreover, a negative experience might discourage them from seeking other treatments in the future. Despite her concerns about the untimely loss of the treatment, Dr. Lee refrains from stating that the termination might interfere with Becky's development and from criticizing the parents' decisions. She attempts gingerly to explore the nature of their resistance, suggesting their disappointment in her refusal to take sides over visitation, but she shifts away from this approach when it appears to fall flat.

PRINCIPLE 4

Premature withdrawal is common in child treatments. Investing in an initial alliance with parents and preparing them for the potentialities of therapy may help prevent untimely terminations. However, parents may still decide to end treatment against the therapist's recommendations due to internal and external pressures. When this happens, it is most important to maintain a positive connection to the family; this means respecting parents' decisions even when they run counter to the therapist's sense of what the child needs.

SUMMARY

In play therapy, termination is foreseeable after the restoration of developmental momentum. Basic criteria for termination involve the child's capacity for fuller and more contented engagement in relationships with peers and adults, as well as in age-salient tasks such as academics or extracurricular interests. When determining readiness to wind down a treatment, the therapist seeks multiple perspectives about the child's functioning and integrates these with the family's particular needs. Mourning is an inevitable component of the termination process, impacting therapist and parents as well as the child; however, a child's developmental pressures and capacities powerfully impact how he or she experiences and manifests the sense of loss. Often, the therapist must deal with situations in which parents prematurely end a child's play therapy; in these situations, the main objective is to advocate for the child's needs but retain an amicable relationship with the family, leaving open the potential for future contact.

KEY POINTS

- Child therapists begin to consider termination when a child's development is back on track; this typically involves a reduction in symptoms, inhibitions, anxieties, and modes of relating that impeded the child's immersion in developmental tasks. Typical indicators of better functioning include age-appropriate seeking of peer relationships, adjustment to school environments, broader interests, and improved autonomous self-regulation.

- The pretermination and posttermination phases are characterized by a sense of loss and process of mourning that affects child, therapist, and parents. Children's developmental status and remaining dependency on their parents affects the way in which they experience and express the loss of the therapeutic relationship.

- The logistics of termination and the plans for possible posttermination contact are flexible, subject to each family's unique needs and preferences.

- When parents' internal and reality-based pressures result in premature terminations, the therapist's main objective is to retain a positive working alliance while advocating for the child's treatment needs.

KEY TERMS

Posttermination phase   The period of time immediately after the treatment has come to an end. During this time the patient experiences a process of mourning and consolidates the previously shared therapeutic functions.

Pretermination phase   The period during which preliminary discussion of termination begins but before an actual date is set for ending the treatment. It allows for a phase in which the goals, shared experience, and potential loss of the therapy can be processed without the looming pressure of an ending date.

Serial treatments   A common phenomenon in childhood therapy in which a clinician treats a child for a period of time during different phases of development.

Termination phase   The period of time, generally of several months' duration, between when an ending date is set and when that date arrives. During this time the patient and clinician process the meaning of the treatment and the sense of impending loss of the relationship. In the psychoanalytic literature, this phase may encompass all three of the termination periods (pretermination, termination, and posttermination).

REFERENCES

Ablon SL: Developmental forces and termination in child analysis. Int J Psychoanal 69(Pt 1):97–104, 1988 3403156

Abrams S: Termination in child analysis, in Child Analysis and Therapy. Edited by Glenn J. Northvale, NJ, Jason Aronson, 1992, pp 451–472

Beiser HR: A follow-up of child analysis: the analyst as a real person. Psychoanal Study Child 50:106–121, 1995 7480399

Bergmann MS: On the fate of the intrapsychic image of the psychoanalyst after termination of the analysis. Psychoanal Study Child 43:137–153, 1988 3227069

Bernstein A: The classical parameters of modern psychoanalytic technique: a review. Modern Psychoanalysis 26(2):125–181, 2001

Bernstein I: On the technique of child and adolescent analysis. J Am Psychoanal Assoc 23:190–232, 1975

Bernstein I, Glenn J: The child and adolescent analyst's emotional reactions to his patients and their parents. Int Rev Psychoanal 15(2):225–241, 1988

Blatt SJ, Behrends RS: Internalization, separation-individuation, and the nature of therapeutic action. Int J Psychoanal 68(Pt 2):279–297, 1987 3583573

Bonovitz C: Termination never ends: the inevitable incompleteness of psychoanalysis. Contemp Psychoanal 43(2):229–246, 2007

Chazan SE: Ending child psychotherapy: continuing the cycle of life. Psychoanal Psychol 14(2):221–238, 1997

Conway PS: When all is said...a phenomenological enquiry into post-termination experience. Int J Psychoanal 80(Pt 3):563–574, 1999 10407751

Craige H: Mourning analysis: the post-termination phase. J Am Psychoanal Assoc 50(2):507–550, 2002 12206542

Craige H: Terminating without fatality. Psychoanal Inq 29(2):101–116, 2009

Deakin E, Gastaud M, Nunn MT: Child psychotherapy dropout: an empirical research review. J Child Psychother 38(2):199–209, 2012

Fabricius J, Green V: Termination in child analysis. A child-led process? Psychoanal Study Child 50:205–226, 1995 7480404

Fosshage JL, Hershberg SG: Epilogue. Psychoanal Inq 29(2):195–200, 2009

Frank KA: Ending with options. Psychoanal Inq 29(2):136–156, 2009

Freud A: Problems of termination in child analysis, in The Writings of Anna Freud, Vol 7. New York, International Universities Press, 1971

Freud S: Analysis terminable and interminable. Int J Psychoanal 8:373–405, 1937

Gabbard GO: What is a "good enough" termination? J Am Psychoanal Assoc 57(3):575–594, 2009 19620466

Glucksman ML: Patients who stay. J Am Acad Psychoanal Dyn Psychiatry 39(1):189–197, 2011 21434753

Kantrowitz JL: A different perspective on the therapeutic process: the impact of the patient on the analyst. J Am Psychoanal Assoc 45(1):127–153, 1997 9112613

Karush RK: Postscripts: reflections on the post-termination phase. Psychoanal Study Child 68:234–247, 2014 26173337

Kogan I: Termination and the problem of analytic goals: patient and analyst, different perspectives. Int J Psychoanal 77(Pt 5):1013–1029, 1996 8933223

Lanyado M: Holding and letting go: some thoughts about the process of ending therapy. Journal of Child Psychotherapy 25(3):357–378, 1999

Loewald HW: Termination analyzable and unanalyzable. Psychoanal Study Child 43:155–166, 1988 3227070

Midgley N, Navridi E: An exploratory study of premature termination in child analysis. J Infant Child Adolesc Psychother 5(4):437–458, 2006

Novick J: Comments on termination in child, adolescent, and adult analysis. Psychoanal Study Child 45:419–436, 1990 2251319

Novick J, Novick KK: Two systems of self-regulation. Psychoanalytic Social Work 8(3–4):95–122, 2001

Novick J, Novick KK: Parent work in analysis: children, adolescents, and adults, part 4: termination and post-termination phases. J Infant Child Adolesc Psychotherapy 2(2):43–55, 2002

Pinsky E: Mortal gifts: a two-part essay on the therapist's mortality, part I: untimely loss. J Am Acad Psychoanal 30(2):173–204, discussion 205–210, 2002 12197250

Poynton M: "We should be playing, not talking": play, self-agency and moving toward depressive moments. Journal of Child Psychotherapy 38(2):185–198, 2012

Shane E: Approaching termination: ideal criteria versus working realities. Psychoanal Inq 29(2):167–173, 2009

Shane M, Shane E: The end phase of analysis: indicators, functions, and tasks of termination. J Am Psychoanal Assoc 32(4):739–772, 1984 6526965

Ticho EA: Termination of psychoanalysis: treatment goals, life goals. Psychoanal Q 41(3):315–333, 1972 5047036

13

Play Therapy, Variations in Child Development, and Serious Psychopathology

Dr. Lee's collaborative relationship with a local mainstream elementary school psychologist led to a number of referrals. Often, these involved children whose adjustment to the early grades was compromised by immature social skills, vulnerable self-regulatory capacities, or inhibitions in self-expression; such developmental challenges posed obstacles to negotiating age-salient tasks but did not necessarily rise to the level of a diagnosable disorder. Six-year-old Ingrid was one such referral. Her sensitive kindergarten teacher noticed that Ingrid was frequently silent in class, sat with other girls but did not necessarily join in their lively discussions at lunchtime, and often spent recess watching rather than participating in her peers' activities. Ingrid did not appear unhappy; when questioned delicately, she shyly reported that she enjoyed watching what her friends were doing. Her peers seemed fond of Ingrid, and a couple of girls favored her company for play dates; one of these girls was a rather dominant child who was more than happy to benefit from Ingrid's diffident attitudes. Ingrid's academic performance was somewhat mixed. She was a talented artist and displayed strong mastery of age-appropriate arithmetic concepts. Her emerging reading and writing skills fell just slightly below age-expected limits, but they were progressing at a satisfactory rate. In class, she was so quiet that the teacher sometimes felt uncertain about Ingrid's comprehension of material; however, although Ingrid had received early intervention services for mild delays in expressive language between ages 2 and 3, a current speech and language assessment indicated average language capacities. The school psychologist was asked to observe Ingrid during the school day; she concurred with the teacher that Ingrid did not seem isolated or unhappy, but did manifest shyness and inhibition.

The school psychologist communicated all of the above information to Dr. Lee, who arranged a series of meetings with Ingrid's parents. They presented themselves as quiet, serious-minded people who were surprised by the school's concern about their daughter's level of reserve; both mother and father asserted that they, too, preferred the quiet of family life and that weekends were often passed contentedly at home. While listening to the child's developmental history, Dr. Lee took note of the following: Ingrid was very shy but not unduly anxious (she willingly attended play dates and went on school trips); she was in the on-level, not the advanced, sections in language arts but her teachers reported good progress; her parents seemed puzzled by Dr. Lee's questions about Ingrid's pretend play (they recalled that she had always preferred a certain stuffed animal and reported that she enjoyed dressing up in her mother's clothes from time to time, but they did not participate with her in imaginary games); and the parents were rather serious, reticent people who enjoyed the quiet of their small family and did not seek out many social outlets themselves. Dr. Lee communicated her sense that Ingrid's development fell within normal limits but wondered aloud with the parents whether, despite her shyness, the girl might actually desire deeper involvement with peers or whether she might experience some frustration about being always seen as the compliant, good-natured friend. Together, the adults decided that Ingrid would have an evaluation with Dr. Lee; given her typically slow-to-warm style, it was agreed that the assessment could proceed slowly and without a designated number of sessions.

Having learned of Ingrid's fondness for drawing and anticipating her bashfulness, Dr. Lee made certain that her art materials were highly visible. After reluctantly leaving her mother, Ingrid followed Dr. Lee to the playroom. She glanced at the assortment of playthings, manifesting no interest, and soon gravitated toward the art table. Without making eye contact with Dr. Lee, she began to draw a well-executed picture of a house, garden, and rainbow. Dr. Lee stayed mostly quiet, facilitating Ingrid's peaceful demeanor and industrious behavior; after a few minutes, she commented briefly, while looking at the drawing, on the girl's use of colors in the rainbow. Ingrid nodded, softly adding, "I saw one like this once." "Oh, so maybe this is a picture of you near your house, seeing a beautiful yellow and orange rainbow," suggested Dr. Lee, careful to modulate her own eagerness to get the child talking. Ingrid smiled and added to the picture a girl holding a stuffed bear. "That looks like you," continued Dr. Lee, "and I can imagine you standing there and thinking…" (she paused). "I'm thinking

'What a pretty rainbow,'" volunteered Ingrid. The two continued to speak about the drawing in quiet voices.

When Ingrid returned for subsequent sessions, Dr. Lee continued to make use of the girl's drawings to facilitate talk about simple scenarios. On one occasion, Ingrid sketched a scene depicting her visit to a zoo; on another, she drew her room at home. Together, she and Dr. Lee briefly discussed the pictures; sometimes this would lead to Ingrid adding in other characters or following Dr. Lee's comments with her own suggestions about what she or one of the animals might be thinking and feeling. Ingrid's art was largely confined to actual lived events, without much embellishment from fantasy. Dr. Lee, who had decided to test out the effect of drawing responsively, attempted a picture that was a more imaginary version of Ingrid's zoo; she then told a brief story about the girl in her drawing who wanted to befriend the animals so much that she taught them how to speak so they could always share their ideas. Ingrid enjoyed the story and asked Dr. Lee for another one. The next time Ingrid drew animals, Dr. Lee asked if she might tell a story about one of them. Ingrid eagerly agreed, and even provided a few details for the therapist's narrative.

When a child between ages 3 and 7 or 8 years—the developmental "high season" for play (see Chapter 3, "Pretend Play")—manifests limited access to pretense, the clinician is confronted with immediate questions: Does the restricted play represent a set of factors or transient conditions that will likely shift over time, allowing for fuller engagement in the psychodynamic play process? Or does the initial presentation signify a true absence of imaginary play, perhaps alerting the therapist to more serious underlying deficits in the necessary symbolic and relational capacities that might impede child–clinician mutuality and ultimately limit the deepening of play treatment? A child's inability to participate fluidly and pleasurably in play with the clinician may reflect temporary reactions to the novel treatment situation (e.g., initial discomfort with the clinician, reluctance to separate from caregivers, or resistance to beginning therapy, as described in Chapter 9, "Getting Started, Creating an Alliance, and Facilitating Play"); normative variations of temperament (e.g., shyness and inhibition); the presence of conflicts that lead to avoidance of or disruption of play themes and affects; mild immaturities in development (e.g., slight delays in language or self-regulation); the deployment of normative defenses (e.g., preference of school-age children for rule-bound games that support recently acquired capacities for self-control); or more serious conditions (e.g., a history of environmental deprivation and trauma, or ego impairments and relational deficits) that derail not only play but also the child's overall developmental progression (Gilmore 2005; Sugarman 2008). Any of these conditions potentially distorts a child's access to play by dampening joy and spontaneity, limiting absorption in pretense, causing disruption as the play elicits intense affective reactions, and interfering with the capacity to achieve a **mutual playing state** with the clinician. The presence of serious psychopathology and developmental delays, discussed in the subsequent sections of this chapter, may result in far greater restrictions and even absence of the child's imaginary capacities. Differentiating among the interrelated developmental systems that impact play— biologically based conditions, unresolved conflicts, defensive styles, and environmental factors—is a complex undertaking that requires the clinician's careful and unhurried assessment (Fonagy and Moran 1991). The evaluation includes the following necessary components: play sessions with the child that help clarify ego functions and relational capacities; the parents' provision of developmental history; the therapist's impressions of their parenting style; and reports from the school and other caregivers.

PRINCIPLE 1

A careful assessment of the child's overall development (including crucial information provided by the parents), play, and relational capacities can help distinguish between temperament-based tendencies and more serious play deficits. Very shy or inhibited children may benefit from therapy that facilitates pretense and encourages self-expression.

As the therapist finds ways to establish trust, name and contain feelings, and attribute meaning to affects and behaviors, young children's play restrictions generally begin to recede. However, not all children actively initiate engagement with the therapist, manifest delight during pretense, and freely assert their creative ideas and pretend scenarios. In the case of Ingrid, inhibitions in both her interpersonal style and her access to imaginary fantasy reflect a number of factors, including temperamentally based shyness, her parents' relative disinterest in pretense, early mild delays in language, conflicts around self-assertion and competition, and anxiety over the expression of spontaneous affects. Moreover, Ingrid's tendency to occupy the role of observer rather than participant with peers further limits her immersion in and practicing of shared dramatic play; she has missed out on myriad, daily development-promoting opportunities with peers to negotiate meanings, narratives, and roles through mutual imaginary play. Dr. Lee's assessment of Ingrid leads the therapist to conclude that the girl's language, social development, and imaginary capacities are not seriously impeded. Ingrid demonstrates pleasure in calm play and in peer interactions and utilizes drawing for self-expression; moreover, her parents report a history of transitional object use and dress-up, and the teachers believe that she is engaged, albeit quietly, in the life of the classroom and making satisfactory academic progress. In the more contained and less chaotic therapeutic playroom, and with the responsiveness of an attentive clinician, Ingrid is able to enter a mutual playing state according to her own pace and preferences. Dr. Lee starts within the child's comfort zone of drawing and gradually expands into potential areas of mutuality and fantasy creation; in addition, she matches Ingrid's soft-spoken tones and accepts long silences, adding in slightly higher levels of conversation and affect without hurrying the girl's adjustment. As she gets to know Ingrid, she also begins to formulate ways in which both she and the parents might foster their daughter's imagination and soften her interpersonal reticence.

> After a few weeks of sessions with Ingrid, Dr. Lee met again with the parents and discussed her impression that their daughter, while not significantly off track in her development, appeared somewhat passive, cautious, and reluctant to initiate her own ideas. She explained that although Ingrid's naturally shy temperament and early language struggles certainly contributed to a lack of assertiveness, there might be additional emotional and developmental pressures that further impacted her confidence, self-esteem, and self-expression. For the moment, she kept to herself various hypotheses, including the impact of the parents' slightly muted affects, lack of natural curiosity about their daughter's imaginary life, and limited desire for sociability; Ingrid's use of avoidance and passivity as defensive solutions to worries about the potentially destructive power of expressing emotions, particularly anger and frustration; and the girl's conflicts over interpersonal competition and assertion. Conversations about these complex

and somewhat abstract issues could wait until she had established stronger rapport with the parents and better understood their vision of their daughter.

The parents, who had been discussing Ingrid between themselves since their original meetings with the school and Dr. Lee, began the meeting with new evidence of Ingrid's social hesitancy. They described a recent event wherein the family encountered a few of Ingrid's friends at a local playground, but she refused to go over and join in the fun despite gazing longingly toward the group. They could now see that Ingrid's inability to participate was causing her some sadness and frustration. In addition, they felt that Ingrid truly enjoyed her sessions with Dr. Lee and would come home eager to make new drawings and tell her parents about them in a slightly more spontaneous and open manner than usual; they were mindful of responding to these overtures with engagement and enthusiasm even though it disrupted the family's usual routines. They asked about additional ways in which they could support Ingrid's development. Dr. Lee praised their responsiveness to Ingrid's drawings and suggested that they work into the routine of family life more time for play and playful activities, consider arranging social afternoons with other families, read Ingrid imaginative stories, speak more freely themselves about affective states, and find ways to gently inquire about their daughter's private thoughts. The decision was made to initiate twice-weekly treatment, with the goals of better understanding all of the issues involved in Ingrid's lack of self-assertion and spontaneity and of helping her feel more comfortable with self-expression. Dr. Lee and Ingrid continued to draw together in therapy; over time, their mutual artwork provided opportunities in which the child used the therapist's narrative scaffolding to develop richer stories and characters.

Although shyness and inhibition may contribute to the restriction of play, the presence of impulsivity and poor emotional self-regulation—even when these conditions do not rise to the level of serious psychopathology—also impedes children's capacity for achieving a mutual playing state with the clinician. Indeed, the ubiquity of aggressive contents and behaviors in child treatment leads to a number of therapeutic challenges (discussed more fully in Chapter 9), including disruptions during play, difficulty with the organization and deepening of pretend narratives, and trouble managing the inevitable affects that are evoked during play (Freud 1972; Gilmore 2005).

The following case vignette, in which parental divorce and the ensuing loss of routines and regularity contribute to a vulnerable child's already shaky self-regulation, serves as another common example of problems faced in play therapy.

Seven-year-old Robby, who had recently begun first grade, was referred to Dr. Lee from the local elementary school psychologist. He had begun the school year shortly after his father's remarriage, which followed 2 years of a contentious divorce process between his parents. The school psychologist described Robby's occasional distractibility and disorderly behavior during music or gym, when the children switched to another classroom and teacher. In addition, trips to the school nurse were frequent, involving vague complaints of headaches and stomachaches. His main teacher perceived Robby as a bright and good-natured student who was making satisfactory academic progress. When Robby was engaged in group or individual tasks, his focus was very adequate, although he tended to seek out the teacher's help a bit more frequently than his classmates. He had a number of friends and was often asked by other children for play dates. The school administration was sympathetic to his difficulties managing transitions and internalizing routines and recognized that the complex family situation contributed to Robby's transient losses of good self-control. However, an incident of disruptive behavior during a game of soccer resulted in a temporary "suspension" from gym class, and the parents were urged to accept a referral to Dr. Lee.

An initial joint parent visit revealed serious discord between Robby's mother and father; each accused the other of embodying the source of the boy's troubles with self-regulation. Through their traded complaints and criticisms, Dr. Lee gleaned the following: Robby's mother was suffering from depression following the marital separation, and she had significant trouble setting limits and maintaining consistent routines at home (often, she and Robby stayed up very late at night together in bed, watching videos, leading to late arrival at school); his father, newly remarried, frequently canceled visitation dates at the last moment to accommodate his wife's preference to spend weekends outside of the city (Robby was expected to understand and accept these scheduled changes); and neither parent had fully attended to the school's reports and increasing warnings that their son's behavioral self-control was deteriorating. After allowing them a certain amount of time to vent grievances, Dr. Lee directed the parents toward Robby's developmental history. Both described him as a normal, active, sociable baby who had achieved major milestones within expected time frames but who had always evidenced mild self-regulatory vulnerabilities; for example, Robby had always hated changes in routine and tended toward anger and tears when frustrated or disappointed. Moreover, it seemed clear that parental tensions, with much arguing after the child was supposedly asleep, dated back to his earliest years and that Robby's "bad days" (filled with overreactions to minor adjustments in the schedule or with bouts of hyperactivity) often followed nights when the adults had fought. Since his father had moved out, when Robby was age 5, the bad days had proliferated; both parents reported that Robby often appeared to be somewhat sullen or in a state of "perpetual motion." Neither parent reported resources for helping Robby during his periods of frustration; his mother tended to leave him to his own devices, rationalizing that "he calms down faster when I give him some space," whereas his father had simply been absent for much of the past year or so.

At the therapist's first meeting with Robby, he separated easily from his caregiver and followed Dr. Lee into the playroom with an air of confidence and curiosity. He circled the room for several minutes before settling onto the floor with a bin of superheroes. He outfitted one figure with various accessories, including a cape and weapons, and then began to fly the character around the room, asserting that he was "on the lookout for bad guys." He paused over the dollhouse, where he quickly flew the superhero into the living spaces, overturning furniture and sweeping small dolls out of the way. Once he had disrupted each of the spaces, Robby glanced at Dr. Lee and exclaimed excitedly, "Almost done!" Then, he attempted to dismantle the walls of the dollhouse; when he realized that the wood construction would not yield to his attempts, he yanked out one of the windows (designed to be removed and replaced) and flung it across the room. Responding to a distinct and unusually strong urge to save her extremely sturdy playhouse and halt further destruction of property, Dr. Lee moved closer while asserting, "Wow, he really is trying to wreck that house completely." "He *did* wreck it. It's destroyed," responded Robby. He then dropped the superhero figure on the ground, stepped over the debris created by his play, sat down at the art table, and began to search through the drawers. He selected a pair of scissors and scoffed at them ("What are these, safety scissors? These are for babies; look, they can't even cut paper!"). He then began to scrape one edge of the scissors repeatedly against the table, eventually creating a tiny groove in the wood. Once again, Dr. Lee found herself wanting to stop Robby and preserve the table. "I could destroy this whole table if I had enough time!" he asserted. At this point, the therapist became aware of her sadder feelings, and a potential interpretation formed in her mind— "You feel destroyed, and your home has been destroyed, but the destroyers are your parents, who are now confusingly both the good guys you love and the bad guys who wrecked your life"—but she recognized this as premature and not useful to vocalize to Robby, so she kept her thoughts to herself. Soon she was again caught up in Robby's action: armed with scissors, he set about attempting to replicate the indentation he had achieved in the art table; he moved quickly around the room, pressing the scissors edge against various surfaces. As he picked up a wooden train and began to carve a scratch in its brightly colored façade, Dr. Lee touched his wrist and suggested that they could pretend to mark up the table, walls, and toys but not actually do so. Robby complied quickly, returning to the table and beginning to cut paper into small pieces while Dr. Lee commented, "There is so much moving and destroying and cutting going on, it makes me wonder if you have some big feelings you are showing me." Robby smiled and nodded and continued cutting.

In this case, temperamental factors, parenting style, and the situation of divorce contribute to Robby's escalating difficulty achieving age-appropriate emotional self-regulation and behavioral control. He presents as a child with solid intellectual endowment, normal social capacities, and adequate imaginary potential who responds quickly and well to adult attentiveness and structure. After meeting with his parents, Dr. Lee becomes aware of the following conditions: the level of hostility between the parents is palpable, even during moments of superficial cooperation around issues involving their son; they have always fought openly, convincing themselves that their child was protected from hearing their conflicts; and the emotional pressures of their difficult marriage and divorce have left both parents with few resources for understanding Robby's struggles and offering him support. Reflecting on her initial session with the child, Dr. Lee realizes that her countertransference reaction—stronger than usual pressure to halt his whirlwind of activity and sense of destructiveness—may reflect the boy's intense need to elicit adult parameters in the face of his own feared harmful potential ("I could destroy this whole table if I had enough time!"). Her experience corresponds with the reports of his classroom teacher and the school psychologist, who have noted that Robby often seeks adult guidance and benefits from brief moments of contact and feedback; he is at his most vulnerable during certain transitional periods of the day, when his main teacher is absent and when the high levels of classroom structure are missing. The style and content of Robby's pretend play provide further information about his current struggles: the affects elicited by the destruction of the house, where the play draws dangerously close to his own internal experience of the divorce, are overwhelming, leading to a complete disruption of the play narrative; the confusion about good guys (the superhero who destroys) and bad guys (whom the superhero allegedly seeks) speaks to his attempts to maintain idealization of his parents and to resolve loving and dependent feelings toward parental figures with more negative emotions; and his focus on themes of power, destruction, and cutting reflect his sense of helplessness, feelings of injury and diminishment, and efforts to manage his rage. Dr. Lee provides a number of interventions, including containment of affects via limit setting (preventing further use of scissors to deface property), acknowledging overwhelming feelings, linking behaviors with internal states, and beginning to elaborate narratives. As the work progresses, her facilitation of play scenarios, comments about the characters and storylines, and observations about play disruptions will help interest Robby in the workings of his mind and increase his understanding and tolerance of affective states (Sugarman 2008). She will also work with Robby's parents, helping them realize the importance of greater stability and predictable routines.

PRINCIPLE 2

Difficult environmental situations, such as parental conflict or separation, can affect the capacity for play, making it more difficult for the child to focus and sustain emotionally regulated states and increasing the likelihood of play disruptions. The therapist's goals include helping the child label affects and create coherent narratives, as well as reducing stress at home through work with parents.

WORKING WITH SERIOUS PSYCHOPATHOLOGY

Children such as Ingrid and Robby pose challenges in the course of their treatments, related to inhibitions, major life events, or acute dysregulation, but they are suitable candidates for play therapy. Play therapy relies on a certain level of relatedness and age-expected ego capacities to be effective, although it is also able to foster those same capacities in a bidirectional manner. Parent work in such cases is often an important adjunct, but the therapeutic action takes place in play. In contrast, children with certain forms of severe psychopathology may require a range of ancillary interventions and supports either before play therapy can even be considered or in tandem with it. Ancillary modalities may include medication; parent counseling and training; placement in special schools or programs; arranging for a shadow teacher; behavioral therapies; occupational, physical, and speech and language therapies; social skills groups; and others. These are intended to stabilize such children's circumstances to render both home and school more conducive to forward movement, reduce the level of distress and disorganization, provide support for impaired communicative capacities, and ideally allow the child to play or play better. Children with severe psychopathology have a range of potentials and prognoses, from fully adaptive to chronically impaired. They also have the usual array of life experience, facilitating or burdening forward movement. Eric, a child with a relatively severe autism spectrum disorder (ASD) suffered the traumatic loss of a parent at age 4½. He is an example of a complex challenge: a child whose baseline functioning is already compromised by deficits in language and play now must deal with the sudden loss of his father and its reverberations in his family.

> Dr. Vargas had developed a relationship with a special education pre-school during his fellowship. This connection led to a number of difficult referrals, in part because the school director had great confidence in his skill and high hopes that psychodynamic play therapy could be helpful for many of her students. She referred Eric, age 4½ years, whose father had committed suicide 6 months previously. Eric was diagnosed with ASD when he was age 3. His expressive language was very limited and he had numerous stereotypies and repetitive gestures, but he seemed to follow activities and could participate, or at least not disrupt, a group building project. Dr. Vargas had observed him and discussed him with the staff during his first year at the school. Then, over the summer, his father shocked the community by jumping off a high suspension bridge. The entire family was reeling from the father's death; his mother was overcome with grief and anger and overwhelmed by the combined responsibilities of managing both the business she cofounded with her husband and their three children. Eric's behavior declined precipitously; over the previous year, he had learned to sit in a circle with his classmates and engage in practiced interactions with the teacher, such as repeating words from a picture book. His spontaneous language was still quite limited, but he was increasingly interested in the production of words. He had enjoyed music time and would sing with pleasure using words well beyond his spoken vocabulary. Now he seemed angry and oppositional during the classroom routines, he would cover his ears and shout during songs, and he resisted the overtures of the assistant teacher who formerly spent a lot of time

with him. In the initial interview, his mother reported that he screamed "constantly" at home and acted afraid of everything; she herself was clearly overwhelmed, tense, and unhappy.

Dr. Vargas had considerable trepidation about the appropriateness of play therapy with this child, who had never struck him as a good candidate and now was traumatized by his father's death and his family's state. Dr. Vargas told the mother that it might be best to attempt a first meeting at school, which was a familiar place where Eric had actually seen Dr. Vargas in the past. Unfortunately, Eric responded with panic when Dr. Vargas came into the classroom to fetch him; when his teachers encouraged him to follow Dr. Vargas into a little adjoining room, he began to flail his arms and legs and shout. This scenario recurred in three attempts. Dr. Vargas consulted with his suitemate, Dr. Reed, who had expertise in cognitive-behavioral therapy (CBT) and parent training; they decided to propose in-home combined parent training and CBT with Dr. Reed and individual meetings on parenting issues for the mother with Dr. Vargas. Although Dr. Vargas felt the mother desperately needed psychotherapy for herself, he concurred that any intervention in the current crisis needed first to be linked to Eric's care. He knew that reconnecting to her disabled son would allow them both to express their anger and grief and might facilitate the mourning process for the entire family.

Because play therapy supports a universal childhood ego capacity, it is an important component of the treatment plan for a child in distress. Nonetheless, it is not always the first or primary intervention, as Eric's case makes clear. For many children with severe psychopathology, other modalities may take precedence, although even in these instances, support for playing is eventually indicated—be it with a therapist, a parent (as in **Floortime** [Greenspan and Wieder 2009]), or a peer play group. Eric is a child with a significant neurodevelopmental disorder who was confused and overwhelmed by his father's death and its impact on his family, especially his mother. Hard as it was to disappoint the school director, Dr. Vargas knew that play therapy, even with a familiar therapist, would not benefit and might in fact destabilize Eric. In this case, at this time, other kinds of intervention were urgently needed to help a family in crisis. Because he knew Eric from the previous year, before his father's death, Dr. Vargas already had serious doubts about whether individual play therapy was a useful modality for Eric at baseline. Despite the child's capacity to comport himself adequately in the classroom, Eric's development was significantly off track at age 3; he had almost no communicative expressive language development and little play capacity. Dr. Vargas felt that a few years of playful group activities and scaffolding in the classroom might gradually make play therapy a viable option. In this new family crisis, helping Eric's mother work through her anger and grief and offering her techniques for managing her unhappy family came first. Dr. Vargas hoped that this would eventually lead to her doing Floortime with Eric; gradually introducing a clinician in that activity might be very helpful in case elements related to the father's death emerged in the play.

As one of the cardinal developmental systems, play is by nature slowly transforming; certain kinds of disorders become notable only when new capacities are expected to emerge. Although most of the neuro-developmental syndromes are identified early, moderate variants may escape detection for several years. For example, in cases at the milder end of the autism spectrum, an affected child's earliest play forms may not raise alarm, perhaps because parents are reluctant to admit the challenge of engaging their infant. But if pretend play has not appeared by the time the child enters prekindergarten, there is little likelihood that, without intervention, sociodramatic play will be possible in the kindergarten year, with further negative repercussions on development. In such circumstances, an assessment is in order. The absence of private pretend play may have been chalked up to inhibition, idiosyncrasy, or immaturity (i.e., slowed developmental pace), but a child's lack of solo pretend play at age 4 is a typical sign of underlying neurodevelopmental disorder and suggests that symbolic capacities, including language, may be delayed or derailed. The developmentally crucial arena of sociodramatic play, the wellspring of interpersonal communication, negotiation, and shared pleasure, is compromised, with serious repercussions for self-representation, self-esteem, and peer relations. Similarly, the play forms of latency cannot occur without maturation of gross motor skills, a cognitive advance to concrete operations, and the enhanced socioemotional range accompanying the evolution of theory of mind, notions of fairness, and turn taking, not to mention an overall shift to a reality orientation and to a pleasure in achievement required for game playing and school performance.

In contrast, the disorders related to trauma show the dramatic rupture of the ongoing normal developmental sequence of play, with loss of play's adaptive plasticity. A child's capacity to play—especially to play collaboratively, flexibly, and joyfully—is a good indicator of progressive forward development. As a corollary, deviations from age-appropriate play forms usually suggest developmental interference and can serve as a gauge of its severity; restoration to the expected path of play development signals improvement.

It is important for the clinician to remember that most forms of childhood psychopathology are multifactorial: even in cases of severe trauma, the "etiology" of the child's condition is rarely singular; rather, it is in large part indeterminate, and, unlike with many medical disorders, it is not destined to become any clearer through laboratory values or indeed through the success or failure of a given treatment. Genes, environmental provision, historical trauma, early attachment disturbance, intrapsychic conflict, family life, cultural conditions, and the child's resilience all figure into the clinical picture (Chused 2000). The fact of multiple contributing sources, ranging from neurobiological substrate to attachment disturbances to abuse, and their impact on ongoing development means that no singular intervention is likely to be "curative" (Pozzi-Monzo 2012). Treatment approaches must address the whole child and not just the diagnosis. Medication, psychodynamic play therapy, parent–infant/child therapy, parent counseling, and educational remediation may all be indicated to provide the child optimal developmental experience and future opportunities. In this chapter, we apply this systems view to ASD, attention-deficit/hyperactivity disorder (ADHD), and posttraumatic stress disorder (PTSD) (the three disorders that were the focus of Chapter 7), which are not infrequently linked to one another as causal agents, mutual contributory factors, or comorbidities. ADHD, for example, is strongly linked to PTSD by many investigators who point to similar symptom pictures, including hyperarousal, fidgeting, restlessness, inability to listen, and so on (Szymanski et al. 2011).

The child clinician, consulted by anxious parents who request play therapy, is obliged first to sort through the diagnostic questions and then to determine whether the child's developmental trajectory is so off-course as to preclude play as a therapeutic medium. Even some glimmer of play potential is reassuring since the treatment can focus on learning to play through the relationship with the therapist; success in this endeavor provides the child an invaluable arena for the practice of self-regulation and explorations of identity, and offers an asset in the development of peer relationships.

PRINCIPLE 3

Clinicians should approach every child brought for evaluation with an open mind and the recognition that, while diagnoses are essential, they do not predetermine the individual treatment plan. Children who present with moderate to severe psychopathology usually need a range of services and interventions to stabilize their current circumstances and maximize the potential contained in their ongoing development.

Regardless of the child's likely diagnosis, the therapist can use the following as a rough guide to the treatment plan. The introduction of play therapy requires the following considerations:

- *Estimate the child's developmental level.* Does the child use digital pointing? Does the child possess some responsive receptive and expressive language? In other words, does the existing language have relational communication potential, or is it primarily phonetic mimicry without comprehension, a poor basis for dialogic exchange (Shapiro 2009)? For example, Eric's language had never demonstrated the degree of give-and-take communication and comprehension that is necessary for him to benefit from play therapy. A developmental pediatric consultation and/or neuropsychiatric assessment should be considered early in the assessment to clarify diagnosis and support recommendations.
- *Assess relatedness.* Does the child have the capacity to connect to the clinician? Even without eye contact, does the child show a glimmer of interest, even minimal receptivity to playfulness, and a hint of conflict about predominant maladaptive defenses? Even if the child spends early sessions clinging to the caregiver and vociferously rejecting the therapist, does the clinician's intuition suggest that there is something accessible? This may take many months to be sure, but therapeutic optimism is a necessary precondition for play therapy. For Dr. Vargas, the four failed attempts to make personal contact with Eric, even with his prior familiarity, indicated the need to

focus the therapeutic efforts elsewhere, especially in the mother–child relationship.

- *Characterize symbolic function.* Does the child show any evidence of a capacity to play in a way that reveals mental contents? Can the child develop minimal narratives, allow for the existence of alternate subjectivities, and tolerate change in existing play rituals? Ideally, there should be a degree of meaning making and flexibility in play that already exists to make it useful as a therapeutic modality. In the case of trauma, in which repetitive unchanging play is a primary symptom, the child's willingness to engage in such play in the office may be an adequate start. The absence of play with the clinician in cases where the parents insist that the child plays at home may reflect the parents' denial or something about the toys or the clinician. The child can be invited to bring favorite toys or games into the sessions, compelling the clinician to decide whether technological media and certain toys and games are to be admitted into the sessions. In our view, the therapist should meet the child in his or her preferred medium and find a way to use it productively for treatment. Video games or YouTube videos are sometimes the only way to engage certain children with significant psychopathology, such as those with ASD or ADHD who are high-functioning.

- *Consider available support systems and their orientation to treatment.* Are the family's expectations reasonable in regard to the child's prognosis? It is important that psychotherapy not be proposed as a "cure" of an underlying neurodevelopmental disorder but rather as a facilitation or augmentation of the child's capacities. In cases of moderate to severe psychopathology, psychotherapy should be one of a number of recommendations.

- *Recognize the need for a team approach in treating psychopathology with strong neuropsychiatric underpinnings.* A treatment plan is rarely singular; it can include neuropsychiatric testing, medication, parent training, parent–child work, family work, remediation, CBT, and play therapy. Obviously, these recommendations have to be prioritized and paced, but it is often helpful to forewarn parents that a need for additional approaches may be necessary in the future. For example, if academic remediation is indicated but not yet possible because of availability of tutors, summer vacation, or the child's level of agitation, it can be suggested as a likely future intervention.

PLAY THERAPY WITH SPECIFIC SEVERE PSYCHOPATHOLOGY SYNDROMES

In the rest of this chapter, we discuss the use of play therapy for children with three common, potentially severe psychopathological syndromes: ASD, ADHD, and PTSD. ASD and ADHD are neurodevelopmental disorders that encompass a variety of developmental aberrations that affect development from birth (Arkowitz 2000; Dawson 2008; Greenspan 2007; Singletary 2015; Voran 2013). PTSD, by definition, is induced by environmental trauma, but its widespread impact on biological stress systems justifies thinking of it as "an environmentally induced complex developmental disorder" (De Bellis and Zisk 2014, p. 187). Optimal development requires environmental nutriment, beginning with maternal attunement and playfulness and sustained by the parental interaction in the **zone of proximal development** that serves to draw the child forward. From the first months of life, this is a transactional process (Dawson 2008). Environmental nutriment also must be sustained by the emerging developmental capacity of the infant, such as through eye contact, smiling, social referencing, soothability, and so on. For some babies with developmental disorders, the **average expectable mother** is simply not adequate to stimulate, regulate, comfort, and nurture the cascade of emerging ego capacities and the evolution of positive internalizations. The parent–infant dynamic is askew from the beginning, creating a prehistory of deviant development in children long before they reach the attention of child professionals. Treatment of these disorders is necessarily framed both by the degree of deficit and by the historical failure to successfully traverse prior sensitive periods of development that depend on parent–infant interaction, which cannot be overcome (Dawson 2008; Shapiro 2009). At this moment in developmental science, it is important to add that there are individuals within a diagnostic category, particularly a broad, overinclusive one like the new category of ASD, whose neurobiological equipment is so impaired or deficient that they cannot be expected to progress in play therapy beyond a certain point or at all. Careful assessment and a comprehensive awareness of other available resources are crucial in consulting on these cases.

AUTISM SPECTRUM DISORDER

Victor was diagnosed as being on the autism spectrum at age 3 years, 5 months and began attending the therapeutic nursery where Dr. Vargas consulted. The child's mother and father both traveled for work, so he was mostly taken care of by a devoted but relatively undemonstrative and laconic nanny. After Victor had attended the nursery for 1 year, including the summer program, Dr. Vargas was discouraged about the child's progress, even though the meltdowns that occurred several times in the first year seemed to have disappeared. Dr. Vargas was concerned that this achievement was primarily the result of avoidance. Victor had minimally delayed language, but his prosody was mechanical and affectless. His receptive language was solid, but he spoke and interacted very little in the classroom or with other children. For example, during reading readiness, he was silent while the class recited each word in a chorus. However, in one-on-one situations, such as when he was taken out of the classroom to work with the reading specialist, he was able to connect sounds and letters and even had some sight words. His classroom behavior was confined primarily to solitary repetitive play with a large (real) key ring holding several keys that he jingled; his mother reported that this "toy" originated when his demand for her keys was so relentless that she finally made him his own set.

Dr. Vargas told the parents that it would help Victor if they could stagger their travel schedules so that at least one of them was home at all times. He said that Victor needed Floortime every day with one of them. He also suggested that play therapy was indicated to see if the child's social skills could be advanced and referred them to a colleague, Ms. Fink, who worked on site at the nursery as a social worker and child clinician. Ms. Fink, who was familiar to all the children at the school, observed Victor in the classroom for several days, gradually approaching him directly and asking if he would be willing to come to her office where she also had some keys, including one that worked to open her special cabinet. He followed her willingly, saying, "Keys please" over and over. In her office, she had locked the toy cabinet and placed the door and cabinet keys with a few others on a large key ring. She allowed him to jingle this key ring for a while and then said with animation, "Uh-oh! I need something I locked in that cabinet! It's a special bicycle lock and key I think you would love. Can you help me get it out?" She led him over and they achieved some form of awkward collaboration as they tried each key. Victor was highly distractible and agitated throughout this endeavor, pacing around the room and shouting, "Keys please!" Ms. Fink described this behavior to him as a reflection of his mood state: "You are really excited to see that bicycle lock and key—it would be fun to use it to lock up all kinds of big things," and then she regaled him with naming these "things" in a lively manner, which ultimately refocused him.

When they got the cabinet door open and the lock and key out, there was a big display of enthusiasm, led by Ms. Fink. Then she said, "What should we lock up?" Victor was unresponsive, so she continued leading the activity: "I love my key ring and don't want to lose it. Can I use this bicycle lock to lock it up? Where do you think I can do it?" He observed her locking up her key ring in a file cabinet and then exclaimed, "You need the ring to keep the key!" Ms. Fink smacked her forehead and said, "What a silly idea! I am locking up the key that I need to unlock the lock!" This dynamic was played out over the next few months in a number of different places in her office, and it became a joke between them. Questioning "Where's the next place?" also became a part of the playful exchange.

Victor is a child who meets some of the requirements for play therapy. He had an average vocabulary and appeared to have average intelligence, definitely showed improvement over the course of the previous year in the school in regard to overall self-regulation, and, despite his classroom isolation, was able to engage in back-and-forth exchanges in one-on-one meetings with his therapist. Ms. Fink was able to feel and express empathy with his parents' discouragement; perhaps that made it easier for her to strongly urge them to rearrange their busy schedules to give more time to Victor. She felt that Victor was subjected to ongoing deprivation and disrupted primary attachments; his parents left him in the care of a minimally verbal caretaker while they sought more satisfying activities elsewhere. This potentially correctible environmental deficit led Ms. Fink to be more hopeful about the gains that might be possible with play therapy.

Compared with Eric, whose case was described earlier in this chapter, Victor represents a far milder version of ASD and has a potential to benefit, at least modestly, from play therapy, in collaboration with more parental involvement and his excellent therapeutic school. Because children currently diagnosed with ASD using DSM-5 criteria (American Psychiatric Association 2013) present such a range of disturbance, some commentators feel that diagnostic clarity has been compromised. With the DSM-5 shift to a dimensional diagnostic system and the reigning notion of spectrum disorders, these experts believe that the specificity of "autism" has been lost. The autism described in DSM-IV (American Psychiatric Association 1994) is now at one extreme of a spectrum that covers a swath of clinical presentations from the former Asperger's disorder to pervasive developmental disorder variants. According to Shapiro (2009), research and clinical studies suffer as a consequence because such an inclusive approach prevents standardized treatment recommendations based on diagnosis and can unnecessarily stigmatize relatively high-functioning children. Others (Grinker 2010), however, welcome this change, suggesting that Asperger's disorder is an inconsistent diagnosis and, in fact, autism by its very nature runs along a spectrum. Of course, it is always true that every child must be evaluated in his or her own right so an appropriate treatment plan can be devised.

A comparison of Eric, Victor, and Emma (a child with ASD whose case was described in Chapter 7) illustrates the enormous diversity within that spectrum diagnosis. Even though all these children have stigmata that make them recognizably "on the spectrum" and continued to show "certain residua" of their disorder after treatment (Shapiro 2009), their baselines and potentials were significantly different. Emma was a highly intelligent, verbal child whose diagnosis of Asperger's disorder was made in a different diagnostic era; her symptom picture places her at the upper end of the spectrum. Her life course is not rare, given her intelligence, verbal abilities, and relatedness. Indeed, it closely resembles Grinker's (2010) description of his daughter's trajectory. Like her, Emma clearly merited a diagnosis of autism at age 3 years, was special schooled and remediated until high school, and then mainstreamed to an artsy, progressive private school. In that high school setting and by that age, she appeared to be one among many "quirky" teenagers. Emma recently graduated from a prestigious university with honors in mathematics, intending to pursue her interest in the history of mathematics in graduate school in the coming year. She is superficially at ease in social groups, although she has always had some friction with roommates. She has a stable romantic relationship. Her mother observes that "there is still something slightly off" in her interpersonal skills and empathy, making her challenging for her friends and family in certain moments. Victor showed considerable improvement with the combined efforts of school staff, specialists, play therapy, and his parents; he was far more sociable in the classroom and gradually gave up his rigid **functional play**. He was not mainstreamed by fifth grade, but such a change is under consideration for middle school.

Eric is still in grade school, but his level of functioning suggests that he will not progress far in academics and will need a protected environment indefinitely.

Children on the low end of the spectrum with significant stigmata—poor social engagement, low intellectual ability, and low prelinguistic/linguistic ability (Dawson 2008)—have been shown repeatedly to be less responsive, even "impervious" to psychodynamic play therapy (Fonagy and Target 1996), although some experts insist that many of these children have pockets of competence or supercompetence that can be cultivated. Children at the high end of the autism spectrum (formerly referred to as Asperger's disorder) usually meet most of the strict criteria for embarking on a play therapy set forth by Shapiro (2009) and others: at least average IQ, age-appropriate language development, a modicum of play capacity, some indication of interest in the therapist, and the potential to improve adaptation. Even without play at the start, it appears that relatively high-functioning children with ASD can be helped to "learn how to play" if they can engage with the therapist and overcome a variety of inhibitions that prevent it. In Emma's case, the inhibition was thinly disguised by her disdainful rejection of doll play. Her therapist ultimately understood and interpreted the narrative that evolved in play therapy—one that gradually inched toward directly playing with Barbies (via Teletubbies and Barbie's little sister, Skipper)—as Emma's struggle to overcome her shame about her pleasure in playing with the hyperfemale, girly Barbies and her uneasiness about endowing dolls with minds.

Play therapy with children with ASD requires that therapists tolerate their patients' "annoyance" (Greenspan 2007) and engage each child at the level of his or her activity, however random or repetitive it may appear. The therapist must be attuned to the patient's capacity to tolerate stimulation and interruption, and must find entry points where only a glimmer of an opening exists. The idea is to make meaning with the child out of what is usually viewed as meaningless stereotypic play or preoccupations (Slade 1999), to model mentalization by attempting to determine intentions and desires, and to acknowledge the mutual impact of patient and therapist—in other words, to "take it personally." Ms. Fink's focus on Victor's keys as the play theme was informed by his profound attachment to them and her conviction that the keys related to his parents' frequent departures and Victor's wishes to keep them "under lock and key." Ms. Fink gradually introduced higher levels of animation and emphasis, variations on themes, and, perhaps most important, playfulness to convey to Victor that she was finding meaning in his behavior, wanted to connect with him, and wanted to make fun together.

PRINCIPLE 4

The diagnosis of ASD encompasses a wide swath of psychopathology. While most child clinicians and researchers agree about a neurobiological substrate to the clinical picture that more or less limits potential improvement, every child is different, has his or her own complex set of contributing factors, vulnerabilities, and strengths, and should be assessed as an individual.

ATTENTION-DEFICIT/HYPERACTIVITY DISORDER

The Riveras had been worried about Maria for several years when, at age 7, her pediatrician finally referred her to Dr. Green. Mrs. Rivera reported to Dr. Green that Maria had always been somewhat overactive and difficult to settle but had managed fine in her Montessori preschool, where she was even considered a leader. She had showed very little interest in learning to read, but the school's position was "she will do it when she's ready." Now in first grade in public school, she was having trouble; she was unable to make friends, her reading was delayed, and she was disruptive both when the class was reading aloud and when students were reading independently and silently. The teacher reported that Maria often seemed to daydream during lessons and then bothered other children when they were supposed to be working independently. During recess, Maria would interrupt other children's play and was often rejected. She cried after school "three days out of five." At home, she was resistant to doing her homework, would roll around on her chair (as her father said, "like she was on the high seas"), and would typically find any excuse to escape. Sometimes homework, especially reading, devolved into screaming fights when Maria "would just not listen" and ran around the room, provocatively pulling books and other items off shelves. Both parents were at their wits' end; they didn't find this behavior at all funny, even though Maria would laugh a lot in a joyless way. The mother observed that sometimes Maria's father called her "crazy"—admittedly, this was not very helpful. Unfortunately, the Riveras felt she was actually driving them crazy. Many of the behaviors they assumed she would outgrow were getting worse; it was harder to get her dressed in the morning, harder to get her to gymnastics class, and harder to get her prepared for bed.

During the consultation, Maria was initially tentative but then began to move around the room, examining and touching everything, and asking, "What's this? What's this?" like a much younger child and then barely listening to the response. Dr. Green's attempts to confine her to the play area were woefully unsuccessful. Even more importantly, Dr. Green felt that Maria did not take her in as a person; her eyes slid off her face to other sights in the room, and when Dr. Green tried to talk to her, Maria was off and running.

Dr. Green felt immediately that Maria would need neuropsychiatric testing and asked Dr. Lee to put Maria on her waiting list. She then spent some time with the Riveras explaining the benefits of testing: clarification of Maria's symptoms and academic difficulties, development of a clearer picture of her cognitive profile, and initiation of the paper trail necessary to get accommodations should they be needed. She did raise the possibility of dyslexia and/or ADHD based on Maria's presentation and supported by the Rivera's description of a family history of ADHD (i.e., two male cousins were already receiving therapy and medication for ADHD) and on Dr. Green's development form that they filled out before the consultation (for Development Form, see Appendix B). The Riveras, therefore, were somewhat informed and not dead set against medication. Dr. Green said she would want to gather information, and then they would talk about what was going on in terms of diagnosis and recommendations. For a comprehensive and convincing assessment, she asked permission to request school staff to fill out an ADHD rating scale for teachers and raised the possibility of a school observation by Dr. Lee, who was thus far unknown to Maria. She also wanted to see Maria at least twice a week, saying that the child not only was likely to have ADHD and some form of learning disability, but also was very unhappy.

Dr. Green knew she would have to be very inventive to engage this child who whirled through her office like a tornado, speaking but not using words meaningfully and being unreceptive to engagement. Dr. Green also felt a need to protect the integrity of the adult portion of the consulting room and her desk, which might have personal or patient-related items on it. It seemed to Dr. Green that helping Maria develop her play would be an early goal, especially because her recess behavior indicated that her lack of social competence was isolating her and no doubt added to her negative feelings. Dr. Green decided to try what she called an "exercise obstacle course" that Maria had to traverse to get to the play area; to increase the child's motivation, Dr. Green purchased some popular pocket-sized dolls with little play sets that the Riveras said Maria coveted. After describing the "obstacle course" game, she said that Maria had to go through it to get the reward of the play sets; Dr. Green promised she would take a turn and be the exerciser too. The game was played as follows: when the "exerciser" came to the office door to enter, she had to pick four cards, sight unseen, from a deck of 12 (invented by Dr. Green for this purpose); each one demanded that the exerciser complete a silly physical task to gradually advance to the pocket dolls. The task cards included items like the following: perform 10 jumping jacks; stand on one foot with eyes closed and count to 10; twirl around twice and touch a moving target (the other person's finger) five times; hop four times on the right foot and three times on the left foot; take a ride on Dr. Green's revolving desk chair for 30 seconds (with a timer) and then jump up into a pose without losing balance; jump with both feet onto a step stool three times; do three addition problems in your head while circling the chair three times. Trying to read the written cards was very challenging for Maria and threatened her tenuous engagement. Dr. Green had the idea to translate them into pictures, which Maria helped create, albeit reluctantly.

After the cards were fully translated, Maria went through the exercises with enthusiasm, and when she finally arrived at her goal, Dr. Green gave her the entry card that read, "You are permitted into the play area. Welcome!" This game was intended not only to tire her out and recruit her restless energy but also to structure her path, to connect actions to numbers and words, and to see how she managed a complex sequence; her reading deficit was already quite clear. The revised game, which Dr. Green called "Maria's Mayhem and March," used pictures to make words, then used words as actions, and ended with words that were a simple friendly communication.

During the third session playing this entering game, Maria received her welcome card but threw it at Dr. Green, saying that it was stupid because she wasn't welcome anywhere else—she was never allowed to play in the boy's four square game at recess, and the girls never wanted her to play their "how to train your dragon game" (loosely based on the franchise of movies and TV shows) and accused her of breaking the rules. Dr. Green remarked on how well Maria had been following the rules of their Mayhem and March game until today and then asked, "What made it harder to play by the rules today?" Dr. Green said she had a feeling that Maria was frustrated because recess wasn't getting any better and maybe she was mad that Dr. Green wasn't helping her enough. After a few moments of unusual silence, Dr. Green went on to say that maybe Maria was *really* mad at her and at the other kids too—maybe she was so mad and sad that she just wanted to give up trying. That statement seemed to go too far, because Maria started to throw all the cards. Dr. Green ducked and exclaimed, "Oops, I guess my talking so much made you madder!" The game resumed in the next session, but it continued to fray, with Maria breaking the rules and escalating her activity; even reversing roles was not interesting to her. Dr. Green said maybe Maria wanted to make new cards and set the rules so the therapist would have to pass hard tests. Maria was excited by that idea and made cards that were impossible to decipher and, when translated by Maria, were difficult to execute (e.g., do five cartwheels with your eyes closed). Nonetheless, Dr. Green was able to use them as impossible tasks, hard to understand and to follow, that Maria made her do, and act as though her inability made her feel like she was dumb. The slow translation of actions to words and feelings was not a smooth one, and a lot of the hours were spent trying to re-engage Maria when she spun out of control.

After 6 months of play therapy, the neuropsychiatric testing was completed and showed that Maria had dyslexia and considerable attentional disturbance: poor working memory, difficulty attending to details, and poor executive function. Dr. Green made a case for a medication trial, which the Riveras accepted, and Maria began taking a low dose of a long-acting stimulant. Communication with the school led to Maria's getting resource room time three times per week. Both interventions led to improvement. However, the Riveras and Dr. Green were concerned about the degree to which Maria's relationships with other kids in school were permanently damaged. Because Dr. Green was about to begin maternity leave, she raised the possibility of a 3-month course of CBT with Dr. Reed during the break from play therapy. Dr. Reed was familiar with Maria and thought she could help the child with some of her dysregulation, disinhibition, and insensitivity to nonverbal cues that got her in trouble with other kids. She was also starting a social skills group for kids with externalizing disorders and thought Maria might benefit from that as well.

When Dr. Green returned from maternity leave, Maria was moderately improved behaviorally. Dr. Reed said Maria had learned how to inhibit her impulsive intrusions into other kids' activities via alternative activities such as sitting with the teachers at recess. It was evident to Dr. Green that Maria continued to struggle with impulsivity especially when she experienced strong emotions. In their first session back, Maria tore into the office; twirled on the desk chair, frequently colliding with the desk and Dr. Green; and finally hopped on one foot and then the other. After what seemed like many minutes, she finally tired herself out and tried to climb into Dr. Green's lap. Dr. Green said she would make space next to her on the chair; she was glad that Maria remembered their entry game with those bossy cards and guessed that Maria must have missed this activity when Dr. Green was away. She reminisced aloud that when Maria was in charge of the game, the cards were so difficult to understand that it made Dr. Green feel like giving up and just throwing those cards around or jumping ahead and ignoring them; she understood why Maria used to do that. She suggested that when Maria didn't understand what was going on or felt left out, she had the same reaction. Dr. Green wondered aloud if her long maternity leave made Maria feel the same way: confused about what Dr. Green was doing all that time with the new baby and left out of their relationship. She told Maria that she knew from Dr. Reed how hard she had worked on not intruding on other kids at recess; now maybe she and Dr. Green could work on figuring out her feelings at those moments and see if she had any choices other than to go sit with the teachers. This was quickly taken up in play with the pocket-sized dolls: Maria repeatedly enacted scenes of exclusion of one hapless girl, whom she called, disparagingly, Baby Blue.

This vignette about Maria highlights some of the difficulties that can occur in working in play therapy with children with ADHD: 1) the driven level of activity of the child with ADHD becomes a vicious circle, inciting others, who then heighten the child's agitation, and 2) the child's inability to regulate his or her state makes for failures in social exchanges, academic settings, and family life. In Maria's case, hyperactivity regularly escalated with frustration; in her reunion with Dr. Green, she was especially overactive as she grappled with her feelings about the separation. Children with ADHD often rely on the projection of their inner chaos through provocative behaviors that rile up everyone else around them in order to relieve themselves of tension and reduce excitement. Efforts to interrupt the provocations by talking about the emotions that the child seems to be experiencing can lead to more explicitly aggressive outbursts, as occurred early in treatment in Maria's case. This response has been termed **semiotic fragility**; putting feelings and narratives into words, usually a therapeutic mainstay, can be disruptive and threatening to these vulnerable children: words feel like hostile and disorganizing attacks (Salomonsson 2006; Sugarman 2010). Dr. Green had learned to wait to offer what seemed like obvious connections between Maria's level of activity and her affects until Maria was calmer; this had the added benefit of encouraging the girl to work on finding her own ways to self-regulate (although some were clearly of limited usefulness outside the office). The play of children with ADHD is often intrusive, jokey, and off-point, and the effect on other children is that they sink to the level of the child with ADHD. Through equanimity and consistent interpretation of the affect driving the activity, the therapist models reflection and asserts the possibility of ego control over affect and action.

A number of psychodynamic thinkers have offered conceptualizations of ADHD and proposed modifications of standard play technique with or without psychopharmacological therapy. Many invoke the transactional paradigm described in relation to ASD: a vulnerable child cannot be appropriately nurtured by caretakers who may be traumatizing, depriving, mentally ill, or simply not attuned to the child's special needs. Medication is readily prescribed for this disorder in the United States (in contrast to Europe), in part because it can be highly beneficial in terms of taking the urgency out of the current crisis. An approach that flexibly combines psychotherapeutic intervention with medication is often necessary to avert a crisis at home or school and to salvage a child's deteriorating self-esteem (Gilmore 2000). The value of play therapy for children with ADHD lies in the opportunities it provides to link their frenetic activity to feeling states, to derive meaning out of their overwhelming affects, and to offer a therapeutic relationship that promotes mentalization and self-regulation. This orientation toward play is helpful independent of preferred theory of etiology, which varies widely depending on the practitioner and the culture. These theories variously propose that ADHD is a variant of PTSD (Szymanski et al. 2011), a manifestation of agitated depression (Seitler 2008), or an epigenetic process in which a particular gene–environment interaction produces and sustains an ADHD phenotype (Nigg 2012)[1]

It is noteworthy that the retrospective analysis of over 700 cases at the Anna Freud Centre (Fonagy and Target 1994, 1996) suggested that lengthy psychodynamically informed treatments were especially effective in helping children with externalizing disorders like ADHD, even more so when anxiety is present. Maria benefited to some extent from the behaviorally oriented CBT but was able to make more generalizable use of the insights Dr. Green offered in regard to the feeling states that led to her maladaptive defenses; these types of interpretations were particularly useful in regard to Maria's intense emotions stirred up in the transference.

---

[1]The epigenetic process concept can, of course, encompass many different theories involving environmental insult.

Prout et al. (2015) have proposed a manualized, time-limited treatment for externalizing disorders that is informed by psychodynamic principles and that utilizes play therapy as its primary medium, supplemented by parent work. This approach emphasizes the following familiar key concepts: 1) behaviors have meaning; 2) externalizing behaviors (impulsivity, aggressiveness, hyperactivity) are defensive projections of intolerable emotional states; and 3) learning to tolerate and reflect on these emotions is of value to parents and children. The patient's play—its themes and disruptions—is used to develop hypotheses about the specific nature of the child's warded-off affects and conflicts. These hypotheses become part of the dialogue that is intended to enhance children's capacity to recognize warded-off feelings, to help them bear the discomfort of feeling those emotions, and, as a consequence, to self-regulate and self-soothe more effectively. In a study by Laezer (2015), children with ADHD and oppositional defiant disorder were placed in two treatment groups, one with psychodynamic treatment alone and the other receiving CBT and/or medication; after 38 months, both groups showed equivalent symptom reduction and lower scores on parent and teacher measures. The conclusions from this study, that dynamic treatment for ADHD is as effective as CBT and as CBT plus medication, supports the observations of the Anna Freud Centre study and our own experience. Moreover, the fact that the Laezer study produced good outcomes after lengthy treatments of over 3 years corroborates the conclusion from the Anna Freud Centre retrospective analysis: these children do best with longer and deeper therapies.

PRINCIPLE 5

Children with ADHD typically are dysregulated by many stimuli, internal and external. They may respond with agitation or aggression to strong emotional arousal. They are often unable to process words—instructions or interpretations—because of *semiotic fragility*. Work with these children requires inventive strategies to dissipate restless energy, maintain engagement, and prepare them for interpretations that, however gentle, may feel to them like an attack.

TRAUMA AND TRAUMA-ASSOCIATED DISORDERS

Charlotte was 2½–3 years old when she was repeatedly sexually abused by Tom, a local jack-of-all-trades who was well known, well liked, and regularly employed for household jobs in a small suburban community. Many episodes of the abuse took place in a laundry room that Tom constructed for the family. He had surreptitiously placed video cameras in the walls of this room and taped the sexual acts there while other family members were nearby and clearly audible. These videos were discovered by police investigating child pornography when Charlotte was 6 years old; her father easily identified her and the setting from the videos. According to both parents, Charlotte had never been symptomatic and never avoided Tom, who was in and out of their home for months. Charlotte's father, a busy CFO of a large company, was the parent who sought consultation with Dr. Lee; throughout the assessment, she found him easily accessible, sorrowful, and eager to do anything to help, whereas Charlotte's mother was embarrassed, victimized, and avoidant.

During the consultation, Charlotte was extremely inhibited, sad, anxious, compliant, quiet, and almost motionless in the play area. She had never done much pretend play except when her older sisters engaged her to play the baby or a "bad student" in various sociodramatic scenarios. Dr. Lee sat with her, inviting her to play by showing her the dollhouse and some figures she picked out to play with: three little girls, a babysitter, a mother and a father, and some other men and women in different uniforms. Dr. Lee asked where she should put them; getting no response, she placed one little girl in a room with a man in overalls and the rest of the family spread around the house. Charlotte seemed to react to this arrangement and left abruptly to go to the bathroom. When she returned, she asked if she could draw. She and Dr. Lee embarked on a regular pattern in the sessions of sitting quietly and drawing together, which very slowly produced a series of tableaus of the family, eventually including the extra man. Drawings with a workman and a little girl appeared occasionally; in these depictions, the girl watched the man making things, hammering with a big hammer or sawing wood. She often drew a bag of candy in these pictures or a big lollipop in the little girl's mouth. There were no drawings depicting an active relationship to the mother.

Dr. Lee felt intuitively that naming the figures was unnecessary and not conducive to Charlotte's unfolding process. The sessions were always interrupted by one or more visits to the bathroom, such that Dr. Lee wondered aloud if Charlotte was checking to see if everything was okay with her body and especially her "privates"" (the family word for the genital area); Charlotte responded flatly, "I have to pee a lot." After many months, her drawings of the man became more frightening, and sometimes he even wore a peaked hood that hid his face. In one picture, he was grabbing a little girl from behind and had one hand over her mouth; her eyes were closed and her cheeks were colored red. Dr. Lee felt this picture offered her a chance to talk directly about Tom, but she approached this gingerly, first asking permission and reassuring Charlotte that she could stop the conversation at any time. She told Charlotte that she knew he was around a lot, took an interest in Charlotte, and encouraged her to watch him work. Dr. Lee also began to remark on the absence of connection between the mother and little girl in the pictures: the little girl seemed not to notice her and was always turned in a different direction. Dr. Lee suggested to Charlotte that maybe her own mother was not always paying attention to what was happening and therefore didn't realize that Tom was too interested in her daughter. While Charlotte neither confirmed nor denied this commentary, she became more relaxed and began, after 10 months, to play with the dolls in the dollhouse.

Charlotte's case is one extreme example of the myriad ways in which children are traumatized by the adults they know. In her case, the failure of her parents to intervene was an intrinsic part of her injurious experience. The absence of conscious memory, due to the timing of these events, is not unusual in the histories of early traumatization. If the trauma occurs in the child's preverbal or early verbal period, then it may never be possible to verbalize the experience from narrative memory. Unfortunately, because such traumatic events can occur without visible evidence, the child's immediate reaction may not be observed by her caregivers; sleep disturbance, transient setbacks in potty training, and clinging behavior are all reactions that can be explained away.

PTSD is treated using a range of modalities, such as CBT, medication, family therapy, and psychodynamic play therapy. Traumatized children reenact aspects of their traumatic experiences through their affective outbursts and behavioral reactions to certain triggering events or by re-creating them in play (Gaensbauer 2011) in stereotypic scenarios that are rigid and joyless reenactments of their experience. These have been variously called **implicit or procedural memories** of the trauma, a reversal reflecting the operation of the passive to active defense, deferred imitation, or the action of the mirror neuron system that retains the experience as a template (Gaensbauer 2011). This form of playing does not provide relief from anxiety and is often not consciously recognized as a repetition (Paley and Alpert 2003). Most clinicians who treat these children, nonetheless, see this play as their most effective therapeutic modality because it gradually offers opportunities for therapeutic intervention. Despite different emphases, they describe an arc to the therapy that involves similar important elements: the play reenactments, revisions of the child distortions and misunderstandings, and corrections or repairs of the course of events.

Lenore Terr (2013), a specialist who has devoted her career to interviewing and treating traumatized children, delineates an approach to trauma that she suggests "fluidly mix(es) psychoanalytically derived psychotherapy, play therapy, cognitive-behavioral therapy, counseling, and medication" (p. 51). She underscores that, unlike adults, children who have endured trauma are most concerned about the threat to attachment figures and "home"; their cognitive immaturity makes comprehension of the actual threat to life much less salient. Three familiar guiding principles—all of which require that the therapist have a thorough understanding of the events—are abreaction, context, and correction, not necessarily in that or any order because the processes are intertwined and codependent.

Abreaction is the retelling of the story *with feeling*; for children, this may involve a lengthy period of learning the names of feelings and identifying them in others and may follow the process of contextualization (described in next paragraph). In children whose **behavioral memory** is an affective explosion, as in the case of Max (who saw his father kill his mother, as described in the vignette in the "Trauma and Associated Stress Disorders" section of Chapter 7), the work would similarly involve naming the feelings and linking the outburst to the experience. In circumstances involving anticipated trauma (e.g., a future surgical procedure), Terr (2013) suggests that explaining what is going to happen is crucial. In cases like Charlotte's, where the events occurred in early childhood, whatever is known from other informants can be gradually offered as it appears to emerge in her drawings. Telling the child what happened, when such information is available and paced according to the child's tolerance, is a step forward in attaching language to memories that are often experienced symptomatically in the body without verbal representation. This gradual process of articulating the events also requires an attuned ear; the child's subjective version and its elaboration may be different due to distortion and/or details unavailable to others (see below). For a child traumatized as young as Charlotte, the therapist might say, "You were so little and so scared, and this is what you figured out about what happened and even why it happened. May I tell you a little more about the situation that your parents and the policemen described? Maybe that will help you see it and understand it a little differently and not blame yourself so much."

Contextualization (Terr 2009, 2013) refers to the natural process of creating a subjectively coherent narrative following a traumatic event: these narratives inevitably draw in conflicts, self-representations, and emotions from the individual's premorbid psychology. Other experts call this process **reappraisal** (Pynoos and Eth 1985). Traumatized individuals, adults and children alike, inevitably and usually unconsciously work over the events of the trauma, developing a story about "how" and "why" it occurred that is part perception and part unconscious fantasy. The understanding of the individual's role in the events is based on this new construct and usually has already happened by the time a patient seeks help. In children, this is a silent process shaped by the level of their cognitive development and their prior experience; the presence, absence, or active participation of their attachment figures; and the type of trauma and sequelae of the events. The reappraisal that occurs is often imbued with age-related confusion about right and wrong and the child's guilt and fear. Playing with a clinician who has gathered as much information about the events as possible allows children to gradually reveal their version with its misperceptions and distortions against the backdrop of the factual narrative; the therapist's role is to recontextualize the events, addressing the child's sense of responsibility and distortions in the representation of the actual events of the trauma (Terr 2009, 2013). This process is primarily cognitive, with attention to the child's level of understanding. As noted, traumatized children spontaneously "reappraise" their experience (Pynoos and Eth 1985)—that is, they develop narratives that are often shaped not only by the events but also by guilt and preexisting conflicts. It is these narratives that are most important to capture in play because they often contain the kernels of the child's symptomatology (Terr 2009). In Charlotte's case, such a theme was present in her description of the little girl as "greedy" because she always wanted candy.

Gaensbauer (1994, 1995, 2011) has also made important contributions to this literature. He suggests that the reenactments are immensely valuable for therapeutic intervention—for symptom reduction, reprocessing, and conscious narrative building. However, in very young children, he warns that reenacting the trauma in play is potentially problematic; the young child's capacity to understand is developmentally limited and the power of words to gradually erode the grip of the repetitive behavior may be reduced. In such situations, therapeutic work based in nonverbal modalities, such as dance, drawing, and music, may be helpful as an adjunct to play therapy.

In Charlotte's case, because conscious memory was not available, drawing became the medium of therapeutic intervention. Dr. Lee was gradually able to talk through the setting in which the traumatic abuse occurred and then address the parents' lack of awareness (or negligence) and Charlotte's own silence. Dr. Lee offered the following narrative: The little girl was scared and lonely because her parents were so busy with the other girls and their many interesting activities. The parents trusted the babysitter (minimally represented in her drawings) to take good care of the youngest daughter. Dr. Lee did not want to exonerate Charlotte's parents (she was quite aware of and struggling with her anger at their negligence), but she felt that Charlotte herself would rewrite this narrative many times as development proceeded and her thinking deepened.

Correction can emerge spontaneously as the child plays with the clinician and the narrative evolves, but in some circumstances it does not. Terr (2009, 2013) offers suggestions on how to work through problematic narratives, such as those perpetuating self-blame or helpless submission: she creates opportunities in play for the child to "right the wrong" for other traumatized children or to forewarn other children who might encounter a similar danger. Often, if given time, children will arrive at corrective narratives spontaneously; their own righting process may also reveal unconscious fantasies about the traumatic experience that the therapist can address.

PRINCIPLE 6

Traumatized children, including those directly affected and those who bear witness, are usually responsive to and in need of play therapy. Traumatic events are usually (although not always) an abrupt rupture of prior conditions; thus, they presumably occur in a nonsymptomatic child who had adequate play prior to the trauma. Exceptions to this assumption of premorbid normalcy are numerous, especially as a very common type of trauma—that is, abuse committed by an attachment figure—is often associated with ongoing strain trauma or even a pattern of trauma that likely preceded the signal event. Traumatized children benefit from play therapy that provides empathic ego bolstering in the therapy; ancillary parent work that brings the parents into the process; a pace matched to the child's tolerance; and a sensitive attuned therapist who can recognize the child's signals.

SUMMARY

Any child in play therapy may require a modification of technique at certain moments or during certain phases of treatment. Children in crisis; over-excited or overstimulated children; children with severe separation anxiety or other anxieties; those with major inhibitions or oppositional behaviors; children who become silent and/or refuse to engage with the therapist—all these situations and more can create new and different challenges in the ongoing treatment of moderate childhood disorders. Such challenges may compel the therapist to introduce new methods or creative approaches in order to establish or reinstate the therapeutic alliance.

Work with severely disturbed children may, from the outset, require a treatment plan that is specific to the disorder and yet still tailored to the individual child. The plan may prioritize a range of interventions in order to stabilize the child's circumstances and calm the crisis before play therapy can be considered. Medication, parent work, school visits, school change, remediation, and occupational therapy are only some of the measures that may precede play therapy and allow it to be useful. In our view, play therapy remains a central feature of any approach to childhood psychopathology: it is the premiere method to foster a vital developmental capacity and promote the universal activity of childhood. It can be helpful to many troubled children with a range of diagnoses. In cases of more severe psychopathology, its place in the overall treatment plan may need to be carefully articulated in order to underscore its important role in restoring the child to a more adaptive path of development and to achieve the child's true potential.

KEY POINTS

- Technical challenges arise in most play therapies. When behaviors emerge that tax the therapist's tolerance and violate the boundaries of the play space, special techniques may be necessary to manage aggression, sexual excitement, regression, protracted silence, and other problematic moments. These may resemble techniques typically utilized in treatments of more severely ill children, such as physical restraint for safety, introduction of structured play, and leading the play narrative.

- With more severe disorders, consideration of play therapy requires a careful assessment of the child's potential to develop play capacity and a relationship with the clinician.

- Among the severe disorders, play itself is often symptomatic; freeing play from joyless repetition, stereotypies, or arrest at the functional level is a major focus; the therapy is in part an effort to help such children "learn to play."

- Some techniques that might prove necessary include a delineation of rules and boundaries, use of marked affect to illuminate the emotion in the play events, slow interpretive pace, physical maneuvers to work off steam, and reduction of distractions.

- Because trauma is a special case, in which an external event has interrupted expected developmental progression, traumatized children differ along a number of dimensions that can influence the presentation: the nature of the trauma, the interval between trauma and evaluation, whether it was a single or repetitive event, the age of the child, the state of language development and other features of prior development, the safety and stability of attachment figures, and the nature of the events, be they sexual, physical, or environmental (such as catastrophic events, natural or man-made).

KEY TERMS

Average expectable mother   Term derived from Hartmann's (1939) early ego psychology, in which he attempted to establish a developmental trajectory assuming an "average expectable environment" in order to explore the idea of ongoing adaptation—that is, the efforts by the ego to balance internal and external forces. The term was applied to mothers later in the evolution of ego psychology in recognition of their prominent role in the infant's earliest efforts at adaptation (Winnicott 1965, 1971).

Behavioral memory   A type of memory that resembles implicit or procedural memory in that it is not considered a part of the dynamic unconscious, even though it is unconscious and not verbalizable. It is memory that is "recalled action" without awareness that it refers to a past experience or action. The memory is sometimes reversed in the behavior (i.e., the behavior enacted is not the presumed actual experience—the passive experience of victim—but rather the active role of perpetrator). It is invoked in the context of early trauma and is usually repetitive and "an unmistakable reproduction of the traumatic experience" (Shapiro and Inderbitzin 1989, p. 826).

Floortime   A technique developed by Stanley Greenspan in which a parent or therapist sits on the floor with a child and uses the child's idiosyncratic lead to engage the child in action and reaction cycles. This provides the adult the opportunity to pull the child into a higher level of shared playing experience, to develop dynamic interactions, and to build sequences of more elaborate play by action–reaction. Floortime technique has been used with infants and children at risk for ASD in order to nurture and grow their functional, emotional, and developmental capacities (Greenspan and Wieder 2009).

Functional play   A play form appearing in the sensorimotor period that precedes symbolic play but continues onward in development. It is "practicing" play that uses objects as they are intended in a repetitive fashion; there is no imaginative use of objects to represent something else.

Implicit or procedural memory   A type of memory that is acquired slowly and is reliable, inflexible, and inaccessible to consciousness (as in rid-ing a bike) (Cortina and Liotti 2007). Part of a contemporary understanding of the developmental complexity of memory, it is not considered part of the dynamic unconscious, which contains conflictual impulses and is maintained by repression.

Mutual playing state Special shared consciousness or ego state that accompanies play during which reality is suspended and the child and therapist are mutually fully engrossed in pretense.

Reappraisal An alternative, more contemporary term for "omen formation," referring to children's "defensive reworking" of a traumatic experience, marked by temporal alterations and perceptual or intellectual distortions, that fabricates ominous signs in the events preceding the trauma. Sometimes reappraisals produce the conviction that the victim could or should have recognized omens or warnings of the impending trauma, thereby preventing it (Terr 2009, p. 278).

Semiotic fragility Term coined by Salomonsson (2006) to denote the potentially disorganizing impact of the clinician's words on the patient with ADHD, who, according to Salomonsson's thinking, lacks a stable internal object that facilitates the experience of words as symbolic communications rather than dangerous objects. It is a concept that might be applied to children on the autism spectrum as well.

Zone of proximal development Term introduced by Vygotsky (1978) to identify the distance between a child's actual developmental level and the (more advanced) one possible with adult guidance (Kassett et al. 2004). This guidance can be imparted by any older person, such as a sibling, because older siblings are important developmental objects helping to propel the child forward.

REFERENCES

American Psychiatric Association: Diagnostic and Statistical Manual of Mental Disorders, 4th Edition. Washington, DC, American Psychiatric Association, 1994

American Psychiatric Association: Diagnostic and Statistical Manual of Mental Disorders, 5th Edition. Arlington, VA, American Psychiatric Association, 2013

Arkowitz SW: The overstimulated state of dyslexia: perception, knowledge, and learning. J Am Psychoanal Assoc 48(4):1491–1520, 2000 11212198

Chused JF: Discussion: a clinician's view of attachment theory. J Am Psychoanal Assoc 48:1175–1187, 2000

Cortina M, Liotti G: New approaches to understanding unconscious processes: implicit and explicit memory systems. International Forum of Psychoanalysis 16(4):204–212, 2007

Dawson G: Early behavioral intervention, brain plasticity, and the prevention of autism spectrum disorder. Dev Psychopathol 20(3):775–803, 2008 18606031

De Bellis MD, Zisk A: The biological effects of childhood trauma. Child Adolesc Psychiatr Clin N Am 23(2):185–222, vii, 2014 24656576

Fonagy P, Moran GS: Understanding psychic change in child psychoanalysis. Int J Psychoanal 72(Pt 1):15–22, 1991 2050481

Fonagy P, Target M: Who is helped by child psychoanalysis? A sample study of disruptive children, from the Anna Freud Centre retrospective investigation. Bulletin of the Anna Freud Centre 17:291–315, 1994

Fonagy P, Target M: Predictors of outcome in child psychoanalysis: a retrospective study of 763 cases at the Anna Freud Centre. J Am Psychoanal Assoc 44(1):27–77, 1996 8717478

Freud A: Comments on aggression. Int J Psychoanal 53:163–171, 1972

Gaensbauer TJ: Therapeutic work with a traumatized toddler. Psychoanal Study Child 49:412–433, 1994 7809298

Gaensbauer TJ: Trauma in the preverbal period: symptoms, memories, and developmental impact. Psychoanal Study Child 50:122–149, 1995 7480400

Gaensbauer TJ: Embodied simulation, mirror neurons, and the reenactment of trauma in early childhood. Neuropsychoanalysis 13(1):91–107, 2011

Gilmore K: A psychoanalytic perspective on attention-deficit/hyperactivity disorder. J Am Psychoanal Assoc 48(4):1259–1293, 2000 11212190

Gilmore K: Play in the psychoanalytic setting: ego capacity, ego state, and vehicle for intersubjective exchange. Psychoanal Study Child 60:213–238, 2005 16649681

Greenspan SI: Levels of infant-caregiver interactions and the DIR model: implications for the development of signal affects, the regulation of mood and behavior, the formation of a sense of self, the creation of internal representation, and the construction of defenses and character structure. J Infant Child Adolesc Psychother 6(3):174–210, 2007

Greenspan SI, Wieder S: Engaging Autism: Using the Floortime Approach to Help Children Relate, Communicate, and Think. Philadelphia, PA, Da Capo Press, 2009

Grinker RR: Commentary: on being autistic, and social. Ethos 38(1):172–178, 2010

Hartmann H: Ego Psychology and the Problem of Adaptation. New York, International Universities Press, 1939

Kassett JA, Bonanno GA, Notarius CI: Affective scaffolding a process measure for psychotherapy with children. J Infant Child Adolesc Psychother 3(1):92–118, 2004

Laezer KL: Effectiveness of psychoanalytic psychotherapy and behavioral therapy treatment in children with attention deficit hyperactivity disorder and oppositional defiant disorder. J Infant Child Adolesc Psychother 14(2):111–128, 2015

Nigg JT: Future directions in ADHD etiology research. J Clin Child Adolesc Psychol 41(4):524–533, 2012 22642834

Paley J, Alpert J: Memory of infant trauma. Psychoanal Psychol 20(2):329–347, 2003

Pozzi-Monzo M: Ritalin for whom? Revisited: further thinking on ADHD. Journal of Child Psychotherapy 38(1):49–60, 2012

Prout T, Gaines E, Gerber L, et al: The development of an evidence-based treatment: regulation-focused psychotherapy for children with externalising behaviours (RFP-C). Journal of Child Psychotherapy 41(3):255–271, 2015

Pynoos R, Eth S (eds): Posttraumatic Stress Disorder in Children. Washington, DC, American Psychiatric Press, 1985

Salomonsson B: The impact of words on children with ADHD and DAMP: consequences for psychoanalytic technique. Int J Psychoanal 87(Pt 4):1029–1047, 2006 16921669

Seitler BN: Successful child psychotherapy of attention deficit/hyperactive disorder: an agitated depression explanation. Am J Psychoanal 68(3):276–294, 2008 18756317

Shapiro T: Psychotherapy for autism. J Infant Child Adolesc Psychother 8(1):22–31, 2009

Shapiro T, Inderbitzin LB: Unconscious fantasy. Panel report. J Am Psychoanal Assoc 37(3):823–835, 1989 2584605

Singletary WM: An integrative model of autism spectrum disorder: ASD as a neurobiological disorder of experienced environmental deprivation, early life stress, and allostatic overload. Neuropsychoanalysis 17(2):81–119, 2015

Slade A: Representation, symbolization, and affect regulation in the concomitant treatment of a mother and child: attachment theory and child psychotherapy. Psychoanal Inq 19(5):797–830, 1999

Sugarman A: The use of play to promote insightfulness in the analysis of children suffering from cumulative trauma. Psychoanal Q 77(3):799–833, 2008 18686791

Sugarman A: Convergences and divergences in treatments of so-called ADHD children. Int J Psychoanal 91(2):395–398, 2010 20536866

Szymanski K, Sapanski L, Conway F: Trauma and ADHD—association or diagnostic confusion? A clinical perspective. J Infant Child Adolesc Psychother 10(1):51–59, 2011

Terr LC: Using context to treat traumatized children. Psychoanal Study Child 64:275–298, 2009 20578442

Terr LC: Treating childhood trauma. Child Adolesc Psychiatr Clin N Am 22(1):51–66, 2013 23164127

Voran M: The protest of a 6-month-old girl: is this a prodrome of autism? J Infant Child Adolesc Psychother 12(3):139–155, 2013

Vygotsky L: Mind in Society: The Development of Higher Psychological Processes. Cambridge, MA, Harvard University Press, 1978

Winnicott DW: A clinical study of the effect of a failure of the average expectable environment on a child's mental functioning. Int J Psychoanal 46:81–87, 1965 14289319

Winnicott DW: Playing and Reality. New York, Basic Books, 1971

RECOMMENDED READING FOR PARENTS

Greenspan S, Weider S: Engaging Autism: Using the Floortime Approach to Help Children Relate, Communicate, and Think. Boston, MA, Da Capo Lifelong Books, 2009

Hallowell EM, Ratey JJ: Answers to Distraction: The Authors of Driven to Distraction Respond to the Most Frequently Asked Questions About Attention Deficit Disorder. New York, Ballantine Books, 2005

Hallowell EM, Ratey JJ: Driven to Distraction (Revised): Recognizing and Coping With Attention Deficit Disorder. New York, Anchor, 2011

Perry B, Szalavitz MT: The Boy Who Was Raised as a Dog and Other Stories From a Child Psychiatrist's Notebook: What Traumatized Children Can Teach Us About Loss, Love, and Healing. New York, Basic Books, 2007

Terr L: Too Scared to Cry: Psychic Trauma in Childhood. New York, Basic Books, 1992

Terr L: Unchained Memories: True Stories of Traumatic Memories Lost and Found. New York, Basic Books, 1995

Van der Kolk B: The Body Keeps the Score: Brain, Mind, and Body in the Healing of Trauma. New York, Penguin Books, 2015

Conclusion

The two of us, both child clinicians and educators, conceived this volume as a response to conversations with students at all levels of training and from the full array of mental health disciplines. In addition to the students' pragmatic concerns about furnishing their offices, choosing toys, and managing the logistics of a child practice, they expressed uncertainty about what to do when young children enter their offices: How do you make them play? How do you play with them? How is it different from "just playing"? How does it become therapy? Won't their parents be dissatisfied, since they don't believe that playing ever changed anything before? We heard these anxieties as a reflection of the trainees' relative inexperience and lack of confidence in the practice of play therapy; the freedom to play in the therapeutic encounter depends on one's conviction in its potential benefit to the child. These trainees did not yet know the wonder and the wildness of entering a child's "conceptual world" through the theater of play (Cohen and Cohen 1993), where a story can evolve over weeks to months, peopled with developing and familiar characters, and punctuated by the representation of events and experiences, all of which reflect the child's inner life as co-created with the therapist. Here the clinician can share in the discovery of the child's fears, sadness, delights, and anxieties as conveyed through characters, narratives, plot twists, catastrophes, resolutions, and happy endings emerging through the play. Here the therapist can gradually modulate the child's experience by giving voice to the aspects of the patient that are repudiated and the impulses and desires that are denied, in addition to enacting the aspects of others that are frightening, unavailable, or seductive and facilitating the child's comprehension. In displacement in play and in the safety of the therapist's office, the child can slowly reintegrate these elements in a more adaptive way.

Trainees today have little opportunity to learn how to work within children's premiere native medium, pretend play, and how to use any form of playing with a child to therapeutic effect. Training in play therapy in residency, social work, and clinical psychology training programs has sharply diminished in importance with the emphasis on evidence-based interventions, despite the rise of credible research demonstrating the benefits of psychodynamic thinking and therapy and the renewed interest in the importance of play from educators and developmental scientists. Even with sensitive and supportive shepherding of child clinicians through their training, such as the wonderful process of "primary supervision" described by Jellinek (2007), there is little recognition that, besides grappling with the new complexity of having to manage families, immature patients, low status in the hospital hierarchy, and the pervasive depreciation of the care of children (Rosenblitt 2008), trainees must also learn (or relearn) the language of play. They must re-awaken their capacities to hear meaning in play and action and must develop the ability to "regress in the service of the ego" (Kris 1943, p. 397) in order to reconnect with these meanings, make sense of them, and find developmentally attuned language or play action to convey their understanding in the densely packed, fast-paced, and emotionally fraught interaction with a child in distress.

It is noteworthy that despite many years of diminished emphasis, psychodynamic treatments for children are being studied and assessed in a growing body of outcome research (e.g., Midgley and Kennedy 2011). Psychodynamic child treatment is the subject of one of the recent American Academy of Child and Adolescent Psychiatry's official practice parameter statements (Kernberg et al. 2012). The Anna Freud Centre's extensive records of lengthy psychodynamic and psychoanalytic treatments have been reviewed in terms of efficacy and indications (Fonagy and Moran 1993; Fonagy and Target 1994; Fonagy et al. 2005; Target 2010; Target and Fonagy 1994a, 1994b), and new theoretical and technical psychodynamic approaches have been developed both in the United States and abroad, including a range of applications—manualized, short term, transference focused, child and adolescent anxiety psychodynamic psychotherapy, and so on (Abbass et al. 2013; Eresund 2007; Hoffman et al. 2016; Midgley and Kennedy 2011; Odhammar et al. 2011; Silver et al. 2013; Sossin 2015)—highlighting the important role of psychodynamic thinking in the understanding of the child's mind and the methodology of treatment. Play has a more or less prominent position in all of these psychotherapeutic permutations.

In our previous volume, *Normal Child and Adolescent Development: A Psychodynamic Primer* (Gilmore and Meersand 2013), we offered the scaffolding for the young clinician to contextualize children each in their developmental moment, to recognize their challenges and conflicts, and to distinguish the developmental from the disordered. In this book, we add the developmental unfolding of children's play forms and the role of play in optimal development, in disorders, and in the treatment process. We focus on the medium of play as the best way to establish communication with the child's inner life, which is essential to the process of helping a symptomatic child or a child who has deviated from the path of normal development. Our aim is to foster the young clinician's capacity to hear the meanings, discern the subjective experience, and appreciate the developmental challenges as keys to helping children, informed by a lens focused on their play and the invaluable information contained within it.

While not a "phrasebook" or dictionary of play, the current contribution is intended to help clinicians become fluent in the language of childhood and the creative productions of their patients. If trainees are not schooled in the art of play, they struggle to understand children's activities in their offices and often feel poorly equipped to engage with children at their level. Even beyond a method of therapy, the observation of play provides the best access to the evolving mental organizations of the child in the language of childhood. Because young children use the pretend mode as a developmental bridge to consensual reality (Fonagy and Target 1996; Gilmore 2011), it is an invaluable window into their emotional life, unconscious fantasy, struggles with affect regulation, conflicts around gender, self-representation, and evolution of superego constraints in the critical passage from oedipal age to school age. During this crucial phase, and for many years thereafter, as children grapple with "real life" and become students, athletes, artists, and thinkers, they rely on play to ease the process and to consolidate elements of their evolving personalities in action and symbolism, borrowing from contemporary artifacts and cultural themes to build their identities and to create their own autobiographical narratives, comforting daydreams, and real aspirations for their futures.

Child clinicians who are familiar with children's play in contemporary culture are prepared to distill meaning from whatever kind of play appears in their offices, in terms of specific play forms, methods of playing, preferred medium, and narrative elements. Children's current preoccupations, anxieties, conflicts, and joys are to be found in this form of communication, far more than through verbal exchange (Winnicott 1971). This is because most young children do not use verbal language to process their emotional experience; play is their natural medium for grappling with the many complexities of their circumstances and inner life. Furthermore, older children and adolescents continue to use action to express their conflicts and feelings, and there is no better education in interpreting action than studying and distilling meaning from imaginary play. This is one reason that all clinicians benefit from working with at least one child during training; contemplating the communication contained in play enhances the skill of "hearing" meaning in the actions of any patient and the art of "translating" these into useful interventions that are simple and concise (Yanof 1996a, 1996b). In the therapy playroom, the educated therapist can discern recurrent themes in the transference and the organizing unconscious fantasies expressed through action and play.

A therapist thus oriented toward understanding the inner life of young patients can begin to recognize central internal conflicts, characteristic mobilization of defenses, environmental opportunities, as well as failures and deficits. As these central dynamics emerge in play and transference, the clinician can help children to express and modulate them, in order to make sense of their own anxieties and reduce symptomatology. Because so much is communicated in playing, the therapist engages with patients at the level of cognitive organization appropriate to their age and conveys meaning through action, often without the need to formulate a verbal interpretation or speak directly to the patient in the room; speaking "in the game"—that is, as the assigned character in the story unfolding in play—is more readily accepted and understood. Playing with young patients provides an array of insights; diagnosis, trauma, interpersonal relatedness, cognitive development, motor skills, and use and misuse of the adults around them are all evident when playing with a child. This communication in displacement (Neubauer 1994), a normative defense of the playing child, sustains the experience of safety in the clinical setting, no matter how revealing the play may be. In addition, the ways in which the child engages the therapist, manages their interaction, and expresses aggression, competition, love, and longing are illuminations of core conflicts and concerns, in living color in the room and in the patient–therapist relationship.

REFERENCES

Abbass AA, Rabung S, Leichsenring F, et al: Psychodynamic psychotherapy for children and adolescents: a meta-analysis of short-term psychodynamic models. J Am Acad Child Adolesc Psychiatry 52(8):863–875, 2013 23880496

Cohen P, Cohen M: Conceptual worlds: play and theater in child psychoanalysis, in The Many Meanings of Play: A Psychoanalytic Perspective. Edited by Solnit A, Cohen DJ, Neubauer PB. New Haven, CT, Yale University Press, 1993, pp 75–98

Eresund P: Psychodynamic psychotherapy for children with disruptive disorders. J Child Psychother 33(2):161–180, 2007

Fonagy P, Moran GS: Advances in single case methodology, in Handbook of Psychoanalytic Research. Edited by Miller NE, Luborsky L, Barber JP, Docherty J. New York, Basic Books, 1993, pp 63–96

Fonagy P, Target M: The efficacy of psychoanalysis for children with disruptive disorders. J Am Acad Child Adolesc Psychiatry 33(1):45–55, 1994 8138520

Fonagy P, Target M: Playing with reality, I: theory of mind and the normal development of psychic reality. Int J Psychoanal 77(Pt 2):217–233, 1996 8771375

Fonagy P, Roth A, Higgitt A: The outcome of psychodynamic psychotherapy for psychological disorders. Clin Neurosci Res 4(5–6):367–377, 2005

Gilmore K: Pretend play and development in early childhood (with implications for the oedipal phase). J Am Psychoanal Assoc 59(6):1157–1182, 2011 22080503

Gilmore KJ, Meersand P: Normal Child and Adolescent Development: A Psychodynamic Primer. Arlington, VA, American Psychiatric Publishing, 2013

Hoffman L, Rice T, Prout T: Manual of Regulation-Focused Psychotherapy for Children (RFP) Externalizing Behaviors: A Psychodynamic Approach. New York, Routledge, 2016

Jellinek MS: Primary supervision. J Am Acad Child Adolesc Psychiatry 46(5):553–557, 2007 17450045

Kernberg PF, Ritvo R, Keable H; American Academy of Child and Adolescent Psychiatry (AACAP) Committee on Quality Issues (CQI): Practice Parameter for psychodynamic psychotherapy with children. J Am Acad Child Adolesc Psychiatry 51(5):541–557, 2012 22525961

Kris E: Some problems of war propaganda—a note on propaganda new and old. Psychoanal Q 12:381–399, 1943

Midgley N, Kennedy E: Psychodynamic psychotherapy for children and adolescents: a critical review of the evidence base. J Child Psychother 37:232–260, 2011

Neubauer PB: The role of displacement in psychoanalysis. Psychoanal Study Child 49:107–119, 1994 7809278

Odhammar F, Sundin EC, Jonson M, et al: Children in psychodynamic psychotherapy: changes in global functioning. J Child Psychother 37:261–279, 2011

Rosenblitt DL: Where do you want the killing done? An exploration of hatred of children. Annual of Psychoanalysis 36:203–215, 2008

Silver G, Shapiro T, Milrod B: Treatment of anxiety in children and adolescents: using child and adolescent anxiety psychodynamic psychotherapy. Child Adolesc Psychiatr Clin N Am 22(1):83–96, 2013 23164129

Sossin K: A movement-informed mentalization lens applied to psychodynamic psychotherapy of children and adolescents with high functioning autism spectrum disorder. J Infant Child Adolesc Psychother 14(3):294–310, 2015

Target M: Psychoanalytic psychotherapy now: where do we fit in? Psychoanal Psychother 24:14–21, 2010

Target M, Fonagy P: Efficacy of psychoanalysis for children with emotional disorders. J Am Acad Child Adolesc Psychiatry 33(3):361–371, 1994a 8169181

Target M, Fonagy P: The efficacy of psychoanalysis for children: prediction of outcome in a developmental context. J Am Acad Child Adolesc Psychiatry 33(8):1134–1144, 1994b 7982864

Winnicott D: Playing and Reality. London, UK, Tavistock, 1971

Yanof J: Language, communication, and transference in child analysis, I: selective mutism: the medium is the message. J Am Psychoanal Assoc 44(1):79–100, 1996a 8717479

Yanof J: Language, communication, and transference in child analysis, II: is child analysis really analysis? J Am Psychoanal Assoc 44(1):100–116, 1996b 8717480

APPENDIX A

Selected Assessment Measures for Play Therapy

CHILDREN'S PLAY THERAPY INSTRUMENT (CPTI)[1]

Outline of the Children's Play Therapy Instrument (CPTI)

Level One: Segmentation of Child's Activity

Non-Play Activity

Pre-Play Activity

Play Activity

Interruption

Level Two: Dimensional Analysis of the Play Activity

Descriptive Analysis

* Category of Play Activity

* Script Description of Play Activity

* Sphere of Play Activity

Structural Analysis

Affective Components of Play Activity

    * Child's Affects Modulation

    * Affects Expressed by Child While in the Play

    * Therapist's Affective Tone

Cognitive Components of Play Activity

    * Role Representation

    * Stability of Representation (People and Play Object)

    * Use of Play Object

    * Style of Role Representation (People and Play Object)

Dynamic Components of Play Activity

    * Topic of the Play Activity

    * Theme of the Play Activity

    * Level of Relationship Portrayed within the Play Activity

    * Quality of Relationship within the Play Activity

    * Use of Language (Child and Therapist)

Outline of the Children's Play Therapy Instrument (CPTI) *(continued)*

Structural Analysis *(continued)*

Developmental Components of Play Activity

* Estimated Developmental Level of Play

* Gender Identity of Play

* Psychosexual Phase Represented in the Play

* Separation-Individuation Phase Represented in the Play

* Social Level of Play

Adaptive Analysis

Coping and Defensive Strategies

Cluster I — Cluster II — Cluster III — Cluster IV
*Normal   *Neurotic   *Borderline   *Psychotic

*Awareness

Level Three: Pattern of Child Activity Over Time

Continuity and Discontinuity in Play Narrative(s)

---

[1]Kernberg P, Chazan SE, Normandin L: "The Children's Play Therapy Instrument: Description, Development, and Reliability Studies." *The Journal of Psychotherapy Practice and Research* 7(3):196–207, 1998.

TEST OF PLAYFULNESS (VERSION 4.0–5/05)[2]

The Test of Playfulness (ToP; Bundy and Skard 1997) reflects three elements of play: intrinsic motivation, suspension of reality, and internal locus of control. It also incorporates a fourth aspect of play called framing, discussed originally by Bateson (1972). Bateson described play as an important arena in which children frame their play by giving and reading social cues (e.g., "I'm playing now. This is how you should act toward me"). The ability to give and read cues is important to success in play and other situations. Thus, items reflective of framing were incorporated into the ToP. The ToP has yet to be shown to be valid and reliable, required for its wider use as an assessment tool.

REFERENCES

Bundy AC, Skard G: Test of Playfulness. Fort Collins, Colorado State University, 1997
Bateson G: Steps to an Ecology of Mind. New York, Ballantine Books, 1972

---

[2]Reprinted from Skard G, Bundy AC: "Test of Playfulness," in *Play in Occupational Therapy for Children,* 2nd Edition. Edited by Parnum D, Fazio LS. St. Louis, MO, Mosby Elsevier, 2008, pp. 71–93. Used with permission.

Test of Playfulness (Version 4.0–5/05)

ITEM Child (#): Age: Rater: In Out Video Live (Circle)	EXTENT 3 Almost always 2 Much of the time 1 Some of the time 0 Rarely or never NA Not Applicable	INTENSITY 3 Highly 2 Moderately 1 Mildly 0 Not NA Not Applicable	SKILLFULNESS 3 Highly skilled 2 Moderately skilled 1 Slightly skilled 0 Unskilled NA Not Applicable	COMMENTS
Is actively engaged.				
Decides what to do.				
Maintains level of safety sufficient to play.				
Tries to overcome barriers or obstacles to persist with an activity.				
Modifies activity to maintain challenge or make it more fun.				
Engages in playful mischief or teasing.				

Test of Playfulness (Version 4.0–5/05) *(continued)*

ITEM Child (#): Age: Rater: In Out Video Live (Circle)	EXTENT 3 Almost always 2 Much of the time 1 Some of the time 0 Rarely or never NA Not Applicable	INTENSITY 3 Highly 2 Moderately 1 Mildly 0 Not NA Not Applicable	SKILLFULNESS 3 Highly skilled 2 Moderately skilled 1 Slightly skilled 0 Unskilled NA Not Applicable	COMMENTS
Engages in activity for the sheer pleasure of it (process) rather than primarily for the end product.				
Pretends (to be someone else; to do something else; that an object is something else; that something else is happening).				
Incorporates objects or other people into play in unconventional or variable **and** creative ways.				

Test of Playfulness (Version 4.0–5/05) *(continued)*

ITEM Child (#): Age: Rater: In Out Video Live (Circle)	EXTENT 3 Almost always 2 Much of the time 1 Some of the time 0 Rarely or never NA Not Applicable	INTENSITY 3 Highly 2 Moderately 1 Mildly 0 Not NA Not Applicable	SKILLFULNESS 3 Highly skilled 2 Moderately skilled 1 Slightly skilled 0 Unskilled NA Not Applicable	COMMENTS
Negotiates with others to have needs/desires met.				
Engages in social play.				
Supports play of others.				
Enters a group already engaged in an activity.				
Initiates play with others.				
Clowns or jokes.				
Shares (toys, equipment, friends, ideas).				

Test of Playfulness (Version 4.0–5/05) *(continued)*

ITEM Child (#): Age: Rater: In Out Video Live (Circle)	EXTENT 3 Almost always 2 Much of the time 1 Some of the time 0 Rarely or never NA Not Applicable	INTENSITY 3 Highly 2 Moderately 1 Mildly 0 Not NA Not Applicable	SKILLFULNESS 3 Highly skilled 2 Moderately skilled 1 Slightly skilled 0 Unskilled NA Not Applicable	COMMENTS
Gives readily understandable cues (facial, verbal, body) that say, "This is how you should act toward me."				
Responds to others' cues.				
Demonstrates positive affect during play.				
Interacts with objects.				
Transitions from one play activity to another with ease.				

Development Form

Parent Form for Children Up to 18 Years Old

Family Information
Child

Full name: _____

Address: _____

City/zip: _____

Home telephone: _____

Cellular telephone: _____

Date of birth: _____

Gender: _____

Caregiver (if any): _____

Cell phone of caregiver: _____

Child's current school: _____

Grade: _____

School telephone: _____

Parent

Full name: _____

Address: _____

City/zip: _____

Home telephone: _____

Cellular telephone: _____

Date of birth: _____

Occupation: _____

Business address: _____

City/zip: _____

Business telephone: _____

Parent

Full name:

Address:

City/zip:

Home telephone:

Cellular telephone:

Date of birth:

Occupation:

Business address:

City/zip:

Business telephone:

Reason for the Consultation

Family History

Please describe both parents' (and stepparents') families of origin, showing their own parents and siblings and their birth order, in family tree or narrative form.

Parent (name):
_____

Parent (name):
_____

Family Psychiatric History

Parent (name):
_____

List all psychiatric illness(es) (e.g., bipolar, depression, schizophrenia) and please designate family member, medications, other treatments, and dates if known. Indicate biological (B) or nonbiological (N) relative.

Parent (name):
_____

List all psychiatric illness(es) (e.g., bipolar, depression, schizophrenia) and please designate family member, medications, other treatments, and dates if known. Indicate biological (B) or nonbiological (N) relative.

Family Medical History

Parent (name): _____

Please note major medical illness(es) of mother and her family of origin.
If deaths have occurred, indicate date and cause.

Mother _____

_____

_____

Maternal Grandmother _____

_____

_____

Maternal Grandfather _____

_____

_____

Aunts and uncles _____

_____

_____

Parent (name): _____

Please list major medical illness(es) of father and his family of origin. If
deaths have occurred, indicate date and cause.

Father _____

_____

_____

Paternal Grandmother _____

_____

_____

Paternal Grandfather _____

_____

_____

Aunts and uncles _____

_____

_____

Child Medical and Psychiatric History

Please describe medical history and major medical illness(es), including medications.

Please describe prior psychiatric or psychological treatment and treating doctors, medications, and reactions.

Please describe current state of health and current medications.

Family Constellation

Does child live with both biological parents?   Yes   No

If no, please explain (including divorce, separation, foster care, adoption).

Who has legal custody?

If child's time is divided between households, please describe schedule.

Please fill in below. If only one household exists, fill in #1, continue on reverse side if necessary.

Household #1

Parent: _____

Siblings: _____   Age _____

_____   Age _____

Half siblings: _____   Age _____

_____   Age _____

Stepsiblings: _____   Age _____

_____   Age _____

Caregiver: _____

Pets: _____

Household #2

Parent: _____

Siblings: _____   Age _____

_____   Age _____

Half siblings: _____   Age _____

_____   Age _____

Stepsiblings: _____   Age _____

_____   Age _____

Caregiver: _____

Pets: _____

Please list caregivers, nannies, or au pairs and approximate dates of employment.

Temperament	Never	Rarely	Sometimes	Often
The baby was easily upset				
The baby was excessively restless				
The baby cried excessively or in a strange way				
The baby reacted badly to new experiences (new foods, places)				
The baby did not seem to enjoy cuddling				
The baby exhibited frequent head-banging				
The baby was unusually sensitive to bright lights				
The baby was unusually sensitive to loud noises				
The baby was upset when a stranger was present From ___ (age) months to ___ (age) months				
The baby was upset when left with a familiar babysitter.				

Developmental Milestones		Years	Months	
Approximate age when baby first:				
Smiled at a person				
Sat without support				
Crawled				
Spoke words				
Spoke phrases				

Toddler Period

Toilet training was achieved for bowels:

Day _____ (years, months)

Night _____ (years, months)

Toilet training was achieved for bladder:

Day _____ (years, months)

Night _____ (years, months)

The child needed to carry or sleep with a special object (e.g., blanket, stuffed animal). Describe:

The child had certain habits (e.g., thumb sucking). Describe:

The baby spoke in sentences from age _____.

Toddler Period	Never	Rarely	Sometimes	Often
There were difficulties in articulation				
In communicating his/her ideas				
In understanding others				
The child sleeps: Alone				
With sibling				
With parents				
There were sleep problems				
The child had temper tantrums				

Toddler Period (*continued*)	Never	Rarely	Sometimes	Often
The child had night terrors (screaming while asleep)				
The child paid no attention to the word "No"				
The child avoided rough-and-tumble play				
The child disliked quiet activities				
The child seemed clumsy and poorly coordinated				

Preschool Period	Never	Rarely	Sometimes	Often
The child avoided playing with other children and preferred to play alone				
The child was shy with strangers				
The child was fearful				
The child became angry				
The child had specific fears				
Name them:				

	Never	Rarely	Sometimes	Often
The child took a long time to settle down after being upset				
The child was easily distracted from an activity				

The first group experience
was at age:

Nursery school (Name):

Kindergarten (Name):

Specific problems in
adjustment:

School-Age Period

Schools attended (Name) (include religious schools):

School-Age Period	Never	Rarely	Sometimes	Often
The child had academic difficulties				
Reading				
Writing				
Spelling				
Mathematics				
The child is in his/her age-appropriate grade		Yes		No
Skipped a grade Grade:				
Was held back a grade Grade:				
The child needed special class placement		Yes		No
The child needed remedial work		Yes		No

Adolescent Period

Schools attended (Name):

Academic Difficulties	Never	Rarely	Sometimes	Often
English				
Foreign language				
Mathematics				
Science				

Please describe school year and type of difficulty:

Behavioral Problems	Never	Rarely	Sometimes	Often
Aggressive behavior				
Truancy				
Trouble with authorities				
Rebelliousness				
Problems making friends				

Please describe:

Interests and accomplishments (Describe):

Substance Use (Drugs and Alcohol) and Nonchemical Dependencies		
Substance: _____	First usage: _____	Frequency: _____
Substance: _____	First usage: _____	Frequency: _____
Substance: _____	First usage: _____	Frequency: _____
Nonchemical activity:	Gambling: _____	Pornography: _____
Social media: _____	Gaming: _____	Other: _____
Please describe:		

Interpersonal Relationships

Does the child/adolescent have close friends?

How does he/she react to peers?

Does the child get in fights?

How does the child spend time, and with whom, when not in school?

What are the child's strengths and assets (sports, aptitudes, talents, etc.)?

Temperamental traits, characteristics, and symptoms

If any family member exhibits any of the following traits, please place the appropriate number(s) from this list into the designated space in the family member list that follows.

1	Bodily complaints; hypochondriasis	20	Jealousy
2	Dissatisfaction (chronic) or lack of pleasure	21	Labile mood
3	Dysphoria (sadness, tearfulness)	22	Mild irascibility
4	Easy fatigability	23	Opinionated; dogmatic
5	Guilt over minor indiscretions	24	Alcoholism
6	Indecisiveness	25	Arrogance
7	Inordinate examination fear	26	Boastfulness
8	Joylessness in work	27	Compulsive gambling
9	Lack of initiative	28	Distractibility
10	Morbid fear of poverty	29	Extroverted; very "outgoing"
11	Pessimism	30	Heightened self-confidence; overoptimism; mild euphoria
12	Scrupulosity	31	Hypersexuality or promiscuity
13	Self-doubt, excessive worrying	32	Insensitivity or coarseness
14	Suicidal ruminations	33	Lack of insight
		39	Teasing others inordinately
		40	"Wanderlust" (inability to settle in one place; constant need to travel or roam from one place to another)
		41	Blames others
		42	Grudge-holding; unforgiving
		43	Humorless
		44	Hypercritical of others
		45	Litigious
		46	Quarrelsome
		47	Resentful
		48	Suspicious (marked) or intense jealousy
		49	Eccentric
		50	Excessively reserved
		51	"Loner"
		52	Self-consciousness (severe)

Temperamental traits, characteristics, and symptoms (continued)

15 Terrifying dreams	34 Overinvolvement in various schemes	53 Tends to be unsociable
16 Abusiveness	35 Overspending	54 Superstitious
17 Heightened premenstrual irritability	36 Raucous laughter or scatological humor or inveterate punning	55 Withdrawn
18 Impulsivity	37 Stubbornness	56 Overly sensitive
19 Irritability	38 Talking too much, or too loudly	

Family member name	Relationship to patient	Number(s) from list

APPENDIX C

Narrative School Reports

Instructing a young colleague or trainee to write a narrative report can make school visits a possibility even after therapy has begun. The task for the observer is to report on what is happening in the classroom, in terms of teacher and other students, always with an eye on what the patient is doing. It helps to tell the observer that hyperbolic adjectives and evaluative words should be minimized: "the child was active" is preferable to "the child was wild." Similarly, "the teacher called the child's name four times" is preferable to "the teacher yelled the child's name." Just the facts, please!

Here are two examples of observational reports[1] that were very helpful in working with parents:

EXAMPLE 1

SCHOOL OBSERVATION OF PETER, AGE 7 YEARS, 3 MONTHS

Teacher: Joan
Assistant Teacher: Lee
Speech Teacher: Patti
Science Teacher: Carol

---

[1]We are grateful to Katherine Cohen for her excellent reports.

8:50—PETER reading book at table. On task.

9:05—*Morning Meeting*. Joan asks class: "Tell me one thing you did over the weekend?" PETER says: "I played my video games."

Joan reminds PETER to focus several times during meeting. She says: "PETER, are you paying attention?" "PETER, I need your eyes." "I still need your eyes." Lee, the assistant teacher, sits next to PETER to keep him on task.

9:20—*Word Study*. Kids in seats; each has personal dry erase board and marker. Joan: "PETER, we are not writing with these markers right now. Can you let go?" PETER shakes head no and resists. Joan takes marker and reprimands PETER.

PETER and kids at table not paying attention. Joan reprimands table: "This is really disappointing behavior." PETER does not pay attention. Joan constantly reminds PETER to focus. He does not participate with class. Joan helps him with each word after presenting word to class. Joan constantly asks PETER to put pen down and focus. He participates minimally with help from teachers. He constantly rests head on arm.

Joan: "PETER, pen down and I want you to participate with the whole class, not on your own with my help afterward." PETER participates with help of teacher. Joan reminds him for each word.

9:50—*Reading Buddy* (5th graders come to class to read with 1st graders). PETER on task.

10:10—PETER leaves room without asking teacher. Joan reprimands PETER. PETER resists, and then goes back to room.

10:15—*Handwriting*. Lee helps PETER. Joan shows class how to write letter. PETER writes while Joan is teaching. Joan: "PETER, do the right thing and put the pen down." Joan takes pen out of PETER's hand. PETER picks pen up. Joan reprimands PETER. PETER does not focus while Joan writes on board. JOAN punishes PETER and tells him he must practice writing during recess.

10:25—*Speech*. Patti, the speech teacher, asks PETER what he did for weekend. PETER tells her he secretly played *Grand Theft Auto* video game.

He fights with pen and makes fighting noises: "Pow, pow."

Patti has PETER draw pictures for each word. PETER draws picture of mailbox and inside are three men: man with sword through chest, man with head chopped off, and man with broken leg. (Please see attached drawings [*included with the original report but not included in this book*].)

10:50—*Recess*. Joan tells PETER she will give him a second chance and he will not have to practice writing. PETER plays tag. Girl falls, and PETER asks if she is okay. PETER helps her up.

Joan ends recess. Class must form line. PETER listens and is in front of line. Joan: "Great job. I am really proud of you, PETER."

11:00—*Science*. PETER sits facing board. He does not participate. PETER not looking at Carol, the science teacher. Carol reminds PETER to pay attention. PETER sitting at table resting head on arm.

PETER works with boy on experiment. Carol reminds PETER to participate. PETER listens. (Carol briefs me on PETER's usual behavior. She tells me he is normally off task but not disruptive.)

Students silently read science book. PETER very focused on book. On task.

11:55—*Math*. Joan gives math instruction. PETER resting head on hand and leaning on wall. Joan: "PETER, you need to be paying attention." He does for brief period then stares off. Lee tries to keep PETER on task. Joan: "PETER, you are part of this lesson." Joan asks him to do math problem in front of class. He gives wrong answer. Joan thinks PETER is joking. Joan: "PETER, answer the question and don't be silly." He is not able to answer.

12:15—*Math work at table with partner*. Joan sits at PETER's table for entire time. PETER on task with direction of Joan.

12:35—*Board instruction*. Joan reminds PETER to pay attention. Joan says: "You should be sitting in the front, so if I allow you to sit in the back you must focus." Sits with head resting on hand.

12:50—*Lunch*. Andrew and PETER sit next to each other at lunch. Andrew tells PETER that he was trying to build a paradise, but a teenager destroyed it. PETER: "Andrew, do you have a sword?" (I can't hear

Andrew's response. Lunchroom is loud, and I don't want to make my observation obvious.)

PETER asks me: "Do you believe in the cross?" I say "I am sorry, but I can't answer that question because that is something I keep private." PETER: "Andrew says the cross is bad." They talk about religion (hard to hear) and then go outside to play.

1:20—*Outside Play.* Andrew and PETER playfully fight. It is aggressive. They kick each other in the stomach and make fighting noises. PETER grabs Andrew. Andrew punches PETER in mouth (he appears to be bleeding). Both kids reprimanded by staff. Staff tells PETER to drink water. PETER goes to nurse. (Staff asks me to escort him. I tell them I don't work there and I am just observing for the day. They send me anyway and tell me where to go.)

1:55—*Reading Aloud.* Joan tells PETER to go to rug spot. He was in wrong spot for reading. Now sitting in front. On task. Joan asks questions about book. Joan: "Wow, PETER, I am so happy to see your hand up." PETER answers questions. Joan: "Nice job PETER!"

After short while Joan tells him to focus. Joan: "Look up PETER."

2:20—*Writing Workshop.* Kids work independently at table. PETER lies on bench. Joan tells PETER to get up. PETER does not listen. She repeats herself. PETER gets up.

Joan asks Lee to help PETER with writing. Now on task. Lee leaves. PETER continues on task.

2:45—*Pack-up.* Joan reprimands PETER for not following cleanup direction. He follows. PETER part of cleanup crew. Joan keeps refocusing PETER on task. Joan: "PETER, finish your task." Kids pack up. PETER on task through pickup.

EXAMPLE 2

SCHOOL OBSERVATION OF JONNY, AGE 5 YEARS, 4 MONTHS

Teacher: Mary
Assistant Teacher: Mike
Assistant Teacher: Ellen

9:05—*Morning Meeting*. JONNY on task.

9:20—*Free Time*. JONNY and Karl (boy in class) build house with blocks. On task.

10:00—*Playtime on Roof Playground*. Two boys in class get in fight. JONNY sees fight and walks away. Mike, an assistant teacher, says to JONNY: "Good job for walking away and not getting involved."

Class walks down stairs back to classroom. JONNY jumps and skips steps. Mike says: "One step at a time, JONNY, so you don't hurt yourself." JONNY responds: "I will walk how I want to." Mike says: "No, you must do one step at a time." JONNY listens. Now on task.

(During playtime outside the teachers tell me this has been a great day for JONNY so far; they thought this might happen with an observer present. Mike also mentioned how he was really proud that JONNY did not get involved in the fight. Mike said JONNY usually gets himself right in the middle of fights.)

10:35—*Snack*. JONNY screams: "No!" Mary asks: "What's wrong?" JONNY says: "I need five pretzels!" (Mary gives each kid 5 pretzels during snack.) Mary says: "Okay, okay." He takes pretzels. JONNY is last to finish snack. Mike reminds JONNY to finish and JONNY is late for story time.

10:55—*Story Time*. JONNY listens to story. Mary then gives class lesson on how Egyptians built pyramids. JONNY raises hand and answers questions. On task.

11:15—*Free Time*. JONNY plays at table with blocks and builds a kingdom. Mike helps. JONNY finds toy that belongs to different classroom. Mary asks JONNY if he can return it. He returns toy and Mary thanks him.

Mary ties JONNY's shoe and they bump heads. JONNY rubs her head to make it feel better. On task.

JONNY plays with Karl and Ellen, the other assistant teacher, to build house. Brick falls on JONNY's head. Ellen consoles him as she gets ice. On task.

During cleanup JONNY tries to pull toy out of Mike's hand. He keeps pulling and will not let go. He lets go once Mike convinces him of a compromise. Mike says he can look at the toy once more after cleanup. Mike helps focus JONNY on cleanup.

11:45: *Show and Tell*. Julian (boy in class) shows class a few toys and passes them around for the class to see. JONNY gets angry and screams at Sara, the girl next to him, because he thought she was taking too long with the toy. JONNY screams: "She is taking too long, Mary!" Mary replies: "No, she is not." JONNY gets his turn with toy. He holds the toy for a long time. Mary says: "You have to pass the toy JONNY." JONNY says: "No because she took too long!" JONNY throws toy to Sara. Another toy is being passed, and JONNY gets upset with same girl again for taking too long. Mary reprimands JONNY. He gets toy, and she reminds him again to pass toy. JONNY whines to Mary to see second toy, and Mary informs him that he already had his chance. He continues to whine. Ellen consoles JONNY, and she has him sit on her lap.

12:00—*Chapter Book Reading*. Still sitting on Ellen's lap during reading. On task.

12:10—*Goodbye Meeting (this is right before lunch; class splits up; JONNY goes with half the class to a different room)*. JONNY and Julian fight on floor. Mary reprimands both kids and has to pull them apart. They stop. Julian and JONNY shake bookcase. Mike reprimands both kids and they stop.

12:15—*Lunch*. Garret (boy in class) teases JONNY. Garret: "I am going to take your food." JONNY screams: "No, this is mine!" Garret keeps teasing JONNY and ignores his responses. Garret says: "Oh thanks, that food is for me? Thanks for your food, JONNY." As Garret keeps teasing JONNY, JONNY keeps getting more frustrated and keeps responding by saying: "No, this is my food!" JONNY keeps asking Garret to stop. Mike tells boys to stop fooling around and eat their food (he says this several times). Mike finally warns them that he will send them out of the classroom if they don't stop. They stop.

Garret wants to share cubby with JONNY. JONNY screams because he does not want to share. Garret puts his lunchbox in the cubby anyway. JONNY hits the wall. Garret walks away while screaming at JONNY. JONNY removes Garret's lunchbox. Garret screams. Mike tells both boys to go to table and talk it out using words. Garret says: "JONNY, you are my best friend and that is why I want to put my lunchbox in your cubby." JONNY says: "I don't want you to put it in my cubby, but you can put it in the cubby next to mine." Mike facilitated that discussion and helped them come to the conclusion. Garret puts lunchbox in the cubby next to JONNY's.

Garret and JONNY are playing drums. Garret says his dad made the drums. JONNY says: "I don't believe you!" Garret says: "Yes he did!" They continue screaming at each other and then JONNY sits on the drum. Garret is upset because he does not want JONNY to ruin the drum. They keep screaming. JONNY threatens that he is going to tell on Garret. Mike reprimands both boys. Mike reminds JONNY how awful he felt when no one believed that he was in the newspaper and that he was doing a similar thing to Garret. They stop fighting.

JONNY now on task drawing at table. Mike asks class to go to rest spot. JONNY listens.

1:00—*Rest Time.* Kids in rest spots. Mike reminds JONNY to be quiet and rest. JONNY now on task. He falls asleep. Rest time is over, and all kids get ready to go back to classroom. Mary (now in room because Mike went on break) tells kids not to wake JONNY. They woke him by accident. He appeared frustrated and was very quiet after his nap, but this dissipated with time.

2:00—*Art and Playtime.* JONNY playing with clay at table. On task. Ellen and Julian also at table. JONNY says to Julian and Ellen: "Stop annoying me!" He then continues to play, and other kids join table. He plays nicely with other kids and shares his clay. Mike reminds JONNY and other kids to clean the mess.

2:50—*Good-bye Meeting.* Mary reading book. JONNY on task. JONNY and Karl get in physical fight after book reading. Mary must pull them apart and reprimands both kids. It is time to leave for the end of the day. JONNY sees babysitter and gets very excited. He runs to her and gives her a big hug. He packs up and leaves.

Index

Page numbers printed in **boldface** *type refer to tables or figures; page numbers with an internal "n" (e.g., 31n1) refer to footnotes.*

Anna Freud Centre, 393, 394, 408
Annoyance, and autism spectrum
    disorder, 387
Anxiety
    responses to themes of play and,
        330
    role of play in management of,
        41
    verbalizing affects or inner states
        and, 325, 326
Apraxias, and school referrals, 240
ASD. *See* Autism spectrum disorder
Asperger's disorder, 181, 386, 387
Assessment. *See also* Evaluation
    autism spectrum disorder and,
        189
    of development, 370–372, 381
    initial consultation and estab-
        lishment of rapport with
        parents, 226–229
    of play, 174, 175–177
    of readiness for termination,
        353–354
    of relatedness, 381–382
Attachment
    disorganized forms of, 16, 20
    disturbances in, 237, 249
    theory on relationship of pre-
        tending to reality and,
        42–43
Attention-deficit/hyperactivity
    disorder (ADHD)
    case examples of, 190–192,
        388–392
    diagnosis of, 192–193
    early television viewing and, 96
    play and playfulness in, 195–196
    play therapy and treatment of,
        392–394
    posttraumatic stress disorder
        and, 380, 393

psychodynamic understanding
    of, 193–194
Test of Playfulness (ToP) and,
    177
Autism Diagnostic Observation
    Schedule and Autism Diagnos-
    tic Interview, 182
Autism spectrum disorder (ASD)
    case examples of, 179–181,
        377–378, 384–385
    cognitive deficits and pretend
        play in, 185–186
    diagnostic criteria for, 181–182
    empathy and, 187
    metarepresentation and, 185,
        186–187
    object play and, 46n2
    playfulness and social play in,
        187–190
    play therapy as approach to,
        385–388
    psychodynamically inclined
        approaches to, 183–185
    symbolic capacity and, 186
    Test of Playfulness (ToP) and,
        177
    theories and research on,
        182–183
Autobiographical narratives, 125
Autonomy
    adolescents and parent–child
        relationship, 311
    working alliance and, 257
Average expectable mother, 383,
    402
Avoidance
    of anxiety-arousing inner states,
        325
    autism spectrum disorder and,
        184n2
    resistance and, 254

Mourning, and termination of play
therapy, 350. *See also* Grief
Mutual play state. *See also* Playing
state
deepening of play therapy and,
323
definition of, 342, 403
initiation and establishment of,
261–264
variations in development and,
370

Narcissism, and parent work, 302
Narratives. *See also* Autobiographical narratives
childhood trauma and development of, 398
deepening of play therapy and
gradual expansion of, 341
school referrals and reports as,
240, 439–445
Negative therapeutic motivation,
and parent work, 302
Neurodevelopmental disorders. *See
also* Autism spectrum disorder
lack of pretend play as underlying sign of, 379
play capacity and, 173
Neuropsychiatric testing, and
school referrals, 239, 240
Neutrality, and meetings with
divorced or separated parents,
228
New object. *See also* Object relations
child–therapist relationship and,
127, 129–130, 327
definition of, 142, 165, 342
therapeutic action and, 158
9/11 World Trade Center attack,
201–202

"9-month revolution," and forms of
engagement in infants, 67
"Nondirective play therapy," 13
*Normal Child and Adolescent Devel-
opment: A Psychodynamic
Primer* (Gilmore and Meersand
2013), 409

Object play
pretend play of oedipal-phase
children and, 47
toddlers and, 46
Object relations. *See also* Developmental objects; New object
attention-deficit/hyperactivity
disorder and, 194
pretend play in young children
and, 72
therapeutic action and, 150,
158–159, 165
Object representation
definition of, 250
role of parents in child's development and, 228
Observation, of child at school,
240, 439–445
Obsessive-compulsive disorder, and
variants of symptomatic play,
178
Occupational therapy, and treatment plans for childhood psychopathology, 400
Oedipal phase (3 to 6 years). *See
also* Preschool period; Toddlers
definition of, 20
developmental chronology of
play forms in, 46–47
evolution of pretend play during,
70–78, 178–179
insight-oriented interventions
and, 138, 139–140